ECG Core Curriculum

ECG Core Curriculum

Franklin H. Zimmerman, MD, FACC, FACP, FAACVPR
Senior Attending Cardiologist
Director of Cardiac Rehabilitation
Phelps Memorial Hospital
Sleepy Hollow, New York
Assistant Professor of Cardiology
Barbara and Donald Zucker School of Medicine at Hofstra/Northwell
Hempstead, New York

New York   Chicago   San Francisco   Athens   London   Madrid   Mexico City
Milan   New Delhi   Singapore   Sydney   Toronto

ECG Core Curriculum

Copyright © 2023 by McGraw Hill LLC. All rights reserved. Printed in China. Except as permitted under the United States Copyright Act of 1976, no part of this publication may be reproduced or distributed in any form or by any means, or stored in a data base or retrieval system, without the prior written permission of the publisher.

1 2 3 4 5 6 7 8 9   DSS   28 27 26 25 24 23

ISBN 978-0-07-178521-1
MHID 0-07-178521-3

This book was set in Minion Pro by KnowledgeWorks Global Ltd.
The editors were Timothy Hiscock and Christie Naglieri.
The production supervisor was Richard Ruzycka.
Project management was provided by Revathi Viswanathan, KnowledgeWorks Global Ltd.
The cover designer was W2 Design.
The text designer was Mary McKeon.
Graphic Design and Illustrations by Rosalie Peng Designs & Illustrations.
This book is printed on acid-free paper.

Library of Congress Cataloging-in-Publication Data

Names: Zimmerman, Franklin H., author.
Title: ECG core curriculum / author, Franklin H. Zimmerman.
Description: 1 ed. | New York : McGraw Hill, [2023] | Includes
    bibliographical references and index. | Summary: "A conversational,
    reader-friendly, clinical approach to electrocardiography. A how-to-read
    ECG teaching tool that provides lessons from basic to advanced"—
    Provided by publisher.
Identifiers: LCCN 2022052572 | ISBN 9780071785211 (paperback) | ISBN
    9780071785228 (ebook)
Subjects: MESH: Electrocardiography | Heart Diseases—diagnosis
Classification: LCC RC683.5.E5 | NLM WG 140 | DDC
    616.1/207547—dc23/eng/20230328
LC record available at https://lccn.loc.gov/2022052572

McGraw Hill books are available at special quantity discounts to use as premiums and sales promotions, or for use in corporate training programs. To contact a representative please visit the Contact Us pages at www.mhprofessional.com.

This book is dedicated to my wife Laurie,
for her love, support, and patience,
and without whom this project would never have been possible.

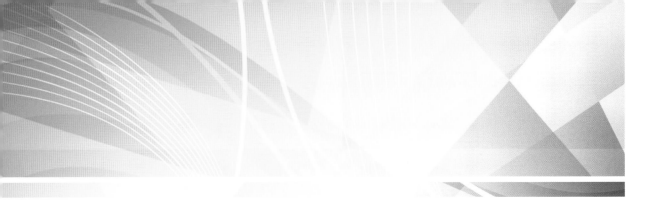

Contents

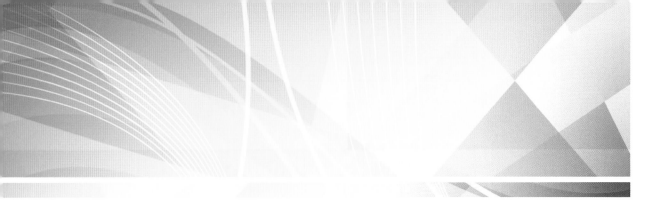

Abbreviations

A	atrium
AEI	atrial escape interval
AH	atrial-His
AN	atrionodal
AP	accessory pathway
APC	atrial premature complex
APD	atrial premature depolarization
ARP	absolute refractory period/ atrial refractory period (pacing)
ARVC	arrhythmogenic right ventricular cardiomyopathy
AT	atrial tachycardia
ATI	atrial tracking interval
ATP	adenosine triphosphate
AV	atrioventricular
AVI	AV interval
AVN	AV node
AVRT	atrioventricular reentrant tachycardia
AVNRT	AV nodal reentrant tachycardia
bpm	beats per minute
COPD	chronic obstructive pulmonary disease
CT	crista terminalis
CTI	cavo-tricuspid isthmus
ECG/EKG	electrocardiogram
ECS	extracellular space
EPS	electrophysiologic study
ER	early repolarization
ERP	effective refractory period
H	His
HBE	His bundle electrogram
HPS	His-Purkinje system
HR	heart rate
HV	His-ventricular
IART	intra-atrial reentry tachycardia
ICD	implanted cardiac defibrillator
IST	inappropriate sinus tachycardia
JPC	junctional premature complex
JT	junctional tachycardia
LA	left arm
LAD	left anterior descending
LAFB	left anterior fascicular block
LAO	left anterior oblique
LB	left bundle branch
LBBB	left bundle branch block
LCx	left circumflex
LGL	Lown-Ganong-Levine
LL	left leg
LM	left main
LPFB	left posterior fascicular block
LQTS	long QT syndrome
LRI	lower rate interval
LRL	lower rate limit
LVE	left ventricular enlargement
LVH	left ventricular hypertrophy
LVOT	left ventricular outflow tract
MAT	multifocal atrial tachycardia
MDP	maximum diastolic potential
MI	myocardial infarction
MTI	maximum tracking interval
MTR	maximum tracking rate
mV	millivolts
N	nodal
NH	nodal-His
PAT	paroxysmal atrial tachycardia
PAVBP	post-atrial ventricular blanking period
PDA	posterior descending artery
PE	pulmonary embolus
PEA	pulseless electrical activity
PMT	pacemaker-mediated tachycardia
POTS	postural orthostatic tachycardia syndrome
PRWP	Poor R wave progression
PVARP	post-ventricular atrial refractory period
PVC	premature ventricular complex
QT	QT interval
QTc	Corrected QT interval
RA	right arm
RB	right bundle branch
RBBB	right bundle branch block
RCA	right coronary artery

RP	resting potential	TdP	*torsades de pointes*
RRP	relative refractory period	TP	threshold potential
RVE	right ventricular enlargement	URL	upper rate limit
RVH	right ventricular hypertrophy	VAI	ventricular-atrial interval
RVOT	right ventricular outflow tract	VEI	ventricular escape interval
SA	sinoatrial	VPB	ventricular premature beat
SN	supernormal period	VPC	ventricular premature complex
SNRT	sinus node recovery time	VPD	ventricular premature depolarization
SQTS	short QT syndrome	VRP	ventricular refractory period
SSRI	selective serotonin uptake inhibitor	VSP	ventricular safety pacing
STEMI	ST elevation myocardial infarction	VT	ventricular tachycardia
SVT	supraventricular tachycardia	WCT	wide complex tachycardia
TARP	total atrial refractory period	WPW	Wolff-Parkinson-White

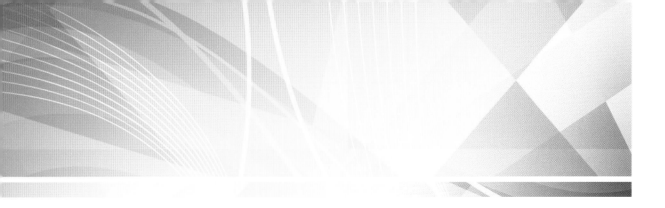

How to Use This Book

If you are completely new to electrocardiography, I suggest you begin at the beginning and read each chapter in sequence. This isn't a novel, so take your time. Depending on your knowledge base and background, the material may be either a quick read or more time-consuming. I have made every attempt to simplify some of the more challenging aspects of electrocardiography, but some topics are more demanding than others. The basic science of the early chapters may be new for some readers, but have no fear, because you are going to become an excellent clinical electrocardiographer without a chemistry or physics degree.

The illustrations are plentiful, designed to enhance and supplement the written material. Make sure you review both the text and illustrations.

Throughout the book, you will find call-out paragraphs with little icons at the side. These are fun little notes that include topics for "history buffs" or "bookworms," who may enjoy a little more detail. Other notes are important for everyone and are identified as a "clinical tip" or a caution to "be careful."

Each chapter introduces a new subject, but deliberately reviews and builds on the previous topics. If you have ever studied music, you know that you need to keep practicing sections you have already mastered as you are learning the new material. When you finish your final lesson, you are prepared to render a virtuoso performance. As you proceed, test your knowledge by answering the questions at the end of each chapter. And for those interested in reading more about specific topics, resources are provided for further study.

Finally, just have fun. I'm confident you are going to enjoy being known as the local ECG expert!

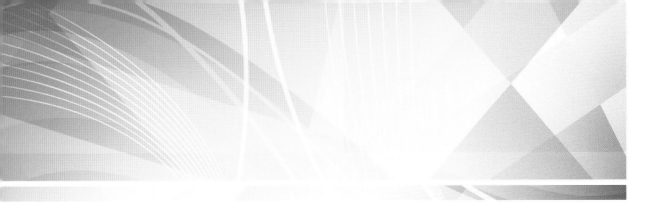

How This Book Is Organized

ECG Core Curriculum is organized into seven sections, each with several chapters. The beginning chapters focus on the basic science and technical aspects of electrocardiography. The middle chapters review ECG findings for a wide range of medical conditions and cardiac arrhythmias. Finally you will learn interpretive techniques you will use every day in clinical practice. We finish up with reference materials and a practice exam.

Section I: Basic Concepts. These chapters establish our foundation. We begin with the history of electrocardiography, followed by chapters devoted to anatomy and electrophysiology. Then the focus is on the technical aspects of recording the information and how to make the measurements essential for interpreting every ECG. Next we review the concept of vectors and the reasons why the deflections on the ECG look the way they do.

Section II: Chamber Enlargement, Bundle Branch Block, and Preexcitation. The first chapter is devoted to the electrocardiographic diagnosis of both atrial and ventricular chamber enlargement. We follow then with intraventricular conduction abnormalities. We finish this section with a review of preexcitation due to atrioventricular bypass pathways.

Section III: Myocardial Ischemia, Infarction, and Pericarditis. In these chapters you will gain the skills necessary to diagnose acute myocardial injury and infarction and differentiate these findings from other medical conditions.

Section IV: The Cardiac Rhythms. You will first learn about laddergrams, a time-honored technique to diagram the cardiac rhythm. Next is a discussion of the mechanisms of arrhythmias. Subsequent chapters are devoted to mastering the gamut of cardiac rhythm disturbances, including supraventricular arrhythmias, ventricular arrhythmias, ectopic complexes, heart block, and aberrant conduction. We then discuss the special challenge posed by wide complex tachycardia. A practical approach to pacemaker electrocardiography completes this section.

Section V: Medications, Metabolic, and More. This section is devoted to miscellaneous topics, items that include the ECG effects of medications and electrolyte disturbances, as well as acquired and inherited QT syndromes.

Section VI. ECG Interpretation. Here you will learn a stepwise and structured approach to interpreting electrocardiograms. An extensive compendium of diagnostic criteria is also provided as a valuable reference.

Section VII: Final Exam. It's time to test your skills with 25 sample tracings, complete with detailed answers and analysis.

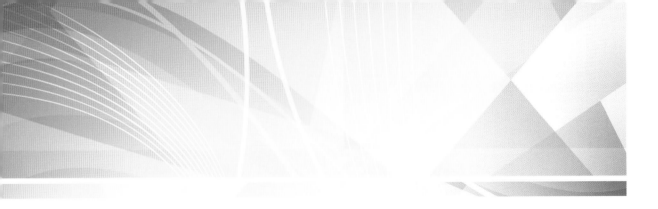

Preface

It's 3 a.m. and you're standing at the bedside of a 64-year-old man with chest discomfort. He's short of breath, covered in perspiration, and frightened. His blood pressure is 90/60 mm Hg and his heart rate is 130 beats per minute.

You have just been handed his electrocardiogram.

At this moment, it doesn't really matter whether you are a paramedic, nurse, medical student, internist, or cardiologist. You have a problem to solve and you have in your hand one of the best diagnostic tools in medicine . . . and you better know how to use it.

That's why you need this book. Because when you finish reading it, you will be well on your way to becoming a master electrocardiographer. And this will be a skill you are going to use for the rest of your professional life.

There are many books devoted to the study of electrocardiography. Some are quick reads and provide you only with the basics. Others are best left on the shelf as a reference. You are going to find that this book is unique. Think of it as a master class in a book, one that's going to make learning electrocardiography easy and enjoyable. Each chapter will quickly help you master fundamental concepts as you progress to more advanced clinical skills. You will learn *why* these funny little "squiggles" look the way they do, and not just memorize patterns. After reading these pages, you will master the techniques necessary to determine whether your patient is having an acute myocardial infarction or if the findings are a normal variant. You will learn how to recognize cardiac chamber enlargement and electrical conduction abnormalities. Complex cardiac arrhythmias and pacemaker electrocardiography will no longer be a mystery.

When you are handed the electrocardiogram of that critically ill patient in the middle of the night . . . you are going to be prepared.

Most of all, you will learn how satisfying and enjoyable interpreting electrocardiograms can be. Like me, I hope that you will find that a career in medicine is a wonderful privilege, and interpreting electrocardiograms will always be an important part of that experience. I believe that one of the best things about a life in medicine is that you never really leave school. You are forever either a student or a teacher. I hope this book will help you to remain both.

—Franklin H. Zimmerman, MD

*"All the advances of modern medicine will never diminish the importance of
a thorough history, a detailed physical examination,
and a well-interpreted electrocardiogram."*

—Franklin H. Zimmerman, MD

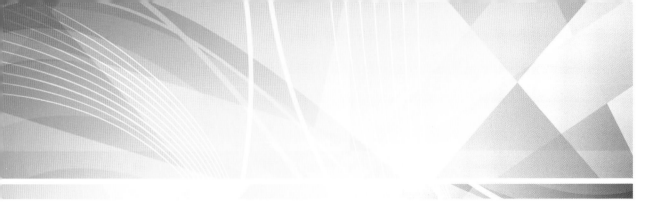

Acknowledgments

I would like to extend special appreciation to Rosalie Peng, my extraordinary and talented illustrator. She endured my endless "tweaks" of the figures and produced some truly unique work.

I owe a debt of gratitude to my friends and colleagues who took time out of their busy schedules to review one or more chapters of the book. This includes Harry Agress, MD; David Blumenthal, MD; Anne Castioni, CCEMTP; Subbarao Choudry, MD; Adam Denker, BS; Sei Iwai, MD; the late Arnold Katz, MD; Michael Lehmann, MD; Stavros Montantonakis, MD; James Reiffel, MD; Arturo Rojas, MD; David Rubin, MD; Carmine Sorbera, MD; Tim Wages, RN; David Wolinsky, MD; and Peter Wong, MD.

I also wish to thank the editorial and production group at McGraw-Hill, originally Karen Edmonson followed by Tim Hiscock, as well as Revathi Viswanathan of KnowledgeWorks Global Ltd., for their stewardship of this project.

SECTION I
Basic Concepts

A Brief History of Electrocardiography

No comprehensive cardiac examination would be complete without performing an electrocardiogram (ECG or EKG). More than 100 years old, the electrocardiograph machine remains the simplest, least expensive, and most valuable tool in cardiology. It's easy to take this bedside instrument for granted. So, before we teach you how to use this vital medical tool, let's take a trip back through history.

The electrocardiograph was first developed in the latter part of the nineteenth century and was the most sophisticated medical device of its time. Even so, not all physicians of that era realized its utility and the lasting success of the ECG as a clinical tool was by no means certain. It was only through a series of brilliant experiments and enhancements did the electrocardiograph reach its full potential as a diagnostic instrument.

▶ THE HEART: AN ELECTRICAL MUSCLE

The potential for living tissue to contain an electric current was recognized in antiquity. Aristotle observed that the electric ray incapacitated its prey with a shock from an organ located in its pectoral fin. Roman physicians in the first century A.D. used such electrically charged sea creatures to treat the pain of headache and acute gout. This phenomenon remained a curiosity of nature until 1787 when Luigi Galvani of the University of Bologna observed that the leg muscle of a frog would contract when stimulated by an electrostatic apparatus. A debate ensued as to whether the frog's muscle was able to react only to an outside influence or whether the electricity was present in the muscle itself. Galvani believed the latter and eventually demonstrated that the stimulating electrical source originated within the living tissue. Galvani's nephew, Giovanni Aldini later expanded on his uncle's theories with a series of sensational

experiments of his own. In 1803 at the Royal College of Surgeons in London, Aldini applied an electrical stimulus to the limbs of an executed criminal, causing the deceased man's muscles to contort.

 FOR HISTORY BUFFS: Many historians believe that Aldini's experiments were the inspiration for Mary Shelley's *Frankenstein*.

By the 1870s, experiments demonstrated that the muscular pumping of the heart was related to an intrinsic electrical impulse. Instruments of the time did not have the capability to further explain the phenomenon, but this launched the search for an acceptable recording device of the heart's electrical current.

▶ THE ELECTROCARDIOGRAPH IS BORN

Two men, Augustus D. Waller of London and Willem Einthoven of Leiden pioneered the path to the modern electrocardiograph machine (**Figure 1-1**). In 1887, Waller used an instrument called a capillary electrometer to take the first surface measurement of the heart's electrical activity that did not require opening the chest and exposing the beating heart. He first termed the recording an "electrogram" and later, a "cardiogram."

By 1901, Einthoven advanced the technique with the use of a measuring device called a string galvanometer (named after Galvani). His improved instrument allowed Einthoven to amplify the electrical signal and record the tracing on a photographic plate. Einthoven published his research in German, introducing the term *electrokardiogram*. This launched a new field of medicine and set the stage for the now familiar abbreviation "EKG."

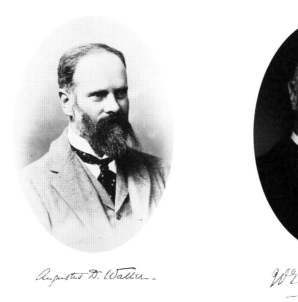

Figure 1-1. Augustus D. Waller (left) and Willem Einthoven (right). (Reproduced with permission from The National Library of Medicine (left); From Photo 12 / Contributor, Getty Images (right).)

CLINICAL TIP: The proper English abbreviation for the electrocardiogram is ECG. I confess in clinical practice I use EKG because I like to pay homage to Einthoven and it's easy to mistake ECG for EEG, which is the abbreviation for electroencephalogram (a test pertaining to a different body system entirely so I'm told). But ECG is correct and the abbreviation my editors prefer, so ECG it is.

The first ECG machines did not resemble today's compact devices. Einthoven's recording apparatus weighed nearly 600 lb, took five people to operate, and required the patient to immerse their arms and legs in a vat of conductive salt solution (**Figure 1-2**). Part of Einthoven's genius was to recognize the clinical potential of using this massive machine to record the heart's electrical activity. He connected his equipment by cable to make recordings from patients at the Academic Hospital in Leiden, located over a mile away. Even his fellow scientist Waller did not appreciate the potential clinical application of the recordings stating, "I do not however imagine that the string galvanometer, however useful and even necessary it may be in the physiological laboratory, is likely to find any very extensive use in the hospital. It can at most be of rare and occasional use to afford a record of some rare anomaly of cardiac action." It was not long before Einthoven proved Waller's prediction wrong, as electrocardiography soon became one of the most valuable diagnostic techniques in medicine.

CLINICAL TIP: One uses an electrocardiograph machine to perform an electrocardiogram.

Einthoven introduced the terminology for the deflections of his string galvanometer, naming the waves "P, Q, R, S, and T," using the convention established by Descartes for labeling geometric points on a curve. In his research paper published in 1906, he reported the descriptions of complete heart block, left and right ventricular hypertrophy, premature complexes, and atrial fibrillation. Einthoven's pioneering accomplishments culminated in his receiving the Nobel Prize for medicine in 1924.

▶ DEVELOPMENT OF THE MODERN ELECTROCARDIOGRAPH

Over time, scientific improvements allowed for the fabrication of a smaller recording apparatus. One of the early manufacturers was the Cambridge Scientific Instrument Company in England, which included among its founders Horace Darwin, youngest son of the legendary evolutionary biologist, Charles Darwin. Noted physicians embraced the new technology, including Alfred E. Cohn of New York's Mt. Sinai Hospital, who in 1909 introduced the first electrocardiograph machine into the United States and William Osler, who purchased a machine in 1912. Another ECG pioneer, Thomas Lewis of University College Hospital in London wrote in 1912, "The time is at hand, if it has not already come, when an examination of the heart is incomplete if this new method is neglected." By 1913, Lewis published the first textbook on the subject entitled, *Clinical Electrocardiography*, where he described the ECG findings of ventricular hypertrophy, heart block, and a variety of other cardiac arrhythmias.

There is much more to the fascinating history of electrocardiography, and I encourage you to explore the suggestions for further reading. Let's now begin our journey into the wonderful world of these "little squiggles."

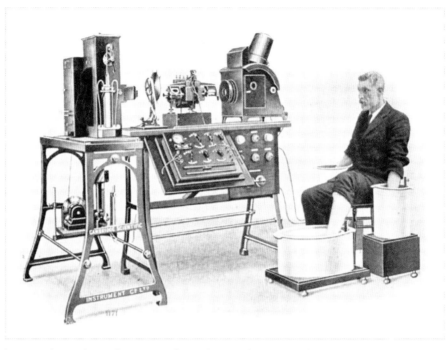

Figure 1-2. Original electrocardiograph machines were large devices that required the subject to place the extremities in a bath of electrolyte solution. (Reproduced with permission from Shade B: *Fast and Easy ECGs: A Self-Paced Learning Program,* 2nd ed. New York, NY: McGraw Hill; 2012.)

Chapter 1 • SELF-TEST

1. What was the original measuring device that Einthoven used to record electrical impulses of the heart called?

2. What letters did Einthoven use to name the deflections he recorded of the heart's electrical activity?

3. Commonly called an EKG, what is the proper English abbreviation for the electrocardiogram?

4. What is the difference between an electrocardiograph and an electrocardiogram?

QUESTIONS

ANSWERS

Chapter 1 • SELF-TEST

1. A string galvanometer.
2. P, Q, R, S, T.
3. ECG.
4. One uses an electrocardiograph machine to perform an electrocardiogram.

Further Reading

Acierno LJ. Augustus Desire Waller. *Clin Cardiol.* 2000;23:307-309.

Barold SS. Willem Einthoven and the birth of clinical electrocardiography a hundred years ago. *Card Electrophysiol Rev.* 2003;7:99-104.

Burch GE, DePasquale NP. *A History of Electrocardiography.* Chicago, IL: Year Book Medical Publishers; 1964.

Burchell HB. A centennial note on Waller and the first human electrocardiogram. *Am J Cardiol.* 1987;59:979-983.

Fisch C. Centennial of the string galvanometer and the electrocardiogram. *J Am Coll Cardiol.* 2000;36:1737-1745.

Fye WB. Disorders of the heartbeat: a historical overview from antiquity to the mid-20th century. *Am J Cardiol.* 1993;72:1055-1070.

Hurst JW. Naming of the waves in the ECG with a brief account of their genesis. *Circulation.* 1998;98:1937-1942.

Kligfield P. The centennial of the Einthoven electrocardiogram. *J Electrocardiol.* 2002;35:123-129.

Kligfield P. Derivation of the correct waveform of the human electrocardiogram by Willem Einthoven 1890-1895. *Cardiol J.* 2010;17:109-113.

Parent A. Giovanni Aldini: from animal electricity to human brain stimulation. *Can J Neurol Sci.* 2004;31:576-584.

Rautaharju PM. A hundred years of progress in electrocardiography 1: early contributions from Waller to Wilson. *Can J Cardiol.* 1987;3: 362-374.

Rivera-Ruiz M, Cajavilca C, Varon J. Einthoven's string galvanometer. *Tex Heart Inst J.* 2008;35:174-178.

Shapiro E. The first textbook of electrocardiography. *J Am Coll Cardiol.* 1983;1:1160-1161.

Silverman ME. Willem Einthoven-the father of electrocardiography. *Clin Cardiol.* 1992;15:785-787.

Functional Anatomy and Physiology

► SURFACE ANATOMY/ORIENTATION IN THE CHEST

A basic knowledge of the anatomy of the heart and conduction system will help you better understand the electrical forces from which the electrocardiogram (ECG) is derived.

First, let's review some anatomical terminology. We are accustomed to looking at the body in three standard anatomical planes—the *frontal* (coronal), *horizontal* (transverse, cross-sectional, or axial), and *sagittal* (longitudinal) (**Figure 2-1**). We can use these planes to describe the direction of electrical forces that comprise the ECG as anterior or posterior (frontal), superior or inferior (horizontal), and right or left (sagittal). Remember that right and left always refer to the patient's right and left, not to the direction viewed from your perspective. Interpreting ECGs would be a lot simpler if the heart conformed to these anatomical planes, but unfortunately, it doesn't. Let's take a closer look.

FOR BOOKWORMS: The midline sagittal plane that divides the body into two equal right and left sides is termed the median plane.

The heart is about the size of your fist and lies in the middle of the thorax. It sits behind the sternum, adjoining the third to sixth costal cartilages, between the lungs and above the diaphragm. The long and short axes of the heart are oriented obliquely compared with the rest of the body such that about two-thirds of the heart's mass actually lies left of the midline (**Figure 2-2**). The geometry of the heart is described as a truncated ellipsoid, with the long axis, from base to apex, rotated 60 degrees leftward from the sagittal plane and 45 degrees inferior from the horizontal plane. "What the heck does that mean?" you ask.

You can understand this orientation more easily by thinking of the heart as shaped like a foam football (**Figure 2-3**). If you were to cut a section off the back end, the intact nose of the football would represent the apex of the heart and the flat end the base. Hold the flat end of the football against your sternum with the nose away from you and the laces facing straight up to the ceiling. Turn the nose of the ball in an arc 60 degrees toward your left, still keeping the laces pointed up. Now tilt the nose of the football in an arc 45 degrees straight down toward your left foot. This is a reasonable approximation of the heart's orientation in the chest. If you now ask a friend to take a knife and (carefully!) slice the football through the laces, the half of the ball you are holding in your right hand would be anterior (in the front) and the half in your left hand would be posterior (in the back). Now you can see why the right-sided chambers of the heart are really **anterior** structures and the left-sided chambers are **posterior**. A lot of confusion results because it's traditional to illustrate cardiac anatomy by showing all four chambers together in a "valentine" view, something we'll be doing for most of the illustrations in this book. This does help you understand many concepts in cardiology, but it's important to recognize that this type of visual aid isn't anatomically correct.

► INTERNAL STRUCTURES (CHAMBERS OF THE HEART AND THE CARDIAC VALVES)

The heart consists of four hollow, blood-filled chambers (**Figure 2-4**). The upper chambers are the **right atrium** and **left atrium**, which are separated by the interatrial septum. The lower chambers are the **right ventricle** and **left ventricle**, which are separated by the interventricular septum. This

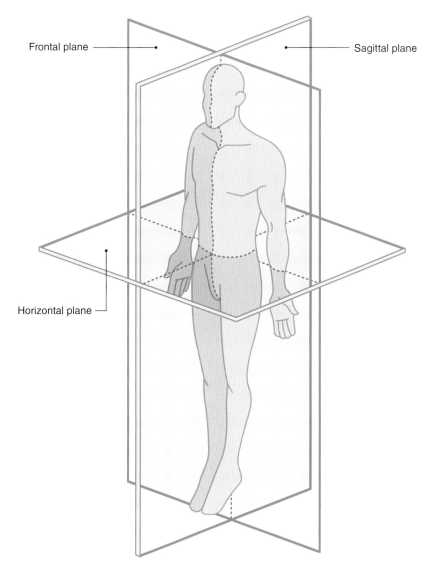

Frontal plane

Sagittal plane

Horizontal plane

Figure 2-1. Anatomical planes separate one half of the body from the other. The frontal plane separates anterior (front) from posterior (back), the horizontal plane separates superior (upper) from inferior (lower), and the sagittal plane separates right from left.

creates a four-chambered, two-sided pump. The atria are relatively thin walled, whereas the ventricles are comparatively thick and muscular.

The cardiac valves provide one-way openings that allow the heart to maintain a continuous circulation of blood. The *atrioventricular* valves separate both atria from their respective ventricles. The **tricuspid valve** lies between the right atrium and the right ventricle. The **mitral valve** separates the left atrium and the left ventricle. The *semilunar* valves (so-called because they are shaped like half-moons) are the **pulmonary valve** and **aortic valve**. The pulmonary valve lies between the right ventricle and the **pulmonary artery**. The aortic valve separates the left ventricle and the **aorta**.

 FOR BOOKWORMS: The twisting process of cardiac embryogenesis makes for the complexity of cardiac anatomy. Unlike the simplified depiction in Figure 2-4, the

ventricular outflow tracts and their corresponding semilunar valves do not all lie in the same anatomical plane. The right ventricular outflow tract lies anterior and rightward of the left ventricular outflow tract. The pulmonary valve is positioned leftward and superior to the aortic valve.

▶ THE CARDIAC CYCLE

The circulatory function of the heart depends on the atria and ventricles alternately filling with blood and then emptying their contents. The *cardiac cycle* represents this action from the beginning of one heartbeat to the next (**Figure 2-5**). It consists of an active (contraction) phase and a passive (relaxation) phase. The contraction phase of the cardiac cycle is called ***systole***, during which blood is ejected from the chambers. This is followed by a relaxation phase, ***diastole***, when blood passively fills the chambers. Atrial systole occurs during

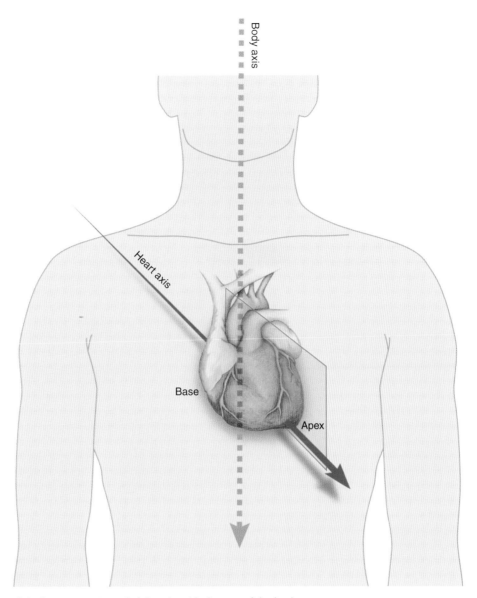

Figure 2-2. The axes of the heart are oriented obliquely with the rest of the body.

ventricular diastole and ventricular systole occurs during atrial diastole, so that one set of chambers is filling while the other is pumping. In clinical medicine the main focus is usually on the pumping action of the ventricles, so from now on we'll use systole to refer to ventricular contraction and diastole to refer to ventricular relaxation. The systolic and diastolic phases of the right and left sides of the heart operate in tandem, creating a simultaneous pulmonary (right-sided) and systemic (left-sided) circuit.

The synchronized timing of systole and diastole allows the heart to circulate blood throughout the body. Let's go through the steps of the cardiac cycle, one chamber at a time.

1. Deoxygenated venous blood returns to the heart via the superior and inferior vena cavae, passively filling the right atrium.

2. The right ventricle relaxes, opening the tricuspid valve and starting the flow of blood. The right atrium then contracts, finishing the job of filling the right ventricle.

3. The right ventricle contracts, pumping blood through the pulmonary valve and into the pulmonary artery, where it flows to the lungs for oxygenation.

4. Oxygenated blood returns from the lungs to the heart via the pulmonary veins, passively filling the left atrium.

5. The left ventricle relaxes, opening the mitral valve and starting the flow of blood. The left atrium then contracts, finishing the job of filling the left ventricle.

6. The left ventricle contracts, pumping blood through the aortic valve and into the aorta, where it circulates to the rest of the body.

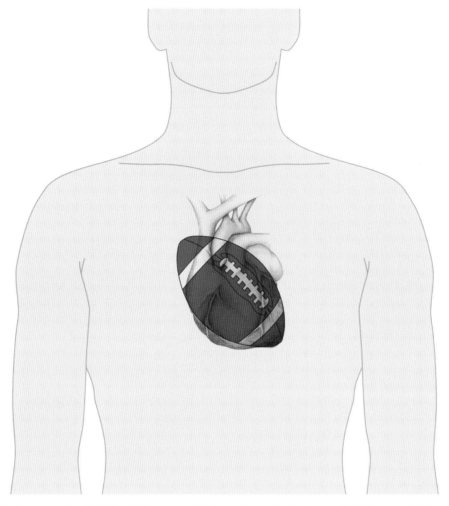

Figure 2-3. Think of the heart as a football tilted 60 degrees left from the sagittal plane and 45 degrees inferior in the horizontal plane related to the normal axes of the torso.

 FOR HISTORY BUFFS: Chinese physicians may have recognized the basic concepts of the cardiac circulation 4,000 years before William Harvey's description in 1628. As stated in the ancient Chinese text *Huangdi Neijing*, "The blood current flows continuously in a circle and never stops. It may be compared to a circle without beginning or end."

▶ THE CORONARY ARTERIES

No muscle, especially one as active as the heart, could function without an ample supply of oxygen-containing blood. The heart derives its own blood supply from the coronary arteries (**Figure 2-6**). The openings (ostia) of the coronary arteries are located in the proximal portion of the ascending aorta, just above the insertion of the aortic valve, and give rise to the **right coronary** (RCA) and **left main** (LM) coronary arteries. The coronary arteries course along the surface of the heart, dividing into major and minor branches that eventually enter the heart muscle to form arterioles and capillaries.

Obstruction of one or more of these blood vessels can result in myocardial infarction (MI). An understanding of basic coronary anatomy will help you recognize ECG patterns of MI, a topic on which we will spend much more time in later chapters. There are many anatomical variants and the anatomy is made more complex because of the oblique orientation of the heart within the chest. Let's go back to the football diagram to clear things up (see Figure 2-6).

The left main coronary artery divides into the **left anterior descending** (LAD) and **left circumflex** (LCx) coronary arteries. The LAD and its branches typically supply the anterior and septal portions of the left ventricle and part of the anterior right ventricle. Think of the LAD as following the same path as the laces of the football. This is the plane that divides the right and left ventricles (interventricular septum). The LCx branches almost at a right angle from the LAD and "circles" around the left (posterior) side of the heart, typically supplying the posterior portion of the left ventricle. It runs in the plane of the AV groove, which divides the atria and the ventricles. In 15% of individuals, the posterior descending artery (PDA) arises from the LCx; a pattern termed a *left dominant* circulation.

The RCA circles around the right (anterior) side of the heart and normally supplies the right atrium, the majority of the right ventricle, and the inferior surface of the left ventricle. Like the

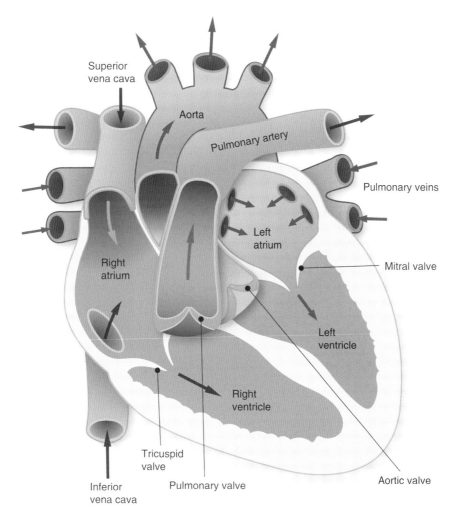

Figure 2-4. Cardiac anatomical structures.

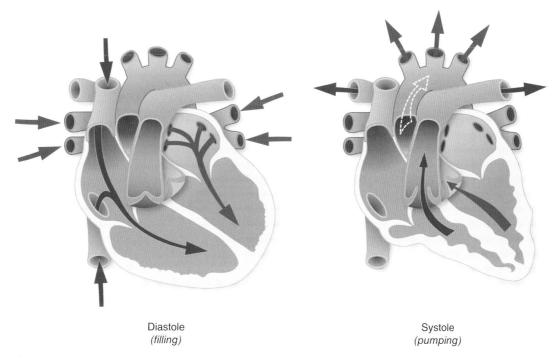

Diastole
(filling)

Systole
(pumping)

Figure 2-5. The cardiac cycle consists of a relaxation phase (diastole) and a contraction phase (systole), during which blood alternately fills and is then ejected from the heart (see text for details).

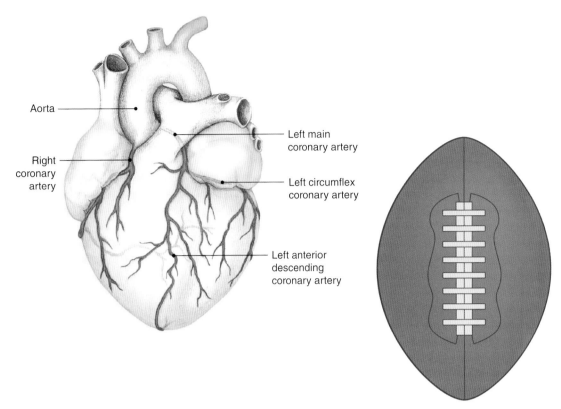

Aorta

Right coronary artery

Left main coronary artery

Left circumflex coronary artery

Left anterior descending coronary artery

Figure 2-6. Blood is supplied to the heart muscle from the right and left coronary arteries, which originate separately from the aorta. The left main coronary artery divides into the left anterior descending artery (LAD) and left circumflex (LCx) artery. (*Note: In this figure, the heart is rotated like the football to show you the relationship of the coronary arteries in a single view*).

LCx artery, the RCA runs in the AV groove. In 85% of individuals, a branch of the RCA becomes the PDA; a pattern termed a *right dominant* circulation.

 CLINICAL TIP: Compression of the coronary arteries during ventricular systole limits blood flow. Therefore, the majority of coronary perfusion occurs during diastole.

▶ THE LAYERS OF THE HEART

The heart is comprised of three layers—the *endocardium, myocardium,* and *epicardium* (**Figure 2-7**). The **endocardium** is the innermost layer that lines the interior surface of the cardiac chambers and the heart valves. The middle layer, or **myocardium**, is the thick muscular layer responsible for cardiac contraction. The thickness of this layer differs depending on the role of each cardiac chamber. The atrial myocardium is thinner than that of the ventricles because the atria have a lower resistance to overcome as they contract. Similarly, the left ventricular myocardium is three times thicker than the right ventricle because of the greater work required to pump blood throughout the systemic circulation compared with the pulmonary circuit. The innermost half of the myocardium, adjacent to the endocardium, is called *subendocardial* and the outermost half, adjacent to the epicardium, is called *subepicardial*.

The outermost layer of the heart is called the **epicardium**. The coronary arteries, capillaries, lymphatics, nerves, and fat are found in the epicardium. A source of confusion is that this layer is also called the *visceral* layer of the *serous pericardium*.

Surrounding the heart is a multilayered protective sac called the **pericardium**. The pericardium is divided into a tough, outer layer called the *fibrous pericardium* and an inner layer termed the *serous pericardium*. The serous pericardium is further subdivided into an outer *parietal* layer and an inner *visceral* layer. As we just mentioned, the visceral layer of the serous pericardium is also named the epicardium. Between the visceral and parietal layers of the serous pericardium is the *pericardial space*, which normally contains a small amount of fluid that acts as a lubricant.

 CLINICAL TIP: Excessive pericardial fluid (pericardial effusion) due to inflammation, trauma, or tumor can cause life-threatening *cardiac tamponade*, where the heart chambers become compressed and cannot maintain circulation.

▶ CELLS OF THE HEART/MICROSCOPIC ANATOMY AND PROPERTIES

The pumping action of the heart requires billions of cardiac cells to coordinate electrical stimulation with muscular action. We can separate cardiac cells into two basic types depending on

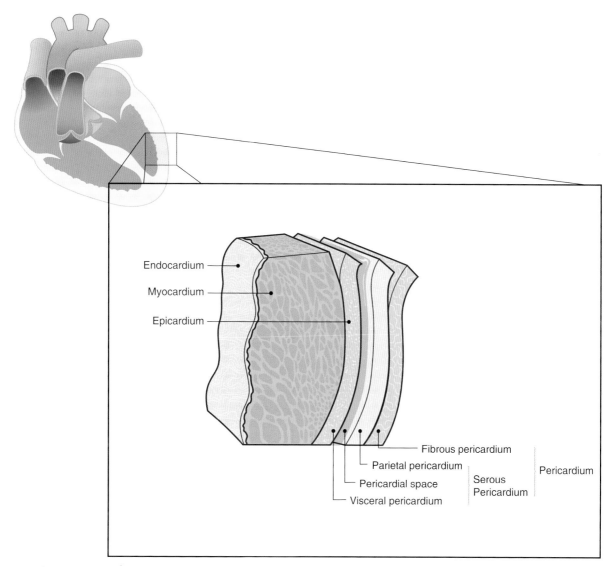

Figure 2-7. The heart consists of three layers of tissue called the endocardium, myocardium, and epicardium. Surrounding the heart is the multilayered pericardium (layers are not drawn to scale). A small amount of pericardial fluid is normally found in the pericardial space between the visceral and parietal pericardium. Note that the visceral layer of the serous pericardium and the epicardium are two different terms that refer to the same anatomical structure.

whether their purpose is either mechanical or electrical. We're going to spend plenty of time in the next chapter explaining the interaction of these cells, but for now, let's just go over the fundamentals.

Myocardial cells (myocytes) are the "working" cells of the heart. They are the muscular cells responsible for mechanical contraction and relaxation in the cardiac cycle. Cardiac myocytes connect in a branching network linked by low-resistance *gap junctions* that can rapidly transmit electrical signals from one cell to another.

Electrical cells include **pacemaker** cells that can initiate electrical signals that ultimately stimulate the myocardial cells to contract. Other electrical cells are those of the **specialized conduction system** whose purpose is to transmit the electrical signals from pacemaker cells to the working myocardium.

▶ ANATOMY OF THE SPECIALIZED CONDUCTION SYSTEM

The heart has an internal "wiring" system that provides for the rapid and coordinated transmission of electrical impulses throughout the heart (**Figure 2-8**). Ultimately, these impulses activate (depolarize) the working cells of the heart and initiate contraction. Knowledge of this system is essential for you to understand electrocardiography. The components of the specialized conduction system include the **sinoatrial (SA) node**, the **interatrial** and **internodal bundles**, the **atrioventricular (AV) junction** (subdivided into the **AV node** and the **bundle of His**), the **bundle branches** (right and left), and the **Purkinje fibers**. Let's take a look at each component individually. For the moment we're going to concentrate on understanding the anatomy. In a

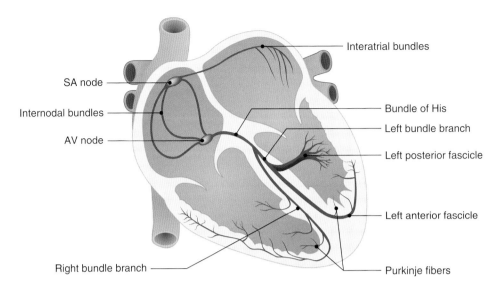

Figure 2-8. The specialized conduction system allows the efficient transmission of electrical impulses throughout the heart muscle.

future chapter, we'll learn how the ECG records the transmission of the electrical impulse through these structures.

Sinoatrial (SA) Node

The SA node is located within the wall of the right atrium near the inlet of the superior vena cava. It is the normal dominant pacemaker of the heart.

Interatrial and Internodal Bundles

On its path from the SA node to the AV node, the electrical impulse first spreads throughout the right atrium, to the interatrial septum, and then to the left atrium. The atrial myocardium rapidly conducts the impulse; however, specialized bundles are postulated to facilitate transmission. The interatrial conduction bundle (Bachmann's bundle) facilitates transmission of the impulse from the right atrium to the left atrium. As a result, the contraction of both atria is virtually simultaneous. Three internodal conduction bundles (anterior, middle, and posterior) are believed to facilitate transmission of the electrical impulse from the SA node to the AV node.

 FOR BOOKWORMS: The interatrial and internodal conduction bundles mentioned in the preceding discussion are not discrete anatomical fibers or tracts. They appear to represent an alignment of atrial myocardial cells that are conduits for preferential electrical conduction. Many authorities do not consider these atrial bundles as true components of the specialized conduction system.

Atrioventricular (AV) Junction

The AV node and the bundle of His comprise the area of the AV junction. Anatomically the AV node is divided into three regions, which have separate electrical properties—an upper junctional area where the three internodal bundles converge; the middle nodal region; and the lower junctional area that comprises the origin of the bundle of His. Electrophysiologists define these regions as the atrionodal (AN), nodal (N),

and nodal-His (NH). The primary purpose of the AV node is to slow the transmission of electrical impulses from the SA node to the ventricles. This allows the ventricles to completely fill with blood before being stimulated to eject their contents. The upper and lower junctional regions contain pacemaker cells, whereas the actual AV node does not.

The bundle of His connects the AV node to the bundle branches. It is a thick bundle of fibers that courses down the interatrial septum to enter the interventricular septum where it divides into the bundle branches.

The Bundle Branches

The right bundle branch and left common bundle branch arise from the bundle of His. The right bundle branch runs down the right side of the interventricular septum, transmitting electrical impulses to the right ventricle. The left common bundle branch divides early into several branches (fascicles). The two major divisions are called the **left anterior-superior** fascicle and **left posterior-inferior** fascicle, which in addition to a smaller **septal** fascicle transmit electrical impulses to the left ventricle and interventricular septum. In reality, this is a simplified description of the left bundle branch because the two major divisions and one minor branch are arranged more as a fan-like array rather than distinct, isolated fibers. In addition, I've chosen to expand the names of the two major divisions of the left bundle, which are more commonly known as the left anterior and left posterior fascicles. As we will learn in a later chapter, this added detail helps to understand the ECG findings present when these fascicles are dysfunctional.

The bundle branches and their divisions divide further into a vast network of Purkinje fibers. These become continuous with the myocytes of the ventricular endocardium.

A term often used to describe the portion of the specialized conduction system distal to the AV node is the *His-Purkinje system*, which refers to the bundle of His, bundle branches, and Purkinje fibers. Transmission of electrical impulses through this system is rapid, allowing efficient stimulation of the entire ventricular myocardium.

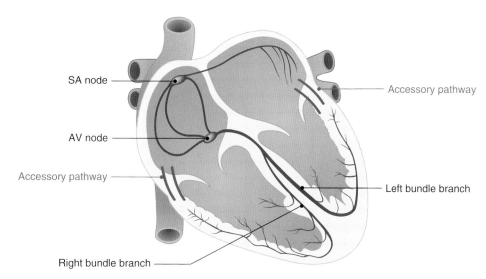

Figure 2-9. Accessory pathways allow electrical impulses to bypass the normal sequence of atrial to ventricular conduction. These may provide a substrate for cardiac arrhythmias.

Accessory Pathways

In the early fetal heart, the atrial and ventricular myocardial chambers are continuous. After the first month of gestation, a layer of connective tissue called the annulus fibrosus forms that anatomically and electrically insulates the atria from the ventricles. Rarely, this separation is incomplete, allowing for a muscular pathway to persist between the atrial and ventricular tissue. Such a corridor is termed an *accessory bypass pathway.* The most common of these are atrioventricular connections (*bundles of Kent*). They are located in a variety of locations around the AV ring, but most often provide an electrical conduit between the right or left atrium to their respective ventricles (**Figure 2-9**).

Accessory pathways have the potential to conduct electrical impulses outside of the normal AV node and His-Purkinje system. The bypass route allows the impulse to proceed directly from the atrial into the ventricular myocardium, which produces a wide and bizarre ECG configuration called the *preexcitation* or *Wolff-Parkinson-White* pattern.

Other, less common types of accessory bypasses include atriofascicular, nodofascicular, nodoventricular, and fasciculoventricular pathways, which represent a variety of possible anomalous links between the atrium, AV node, conduction system, and ventricles. We will spend more time discussing preexcitation and the association of accessory pathways with cardiac arrhythmias in later chapters.

Chapter 2 • SELF-TEST

QUESTIONS

1. The contraction phase of the cardiac cycle is called _____ and the relaxation phase is called _____.

2. The right ventricle is actually a(n) _____ structure and the left ventricle is actually a(n) _____ structure.

3. As blood returns from the great veins to the heart, list the cardiac chambers through which the blood will flow until it is pumped out of the heart through the aorta.

4. Name the coronary arteries that arise directly from the aorta.

5. What are the two main divisions of the left coronary artery?

6. Name the three layers of the heart.

7. What is the name of the primary pacemaker of the heart and where is it located?

8. What anatomical structures comprise the AV junction?

9. List the components of the His-Purkinje system.

10. What are the two major divisions of the left bundle branch?

Chapter 2 • SELF-TEST

ANSWERS

1. • Systole.
   • Diastole.

2. • Anterior.
   • Posterior.

3. Right atrium, right ventricle, pulmonary arteries, pulmonary veins, left atrium, left ventricle.

4. Right coronary artery and left main coronary artery.

5. Left anterior descending and left circumflex coronary arteries.

6. Endocardium, myocardium, epicardium.

7. Sinoatrial (SA) node, located within the wall of the right atrium, near the inlet of the superior vena cava.

8. The AV node and the bundle of His.

9. Bundle of His, right and left bundle branches, and Purkinje fibers.

10. • Left anterior-superior fascicle (left anterior).
    • Left posterior-inferior fascicle (left posterior).

Further Reading

Anderson RH, Razavi R, Taylor AM. Cardiac anatomy revisited. *J Anat*. 2004;205:159-177.

Cook AC, Anderson RH. Attitudinally correct nomenclature. *Heart*. 2002;87:503-506.

Ho SY, Anderson RH, Sanchez-Quintana. Atrial structures and fibers: morphologic basis of atrial conduction. *Cardiovasc Res*. 2002;54:325-336.

Massing GK, James TN. Anatomical configuration of the His bundle and bundle branches in the human heart. *Circulation*. 1967;53:609-621.

Mori S, Tretter JT, Spicer DE, Bolender DL, Anderson RH. What is the real cardiac anatomy? *Clin Anat*. 2019;32:288-309.

Partridge JB, Anderson RH. Left ventricular anatomy: its nomenclature, segmentation and planes of imaging. *Clin Anat*. 2009;22:77-84.

Titus JL. Normal anatomy of the human cardiac conduction system. *Anesth Analg*. 1973;52:508-514.

Uhley HN. The fascicular blocks. *Cardiovascular Clin*. 1973;5:87-97.

Waller BF, Gering LE, Branyas NA, Slack JD. Anatomy, histology, and pathology of the cardiac conduction system: part I. *Clin Cardiol*. 1993;16:249-252.

Waller BF, Gering LE, Branyas NA, Slack JD. Anatomy, histology, and pathology of the cardiac conduction system: part II. *Clin Cardiol*. 1993;16:347-352.

Electrophysiology

▶ AN INTRODUCTION TO CARDIAC ELECTROPHYSIOLOGY

To understand the electrocardiogram (ECG), you need a little background in electrophysiology. After all, it's electricity that makes the heart work. The ECG is nothing more than a recording of the heart's electrical activity. By analyzing the pattern of these recordings, you can diagnose numerous abnormalities of the heart's structure and function. At first you may think this basic science has little to do with "real world" electrocardiography, but have patience. In time you will realize that these concepts come in handy when we start interpreting actual ECG tracings and discussing cardiac medications.

Electrical Properties of Cardiac Cells

There are four inherent electrical properties of cardiac cells: (1) automaticity, (2) excitability, (3) conductivity, and (4) refractoriness. All have important implications with regard to the generation of normal and abnormal cardiac rhythms and each property can vary in health and disease.

Automaticity refers to the ability of cardiac pacemaker cells to initiate electrical activity without an outside stimulus. We read in Chapter 1 that Galvani needed to apply an external electrical stimulus to make his frog leg contract. Nature has provided us with special, self-stimulating, *pacemaker* cells that can start the electrical process on their own.

The SA node is the dominant pacemaker of the heart because its natural rate of discharge is greater than any other potential pacemaker. We're fortunate, however, that the SA node is not the only pacemaker available to maintain cardiac function. If illness or disease causes the SA node to fail, another latent pacemaker can take over, acting like a "backup generator" if the main power goes out. The automatic rates of these subsidiary pacemakers are slower than the SA node, so the heart rate will be lower. For example, the natural automatic rate of the SA node is 60 to 100 bpm, the AV junction 40 to 60 bpm, and the Purkinje system 20 to 40 bpm. Slower pacemakers are

inhibited from firing after stimulation by a faster pacemaker, an effect termed *overdrive suppression*. This is nature's way of keeping these latent pacemakers inactive as the faster pacemaker maintains control.

FOR BOOKWORMS: *Overdrive suppression* is also the term used by electrophysiologists to describe the technique of artificially stimulating the heart at a rapid rate, temporarily suppressing normal cardiac pacemaker activity. Measuring the rate of spontaneous return of the natural pacemaker is used to assess normal or abnormal function. This technique is used to evaluate sick sinus syndrome by determining the sinus node recovery time.

Excitability is the property of all cardiac cells to respond to an outside stimulus.

Conductivity refers to the ability of cardiac cells to transmit an electrical impulse from one cell to another. The speed of conduction is not the same in all areas of the heart. Cells with the fastest conduction are found in the specialized conduction system (bundle of His, bundle branches, and Purkinje fibers). Atrial and ventricular myocardial cells also conduct rapidly, but not as fast as cells of the specialized conduction system. The slowest conduction is found in the AV node. This creates a natural delay in transmitting the electrical signal from the atria to the ventricles, allowing the ventricles time to completely fill with blood before they start contracting.

Refractoriness represents a temporary inability of a cardiac cell to respond to an electrical stimulus. As we will learn later in this chapter, there are times when the cell is either completely or partially refractory.

Charging the Cell

The biochemical electrical activity of living cells is different than household electricity. The electrical current that powers everything in your home results from the flow of electrons through conducting wires. Current across cell membranes

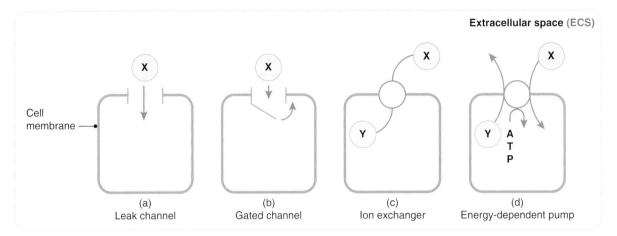

Figure 3-1. Ion transport mechanisms. Means to allow the transport of hypothetical ions, X and Y, across cell membranes. They include pore-like "leak" channels that permit passive diffusion (cell a), gated channels (cell b), exchangers (cell c), and energy-dependent pumps (cell d). All may be present in an individual cardiomyocyte.

derives from the movement of electrically charged particles called **ions**. These particles carry either a positive or negative charge depending on the loss or gain of electrons. Positively charged ions are called *cations* and negatively charged ions are called *anions*.

Cardiac myocytes, like all living cells, are *polarized* at rest. That is, the inside of the cardiac cell is **negatively** charged relative to the outside. This creates an **electrical potential** across the cell membrane, which can be thought of as a type of "pressure" that drives the flow of electrical current. The cell is polarized via a complex system of pumps and channels that modify the relative concentrations of ions inside and outside the cell. Of the many ions involved, sodium (Na^+), potassium (K^+), and calcium (Ca^{2+}) are the most important. The difference between all the positive and negative charges on the two sides of the cell membrane is called the **membrane potential** and is measured in millivolts (mV). Ultimately, it is the electrical charging (polarization) and discharging (depolarization) of the cardiac cells that initiate cardiac contraction and the findings we record with the ECG.

Keep An Eye On Ions

Before we proceed, let's go over a few basic concepts about how ions interact with cell membranes. The cell membrane does not readily allow charged particles to pass into and out of the cell. But nature has provided a number of ways to overcome this barrier (**Figure 3-1**). These include ion-specific channels, ion exchangers, and energy-dependent pumps. Ion channels can act either as open pores that permit the passive diffusion of ions or as "gated" channels that open and close in response to changes in electrical voltage or other factors. Ion exchangers link the transport of two different ions in both directions across the cell membrane. Energy-dependent pumps accomplish the same task but use energy derived from adenosine triphosphate (ATP) to exchange the two ions. There are multiple channels, exchangers, and pumps for all of the key ions involved in cardiac electrical processes including sodium, potassium, and calcium.

To understand how the cell establishes a membrane potential, we need to define a few basic concepts (**Figure 3-2**). When there are more ions on one side of the cell membrane than another, they establish a *concentration gradient*. This exerts a chemical pressure that seeks to passively move ions "downhill" through an open channel and equalize the number of ions on each side (**Figure 3-2a**). But if a positive ion passes through the cell membrane alone without an accompanying anion, it leaves behind a negative charge. This *electrostatic force* tries to maintain electrical neutrality and attract the positive ion back into the cell (**Figure 3-2b**). Eventually, the electrostatic force becomes strong enough to oppose the force of the concentration gradient and the flow of ions stops. This balance determines the *equilibrium potential* for that specific ion (**Figure 3-2c**).

 FOR BOOKWORMS: The equilibrium potential for a monovalent cation can be calculated using the Nernst equation: ($E_m = -61.5 \log [\text{Ion}]_{inside}/[\text{Ion}]_{outside}$).

Who Let the Cation Out of the House?

At rest, a typical cardiac muscle cell has a membrane potential of approximately −90 mV, which means that the inside of the cell has a negative potential of 90 mV compared to the extracellular space. How does the cardiomyocyte establish and maintain this baseline electrical potential, termed the *resting membrane potential*? Let's apply the processes we learned in the preceding discussion to provide an answer (**Figure 3-3**). These include (1) the action of pumps that use energy to actively transport ions across the cell membrane, (2) the balance between the concentration gradient and electrostatic force, and (3) the relative permeability of the cell membrane to passive diffusion of ions through ion-specific channels.

Step one in polarizing the cell depends on an energy-dependent pump called Na^+/K^+–ATPase, which uses ATP to transfer three sodium ions from inside to outside the cell in exchange for two potassium ions (**Figure 3-3a**). This establishes

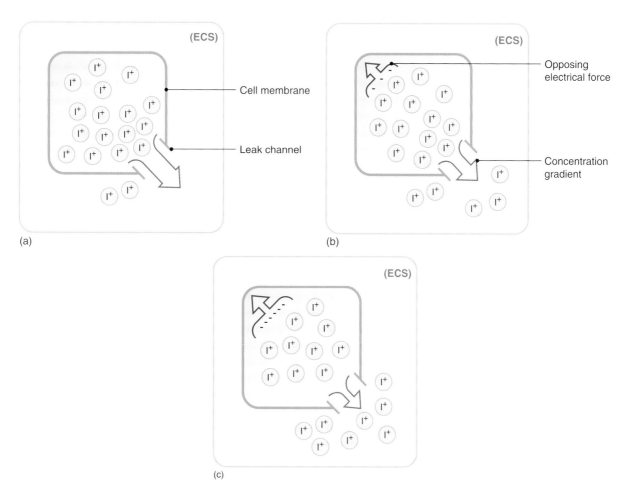

Figure 3-2. Basic concepts of ion movement. The equilibrium potential for a specific ion depends on a balance between the opposing forces of the concentration gradient and the electrostatic force. Inside the cell, each ion is comprised of a positively charged cation (I$^+$) and a negatively charged anion (not shown).

a) Baseline state with more ions inside the cell. A concentration gradient (gray arrow) exerts pressure for ions to move into the extracellular space (ECS).

b) Positively charged cations exit the cell, leaving its anion partner behind. This produces an opposing, negatively charged electrostatic force (purple arrow).

c) A balance between the concentration gradient and the electrostatic force stops the further flow of ions and establishes the equilibrium potential.

a high concentration of potassium ions inside the cell and low outside. Conversely, the pump produces a high concentration of sodium ions outside the cell and low inside. This "three for two" exchange of positive ions generates an ionic current that contributes about −10 mV to the negative electrical potential inside the cell.

CLINICAL TIP: Digitalis is a cardiac medication that interferes with the activity of Na$^+$/K$^+$–ATPase. When the pump is inhibited, less sodium is removed thereby increasing the concentration of intracellular sodium and decreasing the concentration of intracellular potassium. Ultimately, the sodium ions are exchanged for calcium ions, which increase the force of cardiac muscle contraction.

Step two relates to the presence of a concentration gradient across the cell membrane for both sodium and potassium ions,

generated by the action of Na$^+$/K$^+$–ATPase (**Figure 3-3b**). As we mentioned earlier, both sodium and potassium ions are now under chemical pressure to passively reverse the differences in concentration until the opposing electrostatic force stops any further flow of ions. It would appear then that the final membrane potential must be determined by the equilibrium potentials of both sodium and potassium. Not so fast!

It turns out that the cell membrane is much more permeable at rest to the transfer of potassium ions than sodium ions. Yes, both sodium and potassium ions would each like to try and equalize their concentrations across the cell membrane, but to do so, they need to pass through their respective ion channels. Therein lies the issue because there are about 100 open potassium channels for every open sodium channel. This difference in ion permeability is what maintains the high concentration of sodium ions in the extracellular space after they are actively pumped outside the cell and also explains why potassium ions

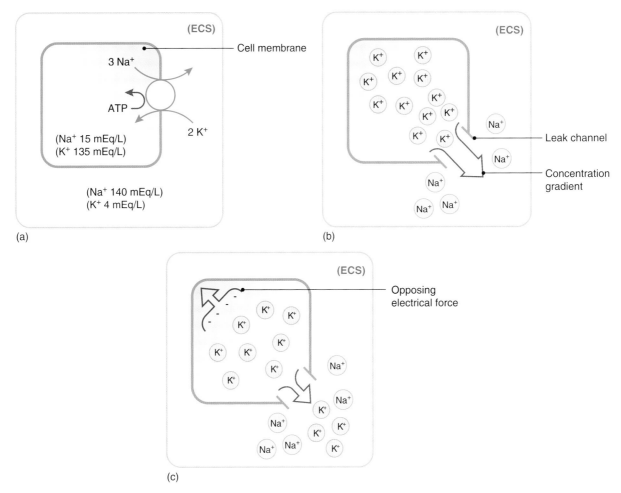

Figure 3-3. Polarizing the cardiomyocyte.

a) Three sodium (Na⁺) ions are exchanged for two potassium ions (K⁺) ions, establishing a high concentration of K⁺ inside the cell.

b) Plentiful K⁺-specific channels allow this ion to diffuse down its concentration gradient back outside the cell.

c) Negatively charged proteins coupled with K⁺ are left behind, producing an electrostatic force. The balance between the concentration gradient and electrostatic force establishes a resting membrane potential of −90 mV.

are the primary determinant of the resting membrane potential. Sodium ions just can't get into the polarization game in resting cells, so potassium ions are the key players.

 CLINICAL TIP: Antiarrhythmic medications exert their effect by modifying cardiac ion channels. Also, hereditary gene mutations of sodium and potassium channels are associated with conditions that predispose individuals to cardiac arrhythmias, including the Brugada and long QT syndromes.

The final step in polarizing the cell is revealed by now following the movement of potassium ions through the cell membrane. We explained that intracellular potassium readily passes through open channels from inside to outside the cell. But as we also learned, a positively charged cation like potassium is partnered with a negatively charged anion. Potassium ions within the cell are primarily coupled with large anionic proteins that are too large to pass through the cell membrane. As the positively charged potassium ions passively diffuse down their

concentration gradient out of the cell, the negatively charged proteins are left behind, creating an opposing electrostatic force (**Figure 3-3c**). When the cell has become about 90 mV more negative inside than outside the cell, the electrostatic force balances the concentration gradient and no more positively charged potassium ions can leave the cell. The net flow of ions ceases and we have established a resting membrane potential of about −90 mV. Now we're polarized!

You may find it helpful to think of the ions in the interior of the cardiac cell as a room full of dancing couples. Each "cute cation" of potassium is dancing with an "overweight anion." It's crowded inside the cell so the ladies want to go outside where there's more room. But the bouncer at the open potassium channel door only allows the slender women to pass, leaving behind one big, angry anion each time. When enough of the ladies exit the room, the angry anions have enough force to intimidate the bouncer and put a stop to the exodus. There are other ions, like sodium, hanging around, but they don't have a pass for this polarization party, so they're not a factor at this point.

▶ DEPOLARIZATION AND REPOLARIZATION

We've just spent a lot of time explaining how the cell becomes electrically polarized. You can think of this as the process by which the cardiac cell becomes an electrochemical battery. But what good is any battery if it doesn't use its energy supply to power a motor? Let's now learn how the heart uses this stored electricity to ultimately stimulate muscle cells to contract (**Figure 3-4**).

Depolarization is the initial electrical event of cardiac cells. The process starts with the flow of positive ions into the cell, which reverses the cell's negative polarity. The wave of depolarization propagates from cell to cell through *gap junctions*, generating an electrical current. It is this process that is recorded by the surface ECG.

Repolarization represents the reestablishment of the baseline electronegative state. Depolarization begins from the endocardium and spreads to the epicardium. Repolarization reverses

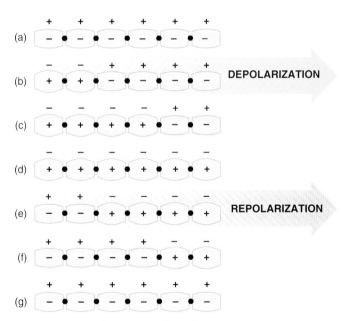

Figure 3-4. Depolarization and repolarization.

a) A muscle fiber with six cells, all in the resting, polarized state (negative inside, positive outside).

b) Depolarization begins.

c) Depolarization continues.

d) All cells are depolarized.

e) Repolarization begins.

f) Repolarization continues.

g) All cells have repolarized and the cell returns to the resting state.

the process but proceeds from the epicardium to the endocardium. This process is also recorded on the ECG.

▶ POTENTIAL FOR ACTION

The cycle of depolarization and repolarization in a single cardiac cell is called the **action potential**. These electrical events can be illustrated graphically as changes in membrane potential over time (**Figure 3-5**). An important concept in understanding the action potential is the **threshold potential**. This is the critical voltage to which a cell must be depolarized before it can generate and propagate an action potential.

There are two general types of action potentials, those of **pacemaker** cells and **nonpacemaker** cells. Pacemaker cells are capable of spontaneous depolarization (automaticity), whereas nonpacemaker cells require an outside stimulus from an adjacent cell. Pacemaker cells are present in the SA node, which we learned in Chapter 2 is the primary pacemaker of the heart. Other cardiac tissues that have potential pacemaker activity include localized portions of the atrium, the proximal and distal portions of the AV junction (not the actual AV node), and the remainder of the His-Purkinje system. Remember that these subsidiary pacemakers are usually latent because of the faster rate of the dominant SA node. Nonpacemaker cells comprise the atrial and ventricular myocardium.

 CLINICAL TIP: Nonpacemaker cells may develop characteristics of pacemaker cells with abnormal automaticity in the setting of inadequate coronary blood flow (ischemia or infarction). Similarly, cardiac diseases may damage normal pacemaker cells and render them ineffective.

The action potential of a typical cardiac muscle cell can be divided into five phases (0, 1, 2, 3, 4). Stage 0 represents depolarization, where the cell loses its negative internal charge. This is followed by repolarization, encompassing stages 1, 2, and 3, where the cell regains internal electronegativity. Phase 4 represents the resting potential. The characteristics of these phases are determined by the flow of ions across the cell membrane, which is different in pacemaker and nonpacemaker cells.

The ion movements responsible for the action potential are referred to as *currents*. By convention, an *inward current* depolarizes the cell and describes the movement of either positive charges (eg, Na^+ or K^+ ions) into the cell, or the outward movement of negative charges (eg, Cl^-). Either action makes the inside of the cell more electropositive. Conversely, an *outward current* repolarizes the cell and describes the exit of positive ions from the cell, or the entry of negative ions. Either action makes the inside of the cell more electronegative.

Let's now look at the different types of action potentials in more detail.

Nonpacemaker Action Potentials

Figure 3-5a displays the typical action potential of a nonpacemaker cell of the ventricular myocardium. Note that there are five distinct phases.

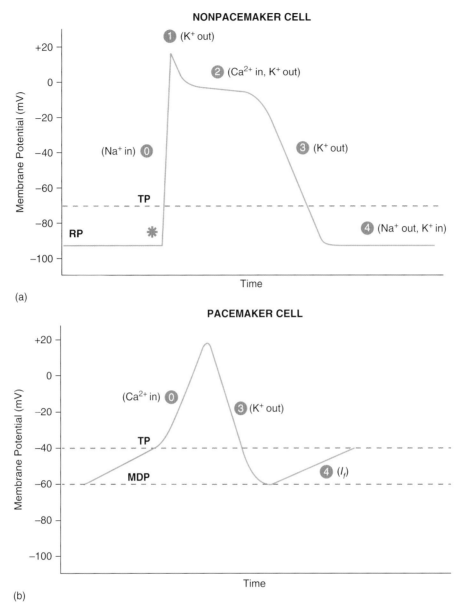

Figure 3-5. Action potential of a nonpacemaker (a) and pacemaker (b) cell. The flow of key ions is depicted during each phase. Abbreviations: resting potential (RP), threshold potential (TP), maximum diastolic potential (MDP), funny current (I_f)

a) Nonpacemaker cells are characterized by a rapid depolarization (phase 0), repolarization (phases 1, 2, and 3), and a true resting potential (phase 4). An outside stimulus (*) is required to initiate depolarization. After reaching the threshold potential, depolarization continues spontaneously.

b) Pacemaker cells have a slow depolarization (phase 0) and repolarization (phase 3), without a phase 1 or 2. These cells do not have a true resting potential, instead exhibiting a gradually upsloping phase 4 from the maximum diastolic potential that represents the property of automaticity.

Phase 0 (rapid depolarization) is the rapid upstroke of the action potential that represents depolarization. The process starts with a depolarizing stimulus from an adjacent cell, which opens gated sodium channels and causes the membrane potential to become less negative. When the voltage reaches the threshold potential, typically in the range of −60 to −70 mV, even more sodium channels open to permit a rapid, self-sustaining entry of sodium into the cell, hence the term "fast response." The rapid influx of positively charged sodium ions reverses the negative polarity of the cell

(depolarization). Note that there is a transient "overshoot" where the membrane polarity actually becomes positive. Separate inactivation gates now interrupt the inward flow of sodium ions, ending phase 0.

Phase 1 (early rapid repolarization) represents the initial repolarization of the cell. It reflects the final closing of the gated sodium channels and opening of outward potassium channels. This results in a net loss of positive ions from the cell, which lowers the transiently positive membrane potential to approximately 0 mV.

Phase 2 (plateau) represents a delay in repolarization. During this phase slow calcium channels open that allow a weak, inward flow of calcium into the cell. Potassium continues to exit the cell as calcium slowly enters. This creates a near balance of inward-flowing calcium ions and outward-flowing potassium ions that produces the plateau. Calcium entry into the cell at this point is a vital trigger in initiating mechanical systole (contraction), which begins at the onset of phase 2. The characteristic plateau in the action potential of cardiac cells has another important physiologic purpose. The electrical delay allows myocardial cells to finish contracting before they can be stimulated again. In contrast, the action potential of skeletal muscle cells lacks this plateau; therefore, rapid stimulation can produce tetanic contraction.

 CLINICAL TIP: Calcium channel blockers, such as verapamil, inhibit the flow of calcium ions during the plateau phase.

Phase 3 (terminal rapid repolarization) restores the negative membrane potential. Potassium ions continue to exit the cell as the slow calcium channels are inactivated. The membrane potential becomes progressively more negative until repolarization is complete.

Phase 4 (resting) represents the time between action potentials. This is when the Na$^+$/K$^+$–ATPase pump is active, which we learned previously is the first step in establishing the resting potential. Here you can see how this pump serves to eliminate the sodium that had entered the cell in phase 0, exchanging it for the potassium that exited during phases 2 and 3. Phase 4 establishes the stable resting membrane potential in nonpacemaker cells of −90 mV using the three-step process we reviewed in the preceding discussion: (1) the Na$^+$/K$^+$–ATPase pump, (2) potassium diffusion out of the cell via open channels, and (3) the balancing of electrostatic and chemical forces. Phase 4 correlates with mechanical diastole (relaxation) and continues until the cell is again stimulated to initiate the next depolarization at phase 0.

Pacemaker Action Potentials

Figure 3-5b displays the typical action potential of a pacemaker cell of the SA node. The action potential of pacemaker cells of the AV junction has a similar configuration. Notice the key differences between this configuration and that of a nonpacemaker cell.

Phase 0 (slow depolarization) in pacemaker cells has a slower upstroke and lower amplitude than nonpacemaker cells, hence the term, "slow response." Depolarization in pacemaker cells is dependent on the slow influx of calcium. The fast sodium channels responsible for the rapid phase 0 response in nonpacemaker cells are inactivated in pacemaker cells.

Phase 3 (repolarization) represents the inactivation of the calcium channel and the opening of potassium channels, which result in repolarization of the cell, typically to a level of −60 mV. The action potential of pacemaker cells does not have a true phase 1 or phase 2.

Phase 4 (diastolic depolarization) in pacemaker cells demonstrates the property of *automaticity*, characterized by a gradual upward slope and **absence of a true resting potential**. This means that these cells can reach their threshold potential, typically −30 to −40 mV, and initiate depolarization on their own **without an outside stimulus**. Compare this with phase 4 in nonpacemaker cells where the resting potential is flat, remaining so until an outside stimulus is applied. As seen in Figure 3-5, both the maximum diastolic (negative) potential and the threshold potential of pacemaker cells are less negative than those of nonpacemaker cells. The ionic mechanism behind the complex process of automaticity in pacemaker cells is not fully understood, but most likely involves two processes that work in concert to depolarize the cell to the threshold potential. One utilizes an unusual channel permeable to both Na$^+$ and K$^+$ ions that results in an inward current. Because of a number of unique characteristics, this primary pacemaker current is termed the "funny current" (I_f). Another current contributing to pacemaker function is mediated by the oscillatory exchange of sodium and calcium ions and is termed the "calcium clock."

A Helpful Analogy

This is pretty complex material, so let me suggest another analogy to help you. Think of the action potential as an old-fashioned Jack-in-the-Box toy. Releasing the clown represents depolarization and pushing the clown back into the box to recoil the spring is repolarization. Each area of the heart has its own type of Jack-in-the-Box, and there are some important differences between a pacemaker and a nonpacemaker toy. You can think of pacemaker cells as having a battery-operated automatic crank that can turn on its own to release the clown. A pacemaker clown is loosely wound and propels the clown slowly upward with "cranky, calcium-dependent coils." Nonpacemaker cells do not have a crank at all and need outside help to open the latch. The nonpacemaker clown is tightly wound that on release, rapidly shoots the clown upward with "swift, sodium-dependent springs."

▶ AUTOMATIC PILOT

The normal automaticity of the SA node can be influenced by outside factors, especially the autonomic nervous system. Sympathetic (adrenergic) or parasympathetic (cholinergic) discharges modify the slope of phase 4 in pacemaker cells, thereby either raising or lowering the heart rate, respectively (**Figure 3-6**). For example, if you take your pulse the next time you are cheering for your favorite team, your heart rate will likely be faster than when you are sitting in the library studying for your next exam. The reason is that when you are excited, your body releases epinephrine from the adrenal glands and norepinephrine from nerve endings, stress hormones called *catecholamines*. These chemicals increase the slope of phase 4 of the action potential, decreasing the time it takes to reach the threshold potential and thereby raising the heart rate. Conversely, if you become nauseated after getting a disappointing exam score because you were watching the game instead of studying for your test, your vagus nerve secretes *acetylcholine*, a

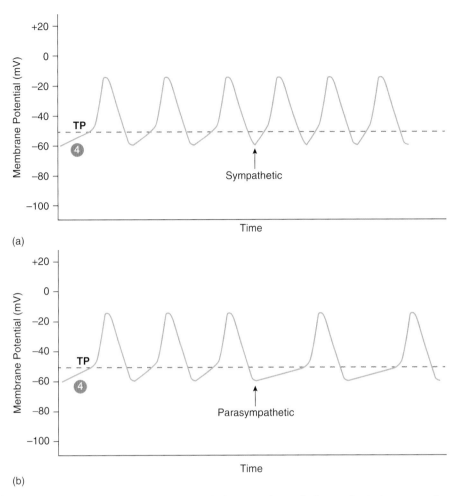

Figure 3-6. Effect of the autonomic nervous system on a typical pacemaker cell. Sympathetic hormones (catecholamines), such as epinephrine and norepinephrine, increase the slope of phase 4 and raise the heart rate (a). Parasympathetic (vagal) hormones, such as acetylcholine, decrease the slope of phase 4 and lower the heart rate (b).

parasympathetic hormone that decreases the slope of phase 4. This increases the time to reach the threshold potential and slows the heart rate. To again use our Jack-in-the-Box model, sympathetic discharges raise the rate you turn the crank, and parasympathetic influences lower the rate.

▶ **REFRACTORY PERIODS**

We've spent a lot of time describing how a cardiac cell is depolarized and repolarized. An equally important concept is *refractoriness*, where the cell is temporarily unable to respond to a new stimulus. This portion of the action potential is called the **refractory period** and primarily reflects the number of fast sodium channels that have entered an inactive state and are temporarily incapable of reopening. Refractoriness helps prevent the heart from being stimulated prematurely before it has finished contracting. As we will learn in subsequent chapters, the concept of refractoriness will play an important role in understanding the genesis of cardiac arrhythmias.

There are different levels of refractoriness during the action potential, called the *absolute, effective,* and *relative* (**Figure 3-7**).

The terminology can be confusing and is used inconsistently between cell physiologists and electrophysiologists, but I'll try to clear things up in the following discussion. In addition, the refractory periods are not the same in all cardiac cells and can even vary within the same cell depending on clinical circumstances. Some of the terms are antiquated, but you are going to see them mentioned in other textbooks of electrocardiography, so I will discuss them all now. The key concept to understand is that during every action potential, there is a period of time when the cell cannot generate or further propagate an electrical stimulus. During other periods of the action potential, the cell can be partially refractory and responds differently.

The *absolute refractory period* (ARP) comprises phases 1 and 2 of the action potential. During this period, the cell **cannot** generate a new action potential, no matter how strong the stimulus is. The reason is that not enough sodium channels have recovered to depolarize the cell again. Think of this as trying to start your car with a completely depleted battery. No matter how many times you turn the ignition, *absolutely* nothing happens.

There is a period comprising the first portion of phase 3 where a stronger than usual stimulus will produce only a very

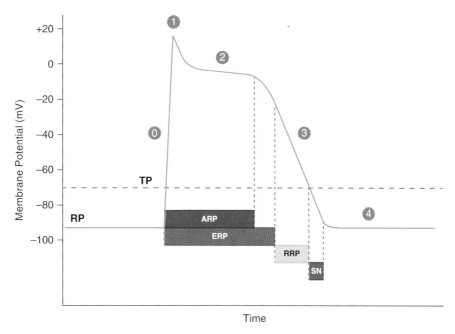

Figure 3-7. Refractory and supernormal periods of the cardiomyocyte. During the absolute refractory period (ARP), the cell is electrically unexcitable. The effective refractory period (ERP) includes the ARP and an additional segment during which a stimulus results in only a local depolarization that cannot be propagated further. During the relative refractory period (RRP), a *greater* than normal stimulus can generate a weak, slowly conducting action potential. During the supernormal period (SN), a *weaker* than normal stimulus can generate a normal action potential.

limited and weak action potential. This unnamed period extends from the end of phase 2 until the membrane potential reaches approximately –25 mV. A stimulus during this time will produce an action potential too weak to propagate further through the conduction system. Some of the sodium channels have recovered, but not nearly enough to propagate a viable action potential. Think of this as a nearly dead car battery where turning the ignition may light the dashboard, but there's not enough power to start the engine.

The term used to describe the **combined** time of the ARP and the additional unnamed period is the *effective refractory period* (ERP). Think of the ERP as that portion of the action potential where a premature stimulus is either absolutely thwarted, or is ineffective. Simply stated, a premature stimulus during the ERP cannot propagate an action potential. To use our automobile analogy, turning the ignition is *effectively* a waste of time because the ultimate goal is to start the engine. You can't do that any time during the ERP. I find it helpful to think of the ERP as the *in*effective refractory period.

 BE CAREFUL: A major source of confusion is that some authors use the terms refractory period, absolute refractory period, and effective refractory period interchangeably. More confusion arises because electrophysiologists use the term *functional refractory period* to describe the minimum time interval in which a delivered premature stimulus will propagate successfully through a specific cardiac tissue. This terminology does not apply to the single cells we are describing here.

There is another period at the very end of phase 3, called the *relative refractory period* (RRP). This occurs after the ERP

when the cell has been repolarized further, approaching the range of the threshold potential. During this period, a **greater** than normal stimulus can depolarize the cell, but the resulting action potential is **weaker** than usual, with a lower amplitude and rate of rise of phase 0. Not all the fast sodium channels have recovered to their fully activated state; therefore, the propagated impulse is limited and has a slower conduction velocity. Think of this period as your lazy "relative" whom you have to berate to help you push your stranded car to the service station (greater than usual stimulus), but he won't put forth much effort (weaker and slower action). He's *relatively* better than nothing, but he doesn't generate the kind of action you would like.

Following the RRP is the *supernormal period* (SN), where a **weaker** than usual stimulus can generate a nearly normal action potential. Here, the cell has been repolarized beyond the threshold potential, but not yet reaching the resting potential. The electrophysiological explanation for this phenomenon is controversial. Think of this as if you are driving a "supercharged" (supernormal) race car, revving the engine close to the starting line. Just a light touch on the pedal and away you go.

The full recovery time, also called the total refractory period, encompasses all of the periods described earlier (ERP, RRP, SN).

▶ EXCITATION-CONTRACTION COUPLING

Depolarization and repolarization are not the same as contraction and relaxation. But these electrical events do trigger the mechanical processes. After all, the ultimate purpose of these electrical actions is to initiate cardiac pumping. The process in the cardiomyocyte that links the action potential with muscle contraction is called *excitation-contraction coupling.*

Excitation-contraction coupling requires the interaction of calcium ions, the contractile proteins *actin* and *myosin*, and regulatory proteins called *troponins*. The complex process begins as calcium ions enter the cell during phase 2 of the action potential. This triggers the release of additional calcium from storage sites within the cardiomyocyte, a phenomenon termed calcium-induced calcium release. Calcium then binds to troponin-C, initiates other steps involving troponin-I, and ultimately allows actin and myosin to interact. Actin and myosin form filaments that slide past each other and shorten, producing muscle contraction (**Figure 3-8**). Relaxation occurs when calcium ions are pumped into an intracellular membrane storage system called the *sarcoplasmic reticulum.* Calcium ions are also removed from the cell during phase 4 via the Na^+/Ca^{2+} exchanger and plasma membrane calcium pumps.

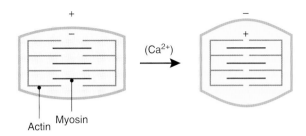

Figure 3-8. Calcium entry into the cardiomyocyte during phase 2 of the action potential activates a complex process that allows the proteins actin and myosin to engage, thereby initiating muscle contraction.

OK, enough with the cell biology. Let's move on to the next chapter where we will learn how to measure these events in a real human being with an electrocardiograph machine.

Chapter 3 • SELF-TEST

1. What are the four inherent properties of myocardial cells?

2. What are ranges of the natural, automatic rates of the following cardiac structures: SA node, AV junction, Purkinje system.

3. At rest, the inside of the cell is electrically negative or positive compared to the outside?

4. The resting membrane potential of the cardiac myocyte is determined primarily by which ion?

5. What is the cycle of depolarization and repolarization of the cardiac myocyte called?

6. What is the critical voltage to which a cell must be depolarized before it can generate an action potential called?

7. In nonpacemaker cells, name the five phases of the action potential and the primary ion movements involved.

8. In pacemaker cells, describe the effect of sympathetic (adrenergic) and parasympathetic (vagal) discharge on the heart rate. They both exert their effect by changing the slope of which phase of the action potential?

9. Define "effective refractory period."

10. The entry into the cell of which ion initiates excitation-contraction coupling and the eventual contraction of cardiac muscle?

ANSWERS

Chapter 3 • SELF-TEST

1. Automaticity, excitability, conductivity, refractoriness.

2. • SA node: 60 to 100 bpm.
   • AV junction: 40 to 60 bpm.
   • Purkinje system: 20 to 40 bpm.

3. Negative.

4. Potassium.

5. The action potential.

6. The threshold potential.

7. • Phase 0: Rapid depolarization—sodium inflow.
   • Phase 1: Early rapid repolarization—potassium outflow.
   • Phase 2: Plateau—calcium inflow and potassium outflow.
   • Phase 3: Terminal rapid repolarization—potassium outflow.
   • Phase 4: Resting—sodium outflow and potassium inflow.

8. • Catecholamines (sympathetic discharge) increase the heart rate.
   • Vagal influences (parasympathetic discharge) decrease the heart rate.
   • Phase 4.

9. The period of time during the action potential when the cell is incapable of generating or propagating an action potential in response to an outside stimulus.

10. Calcium.

Further Reading

Fozzard HA. Ion channels and transporters and cardiac arrhythmias. *Dialog Cardiovas Med.* 2000;5:199-212.

Grant AO. Cardiac ion channels. *Circ Arrhythmia Electrophysiol.* 2009;2:185-194.

Jaye DA, Xiao Y-F, Sigg DC. Basic cardiac electrophysiology: excitable membranes. In: Sigg DC, Iaizzo PA, Xiao Y-F, He B, eds. *Cardiac Electrophysiology Methods and Models.* New York, NY: Springer; 2010:41-51.

Katz A. The cardiac action potential. In: *Physiology of the Heart.* 5th ed. Philadelphia, PA: Wolters Kluwer Lippincott Williams & Wilkins; 2011:369-397.

Klaubunde RE. Electrical activity of the heart. In: *Cardiovascular Physiology Concepts.* Philadelphia, PA: Lippincott Williams & Wilkins; 2005:9-39.

Lin KY, Edelman ER, Strichartz G, et al. Basic cardiac structure and function. In: Lilly LS, ed. *Pathophysiology of Heart Disease.* 5th ed. Philadelphia, PA: Wolters Kluwer Lippincott Williams & Wilkins; 2011:1-27.

Vassalle M. The relationship among cardiac pacemakers: overdrive suppression. *Circ Res.* 1977;41;269-277.

Whalley DW, Wendt DJ, Grant AO. Basic concepts in cellular cardiac electrophysiology: part I: ion channels, membrane currents and the action potential. *PACE.* 1995;18:1556-1574.

From Electrophysiology to Electrocardiography

4

In Chapter 3 we discussed the electrophysiology of a single cell. We learned how an individual cardiomyocyte becomes polarized, depolarized, and repolarized. Now let's see how those electrical events apply to multiple cells, complete muscle fibers, and the entire myocardium. The graphical representation of this process is what we have come to know as the electrocardiogram (ECG).

The ECG does not actually directly measure the electrophysiologic activity of the heart. It gives us no information about anything we learned about membrane potentials in the previous chapter. What it does represent is a graph of the *differences* in electrical potentials as each wave of depolarization travels throughout the myocardium as recorded by electrodes (leads) on the body surface. Depolarization and repolarization of millions of myocardial cells create local regions with various potential differences. As portions of the heart become alternately depolarized and repolarized, the wave of depolarization moves through the myocardium. Because the body contains fluids and electrolytes that can conduct electricity, we can place electrodes on the skin surface and make a recording of this depolarization wave with a galvanometer. The modern electrocardiograph machine is today's evolution of the galvanometer that Einthoven invented more than a century ago.

 FOR BOOKWORMS: A source of confusion is that cellular electrophysiologists view the cell from inside and consider the resting potential as negative. Clinical electrocardiographers view the cardiomyocyte from the outside and consider resting cells as positively charged.

▶ MAKING THE MEASUREMENTS

The concept of measuring potential differences is illustrated in **Figure 4-1**. Think of a galvanometer as a form of balance scale that measures the difference between weights placed on the right and left sides of the apparatus. (Don't forget that in medicine, we refer to the right and left sides of an image as if the patient were facing us, so we'll use the same approach here). In this example, we will define the left side of the scale as positive and the right side as negative. At baseline there are three, 1-kg weights placed on each side of the scale. There is **no difference** between the two sides; therefore, the measurement is recorded as **zero**. If we now take away two of the weights from the right side of the scale, the measured difference has a value of +2 kg (3 minus 1). Using the same convention, if we had initially taken away two weights from the left side leaving three on the right, the measurement would have been recorded as −2 kg (1 minus 3).

Now let's replace the weights with a single cardiac muscle fiber containing six cells (**Figure 4-2**). The weighing pans are replaced with two electrodes, a negative pole on the right and a positive pole on the left. This time instead of weight in kilograms, we'll measure electrical charge differences in millivolts (mV). Note that the measurements reflect the charge **outside** the cell, not inside. At rest, all the cells are polarized with an electrical potential that is negative inside and positive outside (see **Figure 4-2a**). All six cells have the same positive outside charge, so there is **no potential difference** between the right and left sides of the fiber; therefore, the measurement is **zero mV**. If we now depolarize two cells on the right, we leave one polarized cell on the right half of the fiber and three on the left, a difference of two (see **Figure 4-2b**). This potential difference is recorded as +2 mV on the galvanometer. If we continue the process until all the cells have depolarized, there is no potential difference and the galvanometer once again measures zero mV (see **Figure 4-2c**). By the same convention, when two cells on the right have repolarized, there are now two polarized cells on the right and none on the left so a charge difference of −2 mV is recorded (see **Figure 4-2d**).

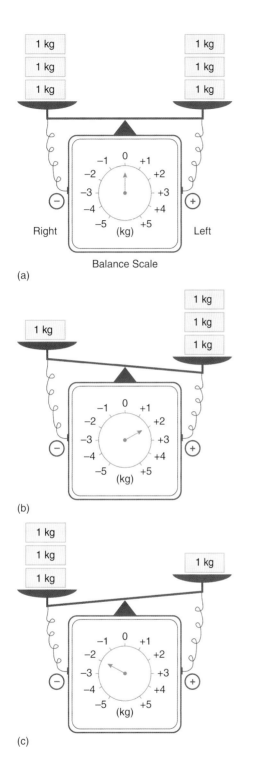

Figure 4-1. A galvanometer is like a balance scale that measures potential differences. Here the recordings are (a) zero, (b) +2, and (c) −2. The right and left sides of the image are depicted from the perspective of a patient facing you.

 FOR BOOKWORMS: This concept also applies to the depolarization and repolarization of a single cardiac cell. I find it easier to illustrate with a cardiac fiber comprised of multiple cells.

Now let's visualize how measurements made from a cardiac muscle fiber produce the deflections we see on the ECG. **Figure 4-3** again shows an isolated strip of myocardium comprised of six individual cells. The fiber is placed on top of a balance scale that is connected to a galvanometer. Also shown is a graphical representation that records the measurements of the galvanometer over time. This is the fundamental concept behind the ECG. According to conventions introduced by Einthoven, an approaching wave of *depolarization* produces a **positive** (upward) deflection and a receding wave of depolarization inscribes a **negative** (downward) deflection. Similarly, an approaching wave of *repolarization* produces a **negative** deflection, and a receding wave of repolarization inscribes a **positive** deflection. Recording the direction and amplitude of the waves of depolarization and repolarization generates the deflections we see on the ECG. Let's now see an example of this concept.

Figure 4-3 demonstrates the galvanometer recordings and ECG of an isolated strip of cardiac muscle. The first group of figures represents depolarization (a-e) and the second group represents repolarization (f-i). A balance scale is used to illustrate the concept of measuring the difference in charges between the two sides of the fiber.

In panel (a), the cells are at rest with all the cells on both sides polarized. There is no potential difference.

In panel (b), two cells on the right have depolarized with one remaining. There are three polarized cells on the left for a net potential difference of +2.

In panel (c), all three of the cells on the right have depolarized. There are three polarized cells on the left, resulting in a maximum potential difference of +3.

In panel (d), all three of the cells on the right have depolarized. On the left, two cells have depolarized with one still polarized, resulting in a potential difference of +1.

In panel (e), all the cells are depolarized on both sides and there is no potential difference.

In panel (f), two cells on the right have repolarized. None of the cells on the left are repolarized, resulting in a potential difference of −2.

In panel (g), all three cells on the right have repolarized. None of the cells on the left are repolarized, resulting in a maximum potential difference of −3.

In panel (h), all three cells on the right are repolarized. On the left, two cells are repolarized, resulting in a potential difference of −1.

In panel (i), all the cells on both sides are again polarized and there is no potential difference.

Note that the system measures only the differences between electrical potentials and cannot distinguish between a fully polarized fiber (panels a and i) and one that is fully depolarized (panel e). In both circumstances, the potential difference between the two sides is zero.

 FOR BOOKWORMS: You can see from this balance scale analogy that the measurements we make have both a magnitude (numerical value) and a polarity (positive

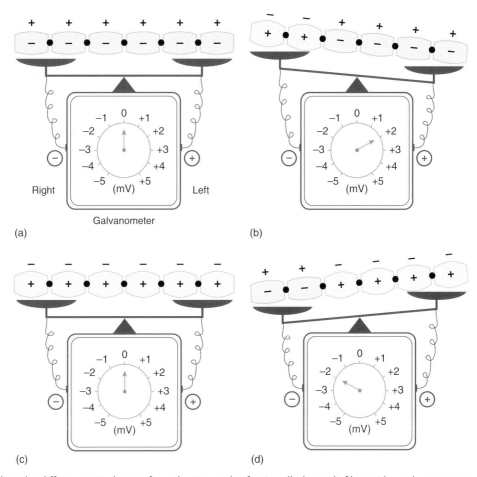

Figure 4-2. Recording the differences in charges from the two ends of a six-celled muscle fiber with a galvanometer.

a) At rest, the number of polarized cells is balanced with no charge difference between the two sides.

b) Two cells on the right have depolarized, resulting in a charge imbalance across the entire fiber of +2 mV.

c) With complete depolarization there is no potential difference between the two sides.

d) Two cells on the right have repolarized, resulting in a charge imbalance of −2 mV.

or negative). This analogy is particularly convenient because the mathematical term *scalar quantity* is used to describe this type of measurement. This explains why you may encounter the term *scalar electrocardiogram* to describe what we now simply abbreviate as ECG (or EKG).

▶ LEADING THE WAY

The electrocardiograph employs a system of leads to analyze cardiac electrical activity from multiple viewpoints. In simple terms, each ECG lead is a pair of terminals that are connected by electrodes to a recording device. One electrode serves as the positive pole and the other serves either as a negative or ground pole. In traditional textbooks of electrocardiography, *bipolar* leads are categorized as those that have two discrete electrodes with opposite polarity, one positive and one negative that record information from different places on the body

surface. *Unipolar* leads are considered to have one positive (also called the "exploring") electrode, but instead of a distinct negative electrode, the electrocardiograph machine uses a mathematically averaged *central terminal* to serve as a negative reference point (also called the "indifferent" electrode). Current recommendations call for the elimination of these terms, recognizing that every ECG lead is essentially bipolar, comprised of electrode pairs that are either physically present or electronically derived.

 FOR HISTORY BUFFS: Traditionally, leads I, II, and III are bipolar. Leads aVR, aVL, aVF, and V1-V6 are assumed to be unipolar.

The conventional ECG allows an analysis in both the frontal and horizontal planes and contains a total of 12 leads. These include the three **standard limb leads (I, II, III),** three **augmented limb leads (aVR, aVL, aVF),** and six **precordial (chest) leads (V1, V2, V3, V4, V5, V6).**

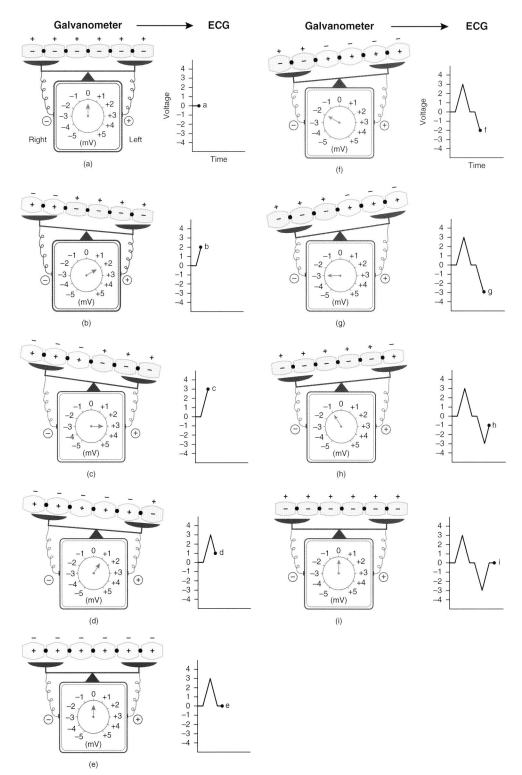

Figure 4-3. Using a galvanometer to measure depolarization and repolarization over time. The connections of the galvanometer are the same as in Figure 4-2. See text for details.

Figure 4-4 demonstrates the standard limb leads (I, II, III) as first envisioned by Einthoven and still in use today. He placed electrodes on the right arm (RA), left arm (LA), and left leg (LL), creating three leads that represent the human body in the frontal plane as an equilateral triangle (Einthoven's triangle). Lead I records the potential difference between the right and left arms, designating the left arm as the positive electrode and the right arm as the negative electrode. Lead II records the potential difference between the right arm and left leg, assigning the right arm as negative and the left leg as positive. Lead III records the potential difference between the left arm and left leg, with the left leg as positive and the left arm as negative. The right leg (ground) electrode serves as a zero reference point, comparing body potentials with the

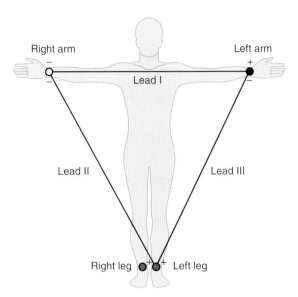

Figure 4-4. Leads I, II, and III are the standard limb leads. The three axes of these leads form an equilateral triangle with the heart at the center (Einthoven's triangle).

surrounding environment and is used to reduce artifacts from electrical interference.

CLINICAL TIP: A major source of technical error in electro-cardiography is misplacement of electrodes. The electrodes are color coded to help with proper positioning: right arm (white), left arm (black), right leg (green), left leg (red). Chest leads are colored brown. A mnemonic I've coined to help you remember limb lead placement is: *"Green and white—on the right, green and red—foot of the bed."*

The augmented limb leads provide information from additional angles (**Figure 4-5**). These three leads record the

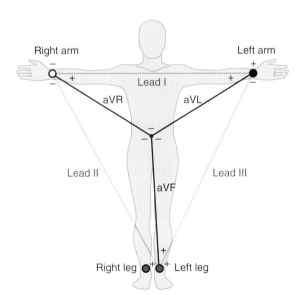

Figure 4-5. Leads aVR, aVL, and aVF are the augmented limb leads. Their axes are from the extremities to a mathematically derived central terminal.

potential differences between the central terminal and the right arm (aVR), left arm (aVL), and left foot (aVF).

FOR HISTORY BUFFS: The augmented limb leads, developed by Frank Wilson in the 1930s and improved on by Emanuel Goldberger in the 1940s, expanded the information provided by Einthoven's standard limb leads. However, the deflections derived between the limbs and the central terminal were of low amplitude and needed a 50% "energy boost" to be better seen, hence the term augmented-voltage, or aV leads.

The six limb leads can be combined to form a **hexaxial** reference system (**Figure 4-6**). This creates a circular reference divided into 30-degree intervals that we can use to describe electrical events in the frontal plane. By convention, the circle is divided into two, 180-degree hemispheres, with positive degrees below the equator and negative degrees above.

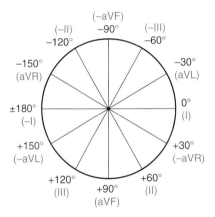

Figure 4-6. The hexaxial reference system combines the limb leads (I, II, III) with the augmented leads (aVR, aVL, aVF), arranging them around a central point. This provides a circular reference that is divided into a positive "southern" hemisphere and a negative "northern" hemisphere.

The precordial leads are utilized to analyze cardiac electrical activity in the horizontal plane (**Figure 4-7**). Six leads are placed across the chest and are identified as V1, V2, V3, V4, V5, and V6. The leads are placed as follows:

- V1—Fourth intercostal space at the right sternal border.
- V2—Fourth intercostal space at the left sternal border.
- V3—Midway between V2 and V4.
- V4—Fifth intercostal space in the midclavicular line.
- V5—In the horizontal plane of V4 at the anterior axillary line, or if the anterior axillary line is ambiguous, midway between V4 and V6.
- V6—In the horizontal plane of V4 at the midaxillary line.

BE CAREFUL: Proper precordial lead placement can be difficult in women with large breasts. Recommendations are inconsistent, with some advocating for placement under and others over the breasts. In most cases, leads can be placed properly by lifting up the breast and placing the electrodes underneath.

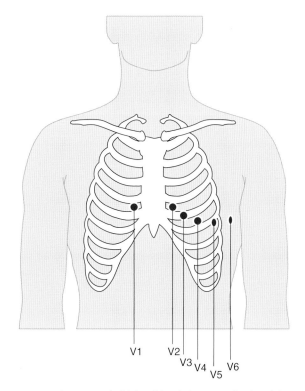

Figure 4-7. The precordial (chest) leads (see text for details).

The geometric relationship of the precordial leads is not as precise as the limb leads, but may be considered such that leads V2 and V6 form a 90-degree angle with V6 at 0 degrees and V2 at +90 degrees. The corresponding approximate angles of the other leads are V1 (+120 degrees), V3 (+75 degrees), V4 (+60 degrees), V5 (+30 degrees).

Combining both the limb and precordial lead systems allows us to analyze the cardiac electrical system in three dimensions (**Figure 4-8**). In the frontal plane, we can describe electrical events in terms of right, left, superior, and inferior. Simultaneous recording using the precordial leads allows us to describe the same events in terms of right, left, anterior, and posterior.

Remember that for any lead we are investigating, a wave of depolarization moving *toward* the positive electrode will produce a positive (upright) deflection. A wave of depolarization moving *away* from the positive electrode will produce a negative (downgoing) deflection (**Figure 4-9**). As we will learn in Chapter 6, a single wave of depolarization will have a different contour and amplitude depending on the location of the recording lead.

Creating a Paper Record

ECG recordings are made on graph paper made up of small and large boxes that are measured in millimeters (mm) (**Figure 4-10**). Each small, light-colored box is 1 × 1 mm and each large, darker box is 5 × 5 mm. Modern ECG machines record 10 seconds of data, with a 2.5-second view of four sets

of three simultaneously recorded leads in the following groups: (I, II, III), (aVR, aVL, aVF), (V1, V2, V3), (V4, V5, V6). To facilitate the interpretation of the cardiac rhythm, a 10-second lead II rhythm strip is also recorded. Alternative displays may be selected from available menu options.

Time is recorded on the horizontal axis. At a standard recording speed of 25 mm per second (mm/sec), each small box represents 0.04 seconds and each large box 0.2 seconds. ECG findings are frequently reported in terms of milliseconds (msec), so by moving the decimal point three places to the right, we can convert the units of each small box to 40 msec and each large box to 200 msec. Regardless of the units we use, adding together five large boxes equals 1 second. To further help with determining time, ECG paper also typically includes 3-second markers either at the top or bottom of the page.

Voltage is recorded on the vertical axis. At a standard calibration, each small, 1-mm box corresponds to 0.1 mV of voltage (1 mV = 10 mm). A 1 mV standardization deflection is recorded either at the beginning or end of every tracing.

 CLINICAL TIP: It is sometimes valuable to adjust the paper speed or voltage standardization to reveal ECG findings that are otherwise hard to visualize. At double standard voltage calibration, 1 mV = 20 mm, which produces deflections that are twice the usual height. At double recording speed, the paper travels at 50 mm/sec, which widens the deflections by a factor of two.

ECG Nomenclature

The deflections recorded by the electrocardiograph machine are described in terms of *waves (waveforms), complexes, segments,* and *intervals.* A **waveform** is a deflection away from the baseline, either in an upward (positive) or downward (negative), direction. The normal ECG has six major waves, named P, Q, R, S, T, and U. A **complex** comprises two or more waveforms (eg, QRS complex). An **interval** is inscribed between two waveforms, measured between the beginning of one deflection and either the beginning (eg, PR) or end (eg, QT) of the next. A **segment** is the time between the end of one waveform and the beginning of the next (eg, PR, ST, TP). Measurements of waves, complexes, segments, and intervals are made from the *baseline,* which is a stable, isoelectric portion of the ECG. Depending on technical factors, either the PR segment or TP segment can serve as the baseline. To correct for the width of the baseline, measurements of upward deflections are made from the upper edge of the baseline to the peak of the wave; downward deflections are made from the lower edge of the baseline to the nadir of the wave.

Let's take a look at each specific component individually in the order they appear on the normal ECG (**Figure 4-11**). Not every interval and segment is routinely reported in electrocardiography, but they are included here for completeness. A good way to analyze each component is to look at each in terms of duration, amplitude, and contour.

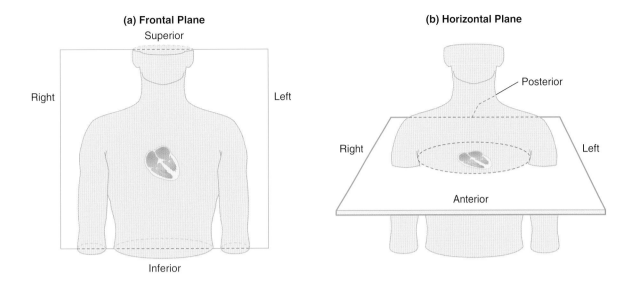

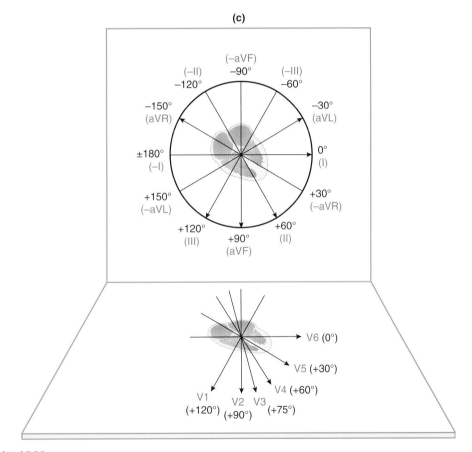

Figure 4-8. The 12-lead ECG.

a) The hexaxial limb lead system analyzes events in the frontal plane.

b) The precordial/chest lead system analyzes events in the horizontal plane.

c) Combining the two systems provides a three-dimensional view of the heart.

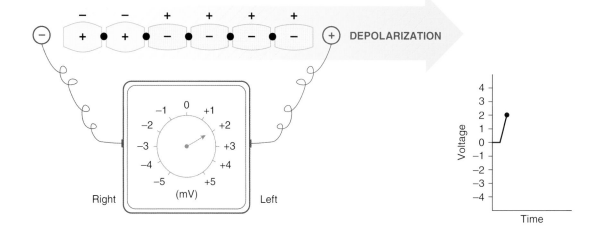

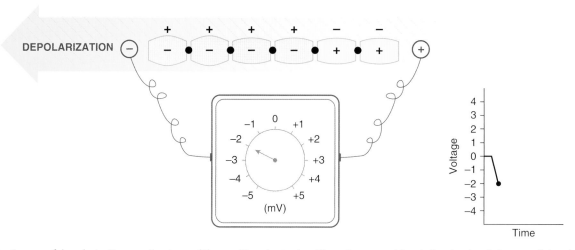

Figure 4-9. A wave of depolarization moving toward the positive electrode will produce a positive deflection (top). A wave of depolarization moving away from the positive electrode will produce a negative deflection (bottom).

 CLINICAL TIP: Voltage abnormalities of segments or waves are traditionally described in terms of millimeters rather than millivolts. For example, an abnormal depression of the ST segment of 0.3 mV below the baseline would be described clinically as "3 mm ST depression."

The **P wave** is the first deflection seen and represents atrial depolarization. Note that the depolarization of the SA node is too small to be visible on the surface ECG. The initial and terminal portions of the P wave represent depolarization of the right atrium followed by the left atrium, respectively. The width of the P wave is measured from where the forward and hind limbs join the baseline. The height of an upright P wave is measured from the upper edge of the baseline to the summit and should not include the thickness of the line. The normal P wave is smooth in contour and is always positive in leads I and II, but may be biphasic in lead V1. The normal P wave has an amplitude of ≤2.5 mm and a duration of ≤0.11 seconds.

The **P-P interval** is the time between two consecutive P waves and is most easily measured from the beginning of one P wave to another. This measurement is utilized to calculate the atrial rate. In sinus rhythm with normal conduction, the atrial rate will equal the ventricular rate.

The **PR segment** is the isoelectric line between the end of the P wave and the beginning of the QRS complex, regardless of whether the initial QRS deflection is a Q wave or an R wave. This segment can serve as a baseline, particularly for measuring the voltages of the QRS complex and ST segment.

The **PR interval** encompasses the P wave and PR segment. This represents the entire time required for the impulse that enters the atria to reach the ventricles, traveling first through both atria, followed by the AV node, bundle of His, bundle branches, and the Purkinje network. The PR interval is measured from the beginning of the P wave to the beginning of the QRS complex, regardless of whether the initial QRS deflection is a Q wave or an R wave. The normal PR interval is 0.12 to 0.20 seconds. The PR interval should be measured in the lead that exhibits the longest interval.

The **QRS complex** predominantly reflects the electrical depolarization of both ventricles (phase 0), but it also includes early repolarization (phase 1). A **Q wave** is the first negative

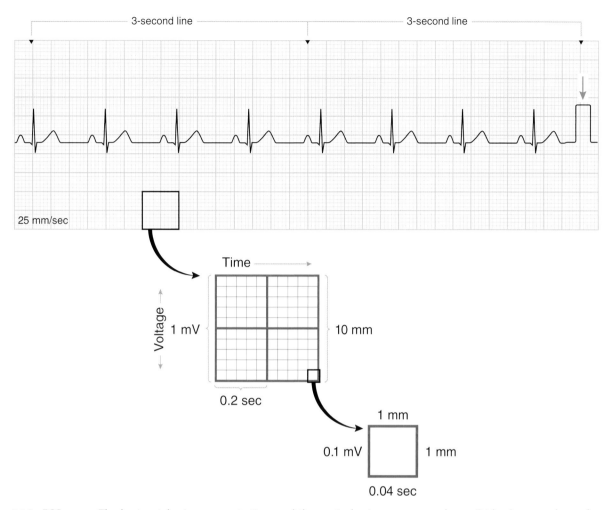

Figure 4-10. ECG paper. The horizontal axis represents time and the vertical axis represents voltage. Grid values are drawn for routine recordings at a paper speed of 25 mm/sec and a voltage standardization of 1 mV = 10 mm (blue arrow).

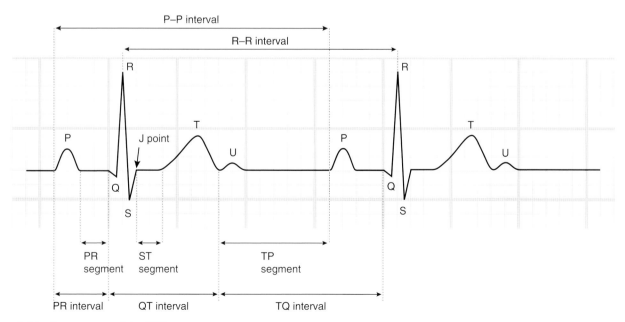

Figure 4-11. Components of the ECG.

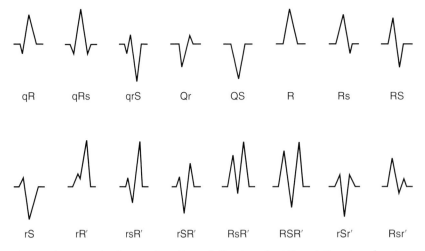

Figure 4-12. The QRS complex can be named using small and large letters to reflect the relative size of each component.

deflection not preceded by an R wave and there can only be one Q wave in each QRS complex. Small Q waves ≤0.03 second related to septal depolarization may be normally found in leads I, II, III, aVL, aVF, and V4-V6. A wider Q wave ≥0.04 second may be a normal finding in lead III, as is a QS complex in leads aVR and V1. An **R wave** is the first positive deflection, with or without a preceding Q wave. Any subsequent positive deflection is called an **R prime (R′) wave**. An **S wave** is the first negative deflection of the QRS complex that extends below the baseline. A subsequent negative deflection is called an **S prime (S′) wave**. A **QS wave** is a QRS complex made up of one large, negative deflection.

Even though this group of deflections is termed the QRS complex, not all will contain an individual Q wave, R wave, and S wave. You will often see a QRS complex that is described as a QR, QS, or RS wave. Capital and lowercase letters can be used to describe the relative sizes of waves comprising the QRS complex (**Figure 4-12**). A QRS complex with three distinct waves is termed *triphasic* (eg, qRs, rSR′), one that has two waves *biphasic* (eg, qR, rS) and a complex with only one discrete wave *monophasic* (eg, R, QS). An additional term sometimes used to describe findings in the QRS complex is a "notch," which is either a small negative deflection in the R wave that does not extend below the baseline or a small positive deflection in an S wave that does not extend above the baseline (**Figure 4-13**). Another descriptor called a "slur" is a localized thickening or smoothing out of a deflection.

The normal QRS complex contains waves that are sharp in configuration. The QRS width is normally 0.06 to 0.10 seconds

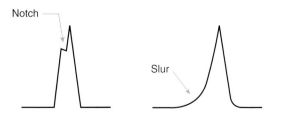

Figure 4-13. The QRS complex may also be described as having a notch or slur.

and is measured in the limb or precordial lead with the longest duration from the beginning of the first deflection (either Q or R wave) to the end of the last deflection. The amplitude of the QRS complex in an individual lead is the sum of the single tallest positive and single deepest negative waveforms of the complex as measured from the baseline. The normal total QRS amplitude should be ≥5 mm in at least one limb lead and ≥10 mm in at least one chest lead, otherwise the QRS is categorized as having *low voltage*. There is a wide variation of the maximum normal QRS amplitude in individual leads. We will be discussing details on abnormalities of maximum voltage in the chapter on ventricular hypertrophy.

The **R wave peak time**, also known as the time to the onset of the **intrinsicoid deflection**, is believed to represent the time it takes for the electrical impulse to travel from the endocardium to epicardium as viewed by that lead (ventricular activation time) (**Figure 4-14**). The actual *intrinsicoid deflection* is the abrupt reversal in the direction that follows the peak of the R wave. The measurement is typically made in the precordial leads from the beginning of the QRS complex to the peak of the R wave (or R′ wave in the presence of bundle branch block). The upper limit of normal R wave peak time is <0.04 second in V1 and V2, and <0.05 second in V5 and V6. The longer R wave peak time in the left precordial leads reflects measurement of the greater mass of the left ventricle compared with the right ventricle, which is recorded by the right precordial leads. Prolongation of the R wave peak time is used in the diagnosis of ventricular hypertrophy and bundle branch block, conditions that increase the activation time from endocardium to epicardium.

The **R-R interval** is the time between two consecutive QRS complexes and is most easily measured from the peak of one R wave to another. This measurement is utilized to calculate the ventricular heart rate (see Chapter 5).

The **ST segment** is the interval between the end of the QRS complex and the beginning of the T wave. The point where the QRS complex and ST segment meet is called the **J point** (J junction). The J point represents the end of early repolarization (phase 1), and the ST segment corresponds to the plateau

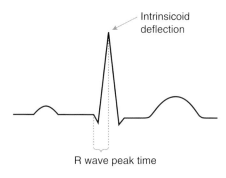

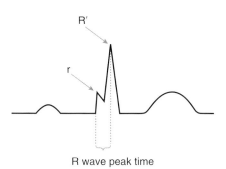

Figure 4-14. The R wave peak time, also known as the ventricular activation time, is measured from the onset of the QRS complex to the peak of the R wave (or R′ wave in the presence of bundle branch block). This measurement is equivalent to the time to the intrinsicoid deflection, which is the reversal of direction at the peak of the R wave.

phase of the ventricular action potential (phase 2). The ST segment is normally isoelectric, but may be slightly elevated or depressed by <1 mm relative to the baseline. Somewhat greater ST elevation may be a normal finding in leads V2 and V3 (<1.5 mm in women and <2 mm in men younger than 40 years). Note that some authors prefer to measure ST segment amplitude 40 to 80 msec after the J point because small differences in membrane potential during repolarization may normally cause slight deviation of the J point and early portion of the ST segment.

The **T wave** represents continuing ventricular repolarization (phase 3). The amplitude of an upright T wave is measured from the upper level of the baseline to the peak of the wave. Inverted T waves are measured from the lower level of the baseline to the nadir of the wave. The amplitude of the T wave should not exceed 6 mm in the limb leads or 10 mm in the precordial leads. The normal T wave configuration is rounded, smooth, and slightly asymmetric, with the terminal portion exhibiting a steeper downslope.

The direction of the T wave usually parallels that of a normal QRS complex in that lead. Accordingly, leads that contain a tall R wave will also have an upright T wave. Similarly, leads with a deep S wave will normally have an inverted T wave. But wait a minute! Didn't we already discuss that repolarization should be recorded in a direction opposite from depolarization? If that were true, then the T wave configuration in each lead should be opposite to that of the QRS (see Figure 4-3). The explanation is that depolarization of the ventricular myocardium spreads

from the endocardium to epicardium, but repolarization begins at the epicardium and ends in the endocardium. Why should that be? One reason is that the action potentials of epicardial cells are shorter than those of the endocardium. In contrast to the hypothetical situation described in Figures 4-2 and 4-3, the *last* ventricular muscle cells to depolarize are actually the *first* to repolarize. The net effect on the ECG is that the direction of the T wave is normally *concordant* with the QRS and not in the opposite direction that we would have expected. And, as we know from looking at the action potential, repolarization is a slower process than depolarization, so the T wave deflection is wider and lower than the QRS deflection.

The **QT interval** is measured from the onset of the QRS complex (start of ventricular depolarization) to the end of the T wave (end of ventricular repolarization). Accurate measurement of the QT interval is particularly vexing because of a variety of issues. These include (1) difficulty in the proper identification of the end of the T wave, (2) accounting for differences in the QT interval in various leads, (3) variability of the QT interval with heart rate and gender, and (4) factoring in the effect of the QRS duration.

The QT interval should be measured in the lead with the longest QT duration. Inspect leads II and V5 initially, but realize that the most accurately determined QT interval may be in another lead. A frustrating fact is that the QT interval may normally vary in different leads by as much as 40 msec, a term called QT *dispersion*. Manual measurements are more accurate than the values derived on automated digital ECG machines, which use a multiple-lead algorithm that can report a QT interval longer than one found in any individual lead. When measuring the QT interval manually, be sure to identify the true end of the T wave and not mistakenly measure a superimposed U or P wave. You may find it helpful to use the tangent method of measurement, drawing a line from the maximum downslope of the T wave until it intersects the baseline (**Figure 4-15**).

The QT interval is normally affected by heart rate. As the heart rate slows, the QT interval normally lengthens; and as the heart rate rises, the QT interval normally shortens. Therefore, the measured QT interval requires a mathematical correction for heart rate called the **QTc**. A variety of methods exist for calculating the QTc. The most common of which is the Bazett formula, which is the QTc = QT interval (measured in seconds) divided by the square root of the R-R interval (measured in seconds). The formula assumes a stable R-R interval and is most valid between the heart rates of 60 and 100 beats per minute (bpm). Other formulas are available that may be reviewed in more detail in the references listed at the end of the chapter.

Tables exist that calculate the normal range of QTc, but these are not always available at the bedside. A quick way to evaluate for QT prolongation, valid between a heart rate of 60 to 100 beats per minute, is to assess whether the QT interval is less than half of the R-R interval. It's easy to use this method by counting the number of small boxes for each interval and doing a simple calculation, checking whether the number of boxes you count for the QT interval is less than half those of the R-R interval. A QT interval of more than half of the R-R interval is

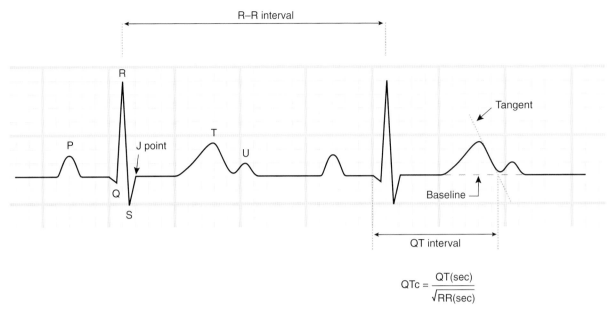

Figure 4-15. Measuring the QT interval using the tangent method and correcting for heart rate. Identify the downslope of the T wave and draw a line until intersecting a baseline derived from the TP segment. The QT interval is the distance from the onset of the Q wave to this point, here measured as 0.38 seconds. Dividing the QT interval by the square root of the R-R interval of 0.8 seconds derives a corrected QT interval (QTc) of 0.425 seconds, which is in the normal range.

potentially abnormal and a more formal mathematical calculation is warranted.

The QTc is also affected by gender. Women normally have a longer QTc than men.

Although there remains a considerable debate, it is reasonable to use the following guidelines for the upper and lower limits of the corrected QT interval (QTc). Values that exceed these require further evaluation for QT prolongation or shortening, either of which may predispose a patient to life-threatening arrhythmias.

Men: >390 msec to <450 msec

Women: >390 msec to <460 msec

Because the QRS complex is part of the QT interval, prolongation of the QRS itself will increase the measurement of the QT interval. In this circumstance, it may be appropriate to measure the **JT** interval. This also requires correction for HR, termed the **JTc**. This measurement is not routinely reported but may become relevant if an apparently prolonged QTc is thought to be due only to QRS prolongation. Readers interested in learning more about this subject should review the supplementary material provided at the end of this chapter.

The **TQ interval** corresponds to the resting potential (phase 4) and is usually close to the baseline. A portion of the TQ segment, the **TP segment**, reflects the time from completion of ventricular repolarization (end of the T wave) to the beginning of the next sinus cycle (P wave). The TP segment is characteristically the most stable, isoelectric segment and, by convention, may be used as the baseline.

The **U wave** is a low-amplitude deflection of controversial origin that may be seen following or partially superimposing the T wave. It is more often present at lower heart rates and may be seen best in leads V2 and V3. The amplitude of the U wave

should be <25% of the T wave in that lead and normally follows in the same direction.

Putting Things Together

Now that we have learned how to name the waves, intervals, and segments, we can correlate the deflections we see on the ECG with the action potentials from various sections of the heart. Let's follow the fate of a single ECG complex from start to finish (**Figure 4-16**).

1. The SA node initiates the sequence of action potentials during each cardiac cycle. Remember this is not detectable on the surface ECG so the recording remains at the baseline.

2. The electrical impulse spreads from the SA node throughout the right atrium and then the left atrial tissue. Before atrial depolarization is complete, the impulse enters the AV node. Transmission continues through the three regions of the AV node (atrial-nodal, nodal, nodal-his), continuing through the common bundle of His, the bundle branches, and the Purkinje network. These events comprise the PR interval.

3. The ventricular muscle fibers are then activated. Depolarization (phase 0) and the first part of rapid repolarization (phase 1) correlate with the QRS complex. The remainder of the QRS complex with the T wave represents completion of repolarization (phases 2-3). The muscle cells of the endocardium depolarize before those of the epicardium. But because they have a shorter action potential, the epicardial cells begin to repolarize before those of the endocardium. The entire QRS complex combined with the T wave represents the collective action potentials of the cells of the ventricular endocardium and epicardium.

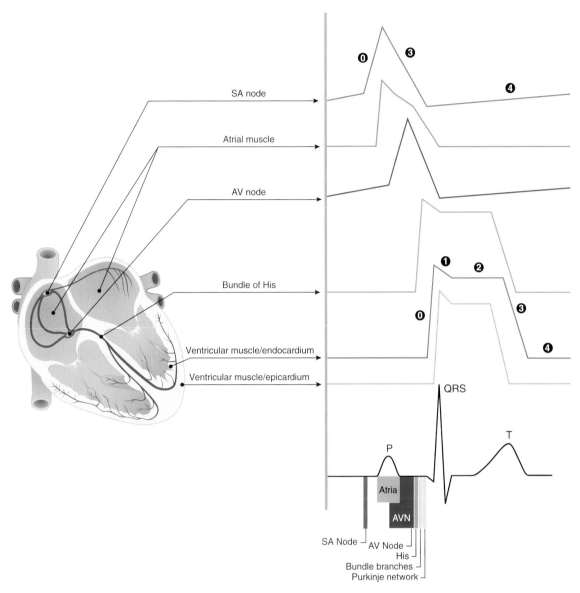

Figure 4-16. The relative timing of action potentials for the SA node, atrial muscle, AV node, bundle of His, ventricular endocardium, and epicardium are shown in relation to the surface electrocardiogram. Action potentials for the bundle branches and Purkinje network are not shown but are noted graphically below the ECG. The circled numbers indicate the phase of the action potential.

4. The ventricular muscle remains electrically at rest following the T wave (phase 4) until the next cycle begins.

Let's now discuss how the electrical events we observe on the ECG correlate with the heart's mechanical action. In Chapter 2 we learned about ventricular contraction and relaxation, also known as systole and diastole. Chapter 3 described the genesis of the action potential, depolarization, and repolarization. In this chapter we learned how to graphically record the electrical events of cardiac cells. Let's see how these items relate to one another.

Figure 4-17 shows an action potential in the lower panel, an ECG tracing in the middle panel, and a pressure curve in the top panel. This allows us to see the relationship of (1) depolarization and repolarization, (2) the ECG waveform, and (3) electrical and mechanical systole and diastole.

 FOR HISTORY BUFFS: This type of diagram is often referred to as a "Wiggers' diagram," named after the noted physiologist, Carl J. Wiggers.

For simplicity, we will focus on left ventricular events. Note that electrical events precede mechanical events. That makes sense because as we learned in Chapter 3, it takes a little time to get the ions working to start the excitation-contraction coupling process. This figure should make it clear that the ECG records electrical, not mechanical events. It should also illustrate that depolarization and repolarization are not identical to mechanical systole and diastole.

Electrical systole encompasses depolarization (phase 0) and repolarization (phases 1-3) of the action potential. On the ECG, electrical systole begins with the Q wave (or an initial R wave)

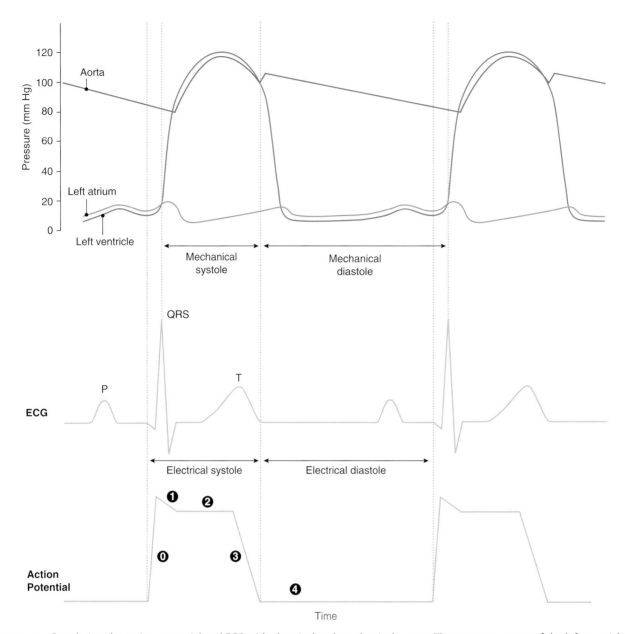

Figure 4-17. Correlating the action potential and ECG with electrical and mechanical events. The pressure curves of the left ventricle, left atrium, and aorta (top) are correlated with the timing of the electrocardiogram (middle). The relative timing of both curves is shown relative to the action potential of a typical endocardial muscle cell (bottom). The circled numbers indicate the phase of the action potential.

and has a duration corresponding with the QT interval. Electrical diastole encompasses the rest period of the action potential (phase 4), which corresponds to the TQ interval of the ECG.

Mechanical systole starts after electrical systole in the left ventricle. It begins with the closure of the mitral valve, which occurs when left ventricular pressure exceeds that of the left atrium, coinciding roughly with the peak of the R wave. The aortic valve opens when left ventricular pressure exceeds that of the aorta, which occurs approximately at the J point of the ECG. Mechanical systole ends with the closure of the aortic valve, which coincides approximately with the end of the T wave. This also marks the beginning of mechanical diastole, which continues until the closure of the mitral valve. The next cycle of mechanical systole now begins.

Technical Troubleshooting

No discussion of the basics of electrocardiography would be complete without mentioning the importance of proper technique and instrumentation. One source of ECG misdiagnosis is technical artifacts. This includes those due to lead misplacements, motion-induced abnormalities, and electrical interference.

Limb lead reversals High on the list of errors is misplacement of the limb electrodes. The most common lead reversal is that of the right and left arms (**Figure 4-18**). This is easily recognized by inspecting leads I and aVR. In lead I, a right arm-left arm lead reversal will turn the normally upright P wave and QRS complex into negative deflections.

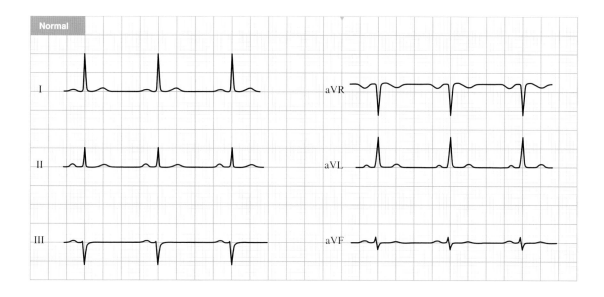

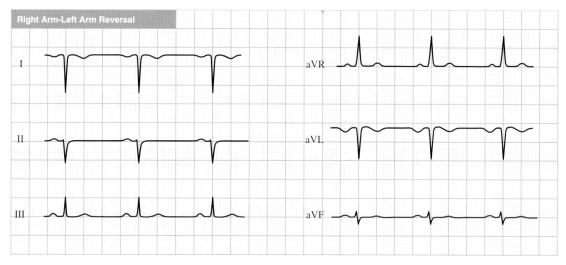

Figure 4-18. Right arm-left arm lead reversal. In a normal tracing (top) the P wave and QRS complex are positive deflections in lead I and negative in lead aVR. With an arm lead reversal (bottom), the P wave and QRS become negative in lead I and upright in lead aVR.

Similarly in lead aVR, the normally inverted P wave and negative QRS complex will become upright. The precordial leads will appear normally, which differentiates this lead reversal from mirror-image dextrocardia.

Limb lead reversals involving a switch between the right leg (ground) and either of the arm electrodes are identified using a different clue. In this situation, the tracing contains a lead with an unusually low voltage that resembles a "flat line." Why should that be? A look back at Figure 4-4 provides the answer. For example, if the right arm and right leg electrodes are exchanged, lead II now measures the potential difference between the right and left legs, which is virtually zero (**Figure 4-19**). Remember, the electrocardiograph machine doesn't know that the electrodes are misplaced and can only record what it "sees." Similarly, a left arm-right leg exchange will now record a flat line in lead III. And if both arms and both legs are reversed, lead I now appears isoelectric.

A left arm-left leg electrode reversal is more challenging and is best recognized by comparing serial tracings that demonstrate an unexplained axis shift (**Figure 4-20**). The same is true with the more uncommon right arm-left leg exchange. A right leg-left leg lead reversal does not alter the ECG, because there is no effect by switching the ground electrode from one leg to the other.

A frequently unrecognized limb lead error is recording a 12-lead ECG using electrodes placed on the shoulders and hips instead of the arms and legs. Such "torso-positioned" electrodes are routinely used for exercise testing as well as for hospital-based telemetry monitoring. This positioning is **not** acceptable for diagnostic electrocardiography. Such nonstandard lead positioning often results in important amplitude and waveform changes caused by a vertical and rightward shift of the frontal plane axis. Q waves related to inferior myocardial infarction may disappear. Other QRS alterations may suggest infarction where none exists. It is acceptable to record an ECG with the

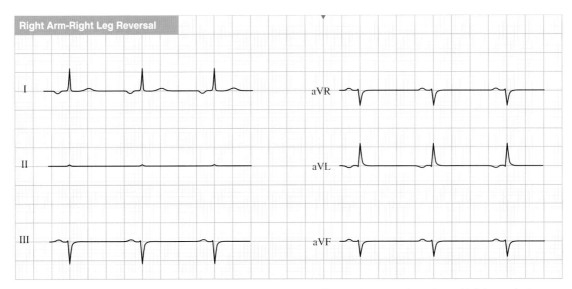

Figure 4-19. Right arm-right leg reversal. Lead II now measures the potential difference between the right and left legs, which is essentially zero.

electrodes placed on the proximal arms and legs rather than near the wrists and ankles, but torso-placed electrodes should not be utilized.

Precordial lead positioning Chest lead misplacement may also lead to misdiagnoses. Electrodes should be placed in the proper interspaces, not on the actual ribs (see Figure 4-7). Placement of leads V1-V6 in an improper sequence will alter the normal R wave progression that is used to evaluate myocardial infarction and chamber enlargement, topics that we will review in subsequent chapters (**Figure 4-21**). A similar problem emerges if the leads remain in the proper sequence, but are placed either too high or too low on the chest.

Motion artifacts The ECG should be acquired with the patient still and placed in a supine position. Motion artifacts caused

by tremor, shivering, or other movement may imitate cardiac arrhythmias (**Figure 4-22**).

Electrical interference Unacceptably "noisy" ECG recordings may result from a number of sources. These include static electricity, poor skin contact, or dry electrodes as well as those derived from power lines and from muscular activity (**Figure 4-23**). Medical devices such as electrical stimulators and pumps may produce gross ECG artifacts that render the tracing uninterpretable. Electrocardiograph machines contain filters to minimize artifacts and improve the quality of the tracing. The high-pass filter passes through signals with a frequency higher than the cutoff value and attenuates lower-frequency signals. It is routinely set at 0.05 Hz and is used to reduce low-frequency baseline wander. The low-pass filter allows signals lower than the selected value and limits frequencies higher

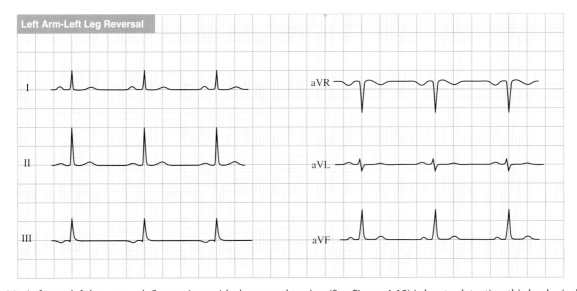

Figure 4-20. Left arm-left leg reversal. Comparison with the normal tracing (See Figure 4-18) is key to detecting this lead misplacement. Note the subtle differences in the QRS complexes. Leads I and II are exchanged as are leads aVL and aVF compared with the original.

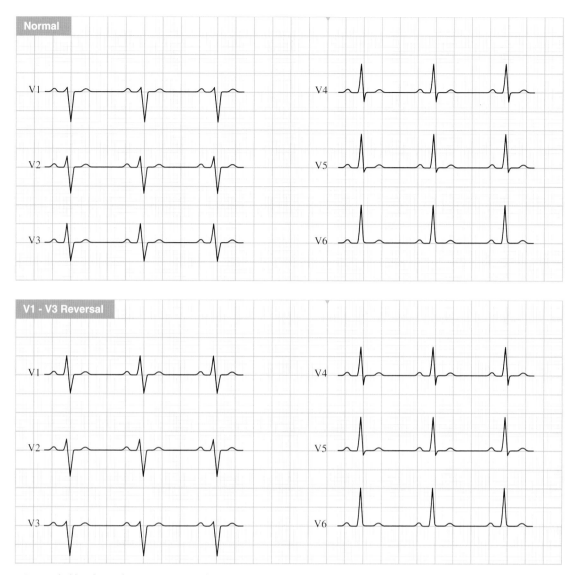

Figure 4-21. Precordial lead misplacement. Normal R wave progression (top) is altered when V leads are misplaced (bottom). Here, the V1 and V3 electrodes are exchanged.

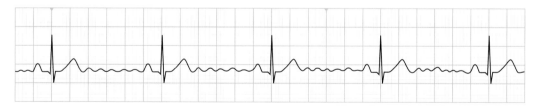

Figure 4-22. Tremor artifact resembling atrial flutter or fibrillation. Normal P waves can be distinguished through the unsteady baseline.

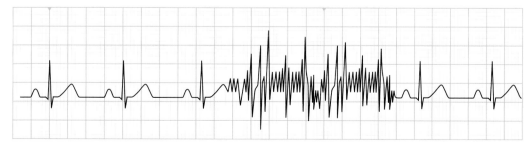

Figure 4-23. Gross electrical artifact resembling ventricular fibrillation.

than the cutoff value. It is routinely set at 150 Hz and reduces high-frequency artifacts from electrical devices and myopotentials. A third "notch" filter targets 60 Hz interference from the main power grid. The high- and low-frequency filters can be adjusted to improve the appearance of the tracing, but runs the risk of reducing diagnostic accuracy. For example, raising the high-pass (low-frequency) filter may eliminate baseline wander, but can distort the ST segment. Lowering the setting of the low-pass (high-frequency) filter may eliminate noise from nearby electrical devices, but will also suppress important high-frequency signals such as pacemaker stimuli or notches in the QRS complex.

Standardization Every ECG records a standardization deflection, normally set at a calibration of 1 mV = 10 mm. Double standardization (1 mV = 20 mm) will produce complexes twice the normal size and half standardization (1 mV = 5 mm) records complexes one-half sized. If the presence of a nonstandard calibration is not recognized, it's easy to make an erroneous diagnosis related to voltage abnormalities.

Chapter 4 • SELF-TEST

1. When moving *toward* the recording (positive) electrode, a wave of depolarization will inscribe what kind of deflection (positive or negative)? When moving *away* from the positive electrode, a wave of depolarization will inscribe what kind of deflection (positive or negative)?

2. What is the potential difference in mV of six muscle cells that are:
   • Fully depolarized.
   • Fully repolarized.

3. The six limb leads are named _____.
   The six precordial (chest) leads are named _____.

4. Recite the mnemonic to help you remember the correct placement of the limb leads.

5. Each small, light-colored box on the ECG represents what unit of time?
   Each large, dark-colored box on the ECG represents what unit of time?

6. The SA node produces what deflection on the surface ECG?

7. The PR interval reflects transmission of the electrical impulse through what portions of the heart?

8. The following items of the ECG correspond with which portion(s) of the action potential?
   • QRS complex.
   • J point.
   • ST segment.
   • T wave.
   • QT interval.
   • TQ interval.

9. How does the QT interval vary with the heart rate? How does the QT interval vary with gender?

10. How can you recognize a right arm-left arm lead reversal?

Chapter 4 • SELF-TEST

1. • Positive (upward).
   • Negative (downward).

2. • Fully depolarized—zero.
   • Fully repolarized—zero.

3. Limb leads: I, II, III, aVR, aVL, aVF.
   Precordial (chest) leads: V1, V2, V3, V4, V5, V6.

4. Green and white—on the right. Green and red—foot of the bed.

5. Small box: 0.04 seconds (or 40 milliseconds).
   Large box: 0.2 seconds (or 200 milliseconds).

6. SA node activity is not visible on the ECG.

7. The PR interval reflects transmission from the sinus node to the ventricles, traveling on the way through the atria, AV node, bundle of His, bundle branches, and the Purkinje network.

8. • QRS interval: Phases 0, 1.
   • J point: End of phase 1.
   • ST segment: Phase 2.
   • T wave: Phase 3.
   • QT interval: Phases 0, 1, 2, 3.
   • TQ segment: Phase 4.

9. The QT interval normally prolongs with slower heart rate.
   The QT interval is normally longer in women than in men.

10. In lead I, the normally upright P wave and QRS complex become negative deflections. In lead aVR, the normally inverted P wave and negative QRS complex become upright.

Further Reading

Al-Khatib SM, Allen-LaPoint NM, Kramer JM, Califf RM. What clinicians should know about the QT interval. *JAMA*. 2003;289: 2120-2127.

CSE Working Party. Recommendations for measurement standards in quantitative electrocardiography. *Eur Heart J*. 1985;6:815-825.

Drew BJ. Pitfalls and artifacts in electrocardiography. *Cardiol Clin*. 2006;24:309-315.

Funck-Bretano C, Jaillon P. Rate-corrected QT interval: techniques and limitations. *Am J Cardiol*. 1993;72:17B-22B.

Garcia-Niebla J, Llontop-Garcia P, Valle-Racero, JI, Serra-Autonell G, Batchvarov VN, Bayes de Luna A. Technical mistakes during acquisition of the electrocardiogram. *Ann Noninvasive Electrocardiol*. 2009; 14:389-403.

Goldenberg I, Moss AJ, Zareba W. QT interval: how to measure it and what is "normal." *J Cardiovasc Electrophysiol*. 2006;17:333-336.

Hodges M. Rate correction of the QT interval. *Card Electrophysiol Rev*. 1997;3:360-363.

Hurst JW. Naming of the waves in the ECG, with a brief account of their genesis. *Circulation*. 1998;98:1937-1942.

Katz AM. The electrocardiogram. In: *Physiology of the Heart*. 5th ed. Chapter 15, Philadelphia, PA: Wolters Kluwer Lippincott Williams and Wilkins; 2011:chap. 15. 401-430.

Kligfield P, Hancock EW, Helfenbein ED, et al. Relation of QT interval measurements to evolving automated algorithms from different manufacturers of electrocardiographs. *Am J Cardiol*. 2006;98:88-92.

Mason JW, Hancock EW, Gettes LS. Recommendations for the standardization and interpretation of the electrocardiogram. Part II: Electrocardiography diagnostic statement list. *J Am Coll Cardiol*. 2007; 49:1128-1135.

Mond HG, Garcia J, Visagathilagar T. Twisted leads: the footprints of malpositioned electrocardiographic leads. *Heart, Lung and Circulation*. 2016;25:61-67.

Mond HG, Haqqani HM. The footprints of electrocardiographic interference: fact or artifact. *Heart, Lung and Circulation*. 2019;28: 1472-1483.

Perez-Riera AR, de Abreu LC, Barbosa-Barros R, Nikus KC, Baranchuk A. R-peak time: an electrocardiographic parameter with multiple clinical applications. *Ann Noninvasive Electrocardiol*. 2016;21:10-19.

Perez-Riera AR, Barbosa-Barros R, Daminello-Raimundo Rodrigo, de Abreu LC. Main artifacts in electrocardiography. *Ann Noninvasive Electrocardiol*. 2018;23;e12494.

Perez-Riera AR, Ferreira C, Ferreira-Filho C, et al. The enigmatic sixth wave of the electrocardiogram: the U wave. *Cardiol J*. 2008; 15:408-421.

Postema PG, DeJong JSSG, Van der Bilt IAC, Wilder AAM. Accurate electrocardiographic assessment of the QT interval: teach the tangent. *Heart Rhythm*. 2008;5:1015-1018.

Rautaharju PM, Surawicz B, Gettes LS. AHA/ACCF/HRS recommendations for the standardization and interpretation of the electrocardiogram. Part IV: the ST segment, T and U waves, and the QT interval. *J Am Coll Cardiol*. 2009;53:982-991.

Rautaharju PM, Zhang Z-M, Prineas, R, Heiss G. Assessment of prolonged QT and JT intervals in ventricular conduction defects. *Am J Cardiol*. 2004;93:1017-1021.

Willems JL, Robles de Medina EO, Bernard R, et al. Criteria for intraventricular conduction disturbances and pre-excitation. *J Am Coll Cardiol*. 1985;5:1261-1275.

Heart Rate

▶ THE HEART RATE: MAKING OUR FIRST MEASUREMENT

It's finally time to start making real measurements, so let's begin by learning how to calculate the heart rate (HR). For every ECG, you should calculate both the ventricular rate and atrial rate. We can calculate the ventricular rate by measuring the time between the QRS complexes (R-R intervals), and the atrial rate by measuring the time between the P waves (P-P intervals). In normal sinus rhythm the atrial and ventricular rates are identical. In patients with cardiac arrhythmias, the atrial and ventricular rates may be very different, something we are going to learn in subsequent chapters. For the following discussion we will concentrate on the R waves to calculate the ventricular rate, but the same principles apply when using the P waves to calculate the atrial rate. There are a number of different methods that you can use, but I will present them in the order I find most practical.

The 6-Second Method

We learned earlier that ECG paper comes with 3-second markers, so two of them represent a total of 6 seconds. By counting the number of QRS complexes within a 6-second period and multiplying by 10, you derive the HR in beats per minute (bpm) (**Figure 5-1**). This is the universal method to calculate HR that you can use with any cardiac rhythm, regular or irregular, fast or slow, and in the presence of premature complexes. Use the following steps for this method:

1. Select an R wave that lines up as close as possible with the first 3-second marker. If you prefer, duplicate the 3-second markers using calipers, a marked note card, or another sheet of ECG paper to line up the first complex exactly with the first marker.

2. Consider the first complex as "zero," counting the subsequent R waves until you reach the end of the 6-second mark.

3. Multiply this number by 10.

That's pretty easy! Yes, I know that the complexes may not line up exactly on the zero and 6-second mark, but the HR you calculate is going to be very close to the actual number and any difference is not likely to be clinically relevant. If the last complex occurs just before the end of the 6 seconds, adjust the HR a little higher. Similarly, if the last complex falls just after the marker, adjust the HR rate lower. Either way, you are going to be in the neighborhood. And if your ECG paper doesn't have 3-second markers, it's easy to mark off the 6 seconds yourself, remembering that 5 large boxes equals 1 second (30 large boxes = 6 seconds).

The Large Box-Triplet Method

For patients with a regular rhythm, it's easy to calculate the HR using only two complexes (**Figure 5-2**). This method is called the large box-triplet method and is by far the fastest. Here we will count the number of large boxes between two R waves. The "triplet" part comes from the series of three numbers **you will need to memorize**. These are **300-150-100**, then **75-60-50**. For most clinical circumstances, these two series are enough. If you are really ambitious, you can memorize one more set of numbers, **43-38-33**. To use this method use the following steps:

1. Select an R wave that lines up as close as possible with the dark line from a large box. If you prefer, duplicate the distance between two complexes using calipers, a marked note card, or another sheet of ECG paper to line up the first complex exactly with the dark line.

2. Count off the large boxes in between two complexes using the sequence: 300-150-100, 75-60-50, etc. until you intersect the next R wave.

3. The number you reach is the HR.

Here again the second R wave may not line up exactly with a dark line and you may need to make an adjustment. For example, if the second R wave falls halfway between the fourth and fifth

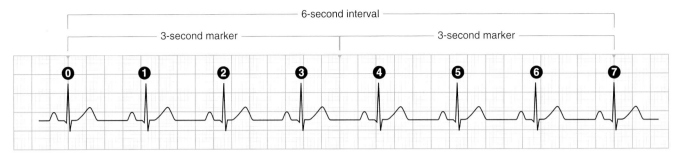

Figure 5-1. 6-second method. Starting with the number "zero," counting seven more complexes within a 6-second interval and multiplying by a factor of ten results in a HR of 7 x 10 = 70 bpm.

boxes, report a rate midway between 75 and 60 (eg, 67). If the R wave falls closer to one number in the sequence than another, make the appropriate adjustment higher or lower. Note in Figure 5-2 that if we had used the 6-second counting method, we would have counted 7½ complexes, which when multiplied by a factor of 10, would have derived the identical HR of 75 found with the triplet method. Until you become confident with your technique, practice calculating the HR using more than one method.

R-R Interval Methods

There are a number of other ways you can use a single R-R interval to calculate the HR in bpm (**Figure 5-3**). All should be used only for a regular, stable rhythm, and not in the presence of cardiac arrhythmias. These methods work well in the presence of rapid heart rates. Here are examples of using different methods to calculate the same HR.

R-R interval method 1 (using large boxes)

1. Select the first R wave.
2. Count the number of large boxes between two consecutive R waves.
3. Divide 300 by this number to derive the HR in bpm.

R-R interval method 2 (using small boxes)

1. Select the first R wave.
2. Count the number of small boxes between two consecutive R waves.
3. Divide 1500 by this number to derive the HR in bpm.

R-R interval method 3 (using time in seconds)

1. Select the first R wave.
2. Measure the interval in seconds between two consecutive R waves. (Remember that each large box equals 0.2 seconds and each small box equals 0.04 seconds).
3. Divide 60 by this number to calculate the HR in bpm.

The Cycle Length Method

The *cycle length* is the term used to describe the length of time between each complex in milliseconds (msec). This method is really the same as R-R interval method 3, but instead of seconds, we convert the time interval between complexes into milliseconds. To use this method (see Figure 5-3):

1. Select the first R wave.
2. Measure the time difference between the first R wave and the next R wave in milliseconds. (Remember that each large box is 200 msec and each small box is 40 msec.)
3. Divide 60,000 by this number to convert the cycle length interval into beats per minute.

Why should we go to the trouble in this calculation to use milliseconds instead of seconds? The reason is that cardiac devices, such as pacemakers and defibrillators, typically report cardiac rhythms in terms of the cycle length in milliseconds. You can convert back and forth from HR in beats per minute to cycle length in milliseconds by using these two versions of the same formula:

$$HR \text{ (bpm)} = 60,000/\text{cycle length (msec)}$$

$$\text{Cycle length (msec)} = 60,000/HR \text{ (bpm)}$$

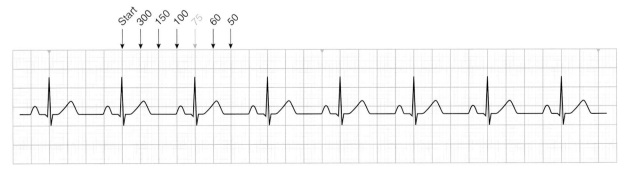

Figure 5-2. Large box triplet method. Counting the sequence of large boxes between two complexes results in a HR of 75 bpm.

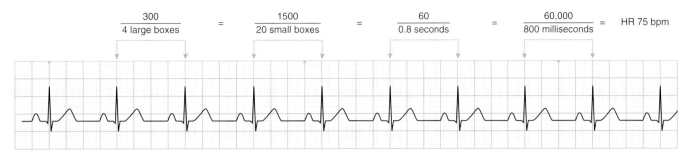

$$\underbrace{\frac{300}{\text{4 large boxes}}}_{} = \underbrace{\frac{1500}{\text{20 small boxes}}}_{} = \underbrace{\frac{60}{\text{0.8 seconds}}}_{} = \underbrace{\frac{60,000}{\text{800 milliseconds}}}_{} = \text{HR 75 bpm}$$

Figure 5-3. R-R interval methods. The heart rate in beats per minute can be derived by four separate methods that measure the distance between two consecutive R waves: (a) 300/#large boxes, (b) 1500/#small boxes, (c) 60/R-R interval in seconds, (d) 60,000/R-R interval in milliseconds. In this example 300/4 large boxes = 1500/20 small boxes = 60/0.8 sec = 60,000/800 msec = 75 bpm.

It's important for you to understand the relationship of cycle length to HR. As seen in **Table 5-1**, the shorter the cycle length, the faster the HR. Conversely, a longer cycle length correlates with a slower HR. It's worthwhile to memorize a few conversions of cycle length to HR as follows:

Cycle length (msec)	= HR (bpm)
1,000	= 60
600	= 100
300	= 200

The Heart Rate Ruler Method

A heart rate ruler is a simple pocket tool that can be used to calculate HR. Use this by lining up the first complex with the indicator arrow. Depending on the design, follow the instructions printed on the ruler to use one, two, or three cardiac cycles to determine the HR. Heart rate rulers should be used with regular, stable rhythms.

Pitfalls

You may encounter a situation where the HR that you measure manually is very different from that calculated electronically by a computerized ECG machine or on a hospital telemetry monitor. Automated calculations can be very accurate, but are subject to a variety of errors. These include failure to identify a QRS complex in patients with low voltage, double counting of the HR in

patients with large T waves, and miscounting of artifacts. When in doubt, rely on a personal, manual calculation of the HR. Computers are valuable, but they cannot replace a human being!

 CLINICAL TIP: Complexes seen on the ECG may not always result in a detectable pulse. This frequently occurs in patients with premature complexes or atrial fibrillation, and is referred to as a "pulse deficit." Pulseless electrical activity (PEA) is the most severe example of this situation, where *none* of the complexes produce a pulse. PEA may occur in patients with severe cardiac conditions such as extensive myocardial infarction, shock, cardiac tamponade, and massive pulmonary embolism. In this critical situation, complexes are present on the ECG, but the heart muscle cannot generate an effective blood pressure or pulse.

Heart Rate Tips and Tricks

We have shown some examples where the complexes line up conveniently with a large grid box, making it easy to calculate the HR. But what do you do if the complexes do not cooperate? We have mentioned earlier that you can use calipers or another piece of paper to help you make your measurement. Let's take a moment to show you the technique (**Figure 5-4**).

Calipers are one of the most helpful tools in electrocardiography and I recommend that you keep one of these inexpensive little instruments handy. To make your calculation, align the two points of the calipers with the R waves of any two complexes. Then lift the calipers and place the first point of the calipers directly on a dark line of a large grid box. Be careful not to change the distance between the caliper points as you make the move. Now use whatever method you prefer described in the preceding discussion to determine the HR.

If you don't have calipers, you can use a blank note card as a substitute. Place the note card along the ECG complexes of interest and make a pen mark to indicate the R-R interval. Then align the marks with a dark line of a large box as discussed earlier.

Determine Both the Atrial Rate and Ventricular Rate

Up until now we have concentrated on using the QRS complex to determine the ventricular rate in the presence of a stable, regular cardiac rhythm. But this is only one step in analyzing

TABLE 5-1	Cycle Length Versus HR
Cycle Length (msec)	**Heart Rate (bpm)**
1,200	50
1,000	60
750	80
600	100
500	120
400	150
300	200
240	250
200	300

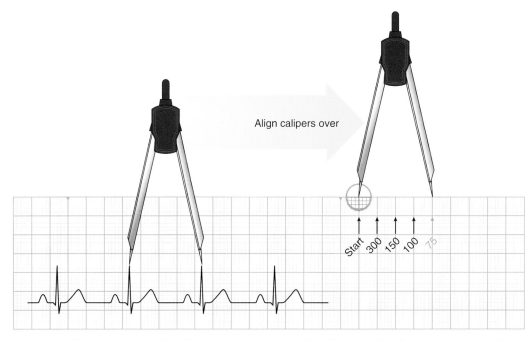

Figure 5-4. Using calipers. Place one point of the caliper on the peak of the R (or P) wave of the first complex. Expand the calipers, placing the second point on the peak of the R (or P) wave of the second complex. Align the calipers with a grid box and use your preferred method to determine the heart rate.

the cardiac rhythm. If P waves are present, you need to report both the atrial and ventricular rates, which may not always be the same. Sometimes the atrial rate will be faster than the ventricular rate; other times it will be slower. You are also going to encounter many situations where the heart rhythm is irregular. Not to worry! You already have all the tools you need to measure the HR accurately in each of these situations. Let's look at a few examples.

 CLINICAL TIP: Remember that only 10 seconds of data are recorded on the standard ECG. Regardless of the method, we ultimately report the average atrial and ventricular rate for those 10 seconds, converting the information into beats per minute. Also, the HR for some of the complexes may be different than the average reported

for the complete tracing. In this situation, it may be more useful to describe the rate of these complexes in terms of their cycle length.

Figure 5-5 shows a situation where the rhythm appears regular, but the atrial rate looks to be very different from the ventricular rate. Let's make sure by measuring both. You can use whatever method works best for each task. I suggest using the large box triplet method to measure the rate between two P waves (P-P interval), where we now determine that the atrial rate is 75 bpm. Using the 6-second method, we determine that the ventricular rate is 40 bpm. Something is very wrong here, isn't it? You can read a little more about this condition in the following clinical tip, but as far as this chapter is concerned, our work is done.

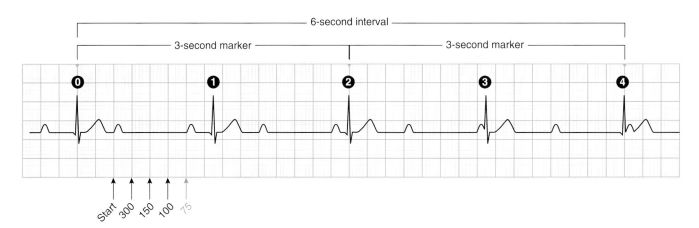

Figure 5-5. Using two methods to determine different atrial and ventricular rates in the presence of complete heart block. Using the triplet method, the atrial rate is 75 bpm. Using the 6-second method, the ventricular rate is 40 bpm.

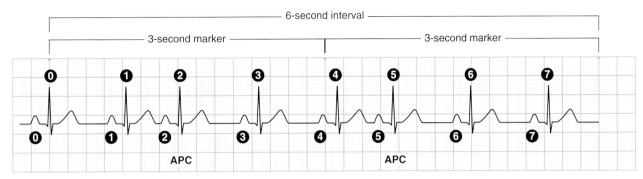

Figure 5-6. Using the 6-second method to determine the atrial and ventricular rates in the presence of atrial premature complexes (APCs) (complexes 2 and 5). The average atrial and ventricular rates are both approximately 75 bpm.

 CLINICAL TIP: Figure 5-5 is an example of *complete heart block*, where there is no relationship between the P wave and the QRS complex. Here the electrical signal generated by the SA node fails to reach the ventricles. A subsidiary pacemaker in the AV junction has kicked in to support life but at a lower rate than the heart's primary pacemaker in the sinus node (see Chapter 3).

What do we do if there is an irregular heart rhythm as shown in **Figure 5-6**? In this situation it's best to use the 6-second counting method. By using this technique, we determine in this example that the average atrial and ventricular rates are both approximately 75 bpm.

 CLINICAL TIP: Figure 5-6 is an example of a tracing with *atrial premature complexes*. A premature depolarization has initiated in the atrium, prior to the usual timing of the sinus node. The electrical transmission travels in the normal fashion through the conduction system, producing a normal-looking QRS complex.

Figure 5-7 shows a different type of irregular rhythm. In this tracing there are some wide, bizarre-looking QRS complexes without a P wave before. By using the 6-second method to include the bizarre complexes, we find a ventricular HR of 70. But what about the atrial rate? If we use

the 6-second counting method, we seem to come up short, counting only five visible P waves. Does this mean the atrial rate is 50? No way! In reality the P waves are present, but are obscured by the wide complexes. You can correct for this by including the P waves you cannot see as you count. Use your calipers to measure the first P-P interval and "march out" the P waves, keeping count from the first P wave. You will find the subsequent P waves arrive on time. If you are unsure that you did this correctly, check yourself by analyzing two complexes with visible P waves and measure the P-P interval, using one of the interval methods described in the preceding discussion to calculate the atrial rate.

 CLINICAL TIP: Figure 5-7 is an example of a tracing with *ventricular premature complexes*. A premature depolarization has initiated in the ventricles, outside of the normal conduction system, producing a wide, bizarre-looking complex. The sinus impulse has actually occurred with normal timing, but the premature QRS complex obscures the P wave.

Normal and Abnormal Heart Rates

By convention, a normal HR is between 60 and 100 bpm. A HR faster than 100 bpm is termed **tachycardia**. A HR slower than 60 bpm is termed **bradycardia**.

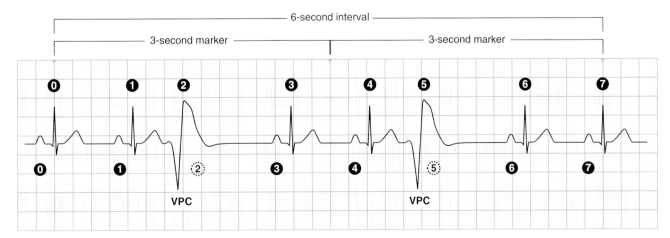

Figure 5-7. Using the 6-second method to determine the atrial and ventricular rates in the presence of ventricular premature complexes (VPCs) (complexes 2 and 5). The shadow numbers represent P waves that are obscured by the VPCs. The average atrial and ventricular rates are both 70 bpm.

Chapter 5 • SELF-TEST

1. Tachycardia is defined as a heart rate of _____.

2. Bradycardia is defined as a heart rate of _____.

3. Describe the 6-second method of calculating heart rate.

4. Recite the first two triplet sequences of the large box triplet method of calculating heart rate.

5. What is the HR in bpm when the R-R interval is four large boxes?

6. Convert the following HR from bpm to cycle length in msec.
   • 60 bpm.
   • 75 bpm.
   • 100 bpm.
   • 160 bpm.

7. Convert the following R-R cycle length in msec to HR in bpm.
   • 300 msec.
   • 480 msec.
   • 750 msec.
   • 1,250 msec.

8. With an irregular heart rhythm, what is the preferred method of calculating heart rate?

Chapter 5 • SELF-TEST

1. >100 bpm.

2. <60 bpm (Note: Some authors define it as <50 bpm.)

3. • Select an R wave that lines up as close as possible with the first 3-second marker.
   • Consider the first complex as "zero," counting the subsequent R waves until you reach the end of the 6-second mark.
   • Multiply this number by 10.

4. 300–150–100, then 75–60–50.

5. 75 bpm (300 ÷ 4).

6. • 1,000 msec (60,000 ÷ HR).
   • 800 msec.
   • 600 msec.
   • 375 msec.

7. • 200 bpm (60,000 ÷ cycle length).
   • 125 bpm.
   • 80 bpm.
   • 48 bpm.

8. 6-second method.

Vectors, Activation, Axis, and Rotation

▶ THE VECTOR CONCEPT

Thus far we've learned the genesis of electrical current in cardiac tissue and how to record their movements on an electrocardiograph. Now it's time to understand why these funny little squiggles look the way they do in health and disease. To do so, we need to be familiar with the concept of vectors.

A wave of depolarization is the driving force behind every cardiac cycle. Over time, this electrical current moves through the entire heart, originating with the primary pacemaker in the SA node, traveling through the atria, the AV node, the specialized conduction system, and ultimately spreading throughout every ventricular muscle cell. At each point in time, we can illustrate the magnitude and direction of the electrical wave as it completes its journey from start to finish as an *instantaneous cardiac vector*. A vector is represented graphically as an arrow that has *magnitude*, *direction*, and *polarity*. The length of the arrow indicates the magnitude (voltage) of the electrical current, the orientation of the arrow indicates the direction of the force, and the tip of the arrowhead indicates electrical positivity (**Figure 6-1**). In electrocardiography, we assume that the galvanometer records the instantaneous cardiac vectors as if they were generated from a single point in the center of the chest.

The direction and magnitude of an instantaneous cardiac vector are not really a single measurement, but represent the mathematical resultant of all the electrical forces moving in every direction at that moment in time. You can understand the concept of combining vector forces by picturing the path of a football as the kicker boots the ball in the presence of a crosswind (**Figure 6-2**). The flight of the ball is the net effect of the combined forces of the "kicking vector" and the "wind vector." Just like the fan whose concern is on the ultimate flight of the football, our interest is the net effect of multiple, simultaneous electrical waves. The same concept applies when we analyze cardiac vectors. Each single vector depicted represents the net resultant of multiple concurrent depolarizations (**Figure 6-3**).

Different Looks from Different Leads

The 12 leads of the electrocardiograph provide a way to analyze the movement of vectors through the heart over time. Each lead provides a different "view" of the same electrical sequence. Recall that a wave of depolarization moving toward the positive electrode will record a positive (upward) deflection. Conversely, a depolarization wave moving away from the positive electrode will record a negative (downward) deflection. The amplitude of the deflection recorded by each lead depends on the projection of the cardiac vector relative to that lead. Whoa, that last statement sounds a little complicated!

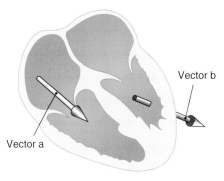

Figure 6-1. Cardiac vectors have magnitude, direction, and polarity. The direction of vector (a) can be described as leftward, inferior, and anterior. The direction of vector (b) is leftward, inferior, and posterior.

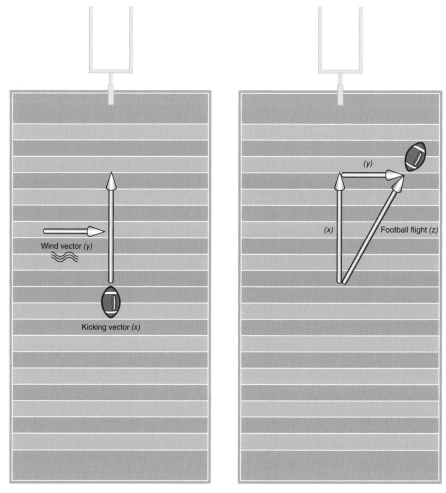

Figure 6-2. The ultimate path of a kicked football (z) will result from combining the "kicking vector" (x) with the "wind vector" (y).

But don't worry about digging out your old high school trigonometry book, because this concept is easier to understand than you may think.

Let's analyze three instantaneous cardiac vectors, x, y, and z, occurring one second apart and see how they might appear on an electrocardiogram (ECG). To make things easy, let's begin with a simplified frontal plane containing only leads I and aVF (**Figure 6-4**). At the start there is no electrical activity. One second later, vector x appears (panel a). It has a magnitude of

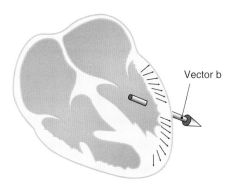

Figure 6-3. Vector (b) represents the net resultant of multiple, simultaneous depolarization waves.

5 and is positioned at a 45-degree angle between leads I and aVF. How will this vector appear as viewed from the perspective of leads I and aVF? We determine this by drawing a line from the tip of the vector perpendicular to the lead of interest (panel b). The point where the line intersects that lead is the magnitude of the instantaneous vector *as recorded by that lead*. It's as if we shined a flashlight on the vector perpendicular to the lead of interest, allowing the vector to cast a shadow (projection). By using this method, we can use simple math to determine that the magnitude of vector x with respect to both leads I and aVF is approximately +3.5. In this example, the value in both leads I and aVF is identical because vector x lies equidistant between the two.

FOR BOOKWORMS: We use the Pythagorean theorem of $a^2 + b^2 = c^2$ and other trigonometry formulas to determine the magnitude of the sides of a right triangle, plugging in the known values for the angles and sides to solve for the unknowns.

One second later vector y appears. It has the same magnitude of 5 as vector x but has a different direction (panel c). If we conveniently place it at a 53-degree angle from the horizontal

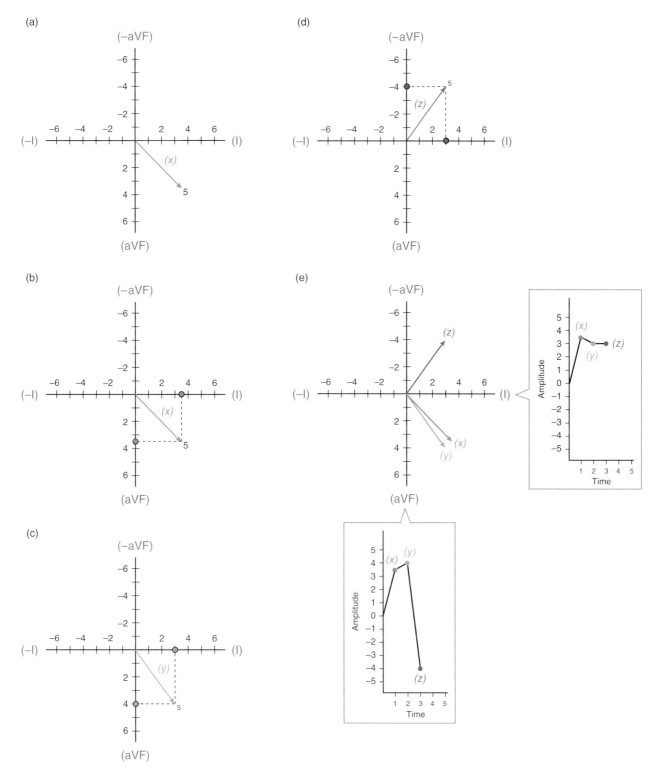

Figure 6-4. The magnitude of a vector as recorded by any lead is found by projecting a perpendicular from the tip of the vector to the lead of interest (panels a-d). Panel e illustrates a recording of the magnitude of the vectors in leads I and aVF over time.

(or 37-degree from the vertical), it projects a magnitude of +3 in lead I and +4 in aVF.

Vector *z* arrives 1 second later (panel d). It has the same relative angles as vector *y* but is now pointing *away* from lead aVF, toward the negative pole (−aVF). In lead I, the magnitude of the vector is still +3. But in aVF, the magnitude is measured as −4.

We can then combine our measurements to construct a graphical record for each lead over time (panel e). By connecting the dots in this graph we have the makings of a rudimentary ECG.

We can use this same process to analyze how the vector would appear in other leads. Let's go back to our hexaxial

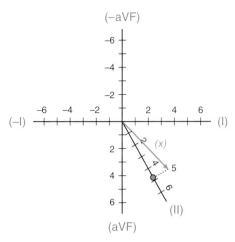

Figure 6-5. The magnitude of vector *x* as recorded by lead II is derived by projecting a perpendicular from the tip of the vector to the lead of interest.

system and analyze the original vector *x* as viewed by lead II (**Figure 6-5**). For this exercise, we draw in lead II and again project a perpendicular to that axis, finding a magnitude of approximately +4.8. This method can be used for every lead in the frontal plane. All you need to do each time is look at the vector with respect to the lead of interest, project a perpendicular, and make your measurement, remembering to consider whether the vector has an orientation toward the positive or negative partner of that lead.

Now let's discuss the precordial leads, which visualize cardiac vectors in the horizontal plane (**Figure 6-6**). Unlike the hexaxial lead system in the frontal plane, which easily describes the cardiac vectors in terms of 30-degree angles, the chest leads are less precise. Still, the same basic principles apply. You derive the magnitude of a vector in each lead, V1-V6, by projecting a perpendicular from the vector tip to the lead of interest.

A Moving Target

We can diagram the spread of the electrical impulse through the heart as a series of cardiac vectors. To use a baseball analogy, think of this electrical wave as a batter racing around the bases (**Figure 6-7**). At each point in time, we can describe the base

runner's position as an instantaneous vector. Now let's consider how we would use vectors to graph the path of the base runner in the horizontal plane from the perspective of two fans, one sitting in the stands behind home plate (eg, lead V2) and the other seated perpendicular behind the on-deck circle (eg, lead V6). Hmmm, that looks a little like a QRS complex doesn't it?

Getting Loopy

If we connect the tips of every individual vector in sequence, we create a diagram called a *vector loop*. This gives us a representation of the continuous movement of vectors as the electrical impulse spreads through the heart. Think of this as if our base runner were leaving little drops of paint behind him to record his path around the bases (**Figure 6-8**).

FOR BOOKWORMS: Cardiac electrical activity can be illustrated with a vectorcardiograph, which derives vector loops in the frontal, horizontal, and sagittal planes. A directional arrow indicates the sequence of vectors over time and can characterize the loop as either clockwise or counterclockwise. The information contained in a vectorcardiogram is identical to that of the scalar ECG, but presented differently. At one point this technique rivaled that of electrocardiography, but it was not considered practical for clinical use and fell out of favor. Also, vectorcardiography is not useful for analyzing arrhythmias.

Why bother with all this business about vectors and loops? The reason is that by understanding the vector-ECG relationship you will understand *why* ECG tracings look the way they do. Don't fall into the trap of memorizing patterns and then trying to match the diagnoses! Combining the vector pattern recorded with the limb leads in the frontal plane with those recorded by the precordial leads in the horizontal plane will allow you to understand the three-dimensional relationship of the electrical events occurring within the heart and become a master electrocardiographer.

Sequence of Activation

Now that we understand the basics of vector theory, it's time to apply these principles to describe the flow of electricity

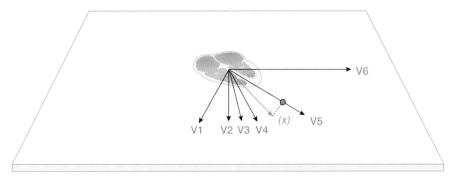

Figure 6-6. Depiction of a cardiac vector in the precordial leads. The magnitude of vector *x* as recorded in lead V5 is found by drawing a perpendicular from the tip of the vector to the lead of interest. The spatial relationship between the precordial leads is not as precise as those of the chest leads, but the principles as previously described still apply.

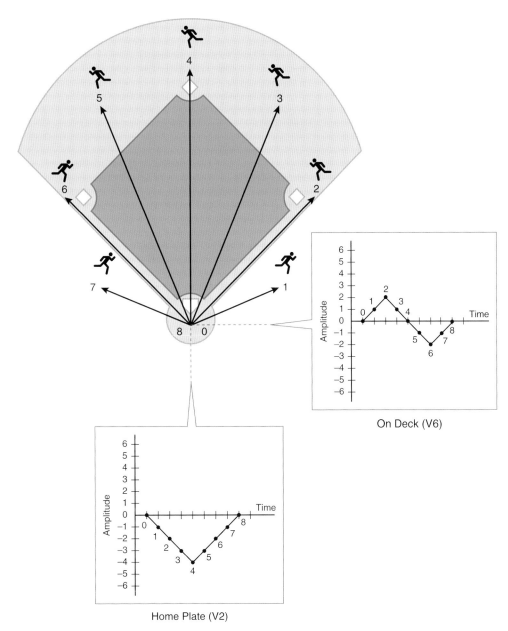

Figure 6-7. The movement of the electrical vectors throughout the heart in the horizontal plane is similar to that of a batter circling the bases. The viewpoint of the base runner's path from a fan sitting behind home plate and one behind the on-deck circle is analogous to leads V2 and V6 of the ECG. The magnitude and direction of each vector record the path of the batter from the perspective of each lead.

traveling through the normal heart. Let's start in order, beginning with the atria and following with the ventricles.

Atrial depolarization After originating at the SA node, the electrical current spreads first through the right atrium, followed by the left atrium (**Figure 6-9**). For simplicity, it's reasonable to divide the normal P wave into two vectors. This is an arbitrary distinction because the spread of electricity is continuous throughout the atrial myocardium. Figure 6-9 shows the vectors, loops, and corresponding ECG representation of atrial activation in the frontal and horizontal planes. Vector 1 represents right atrial depolarization, which is directed leftward, inferior, and anterior. Vector 2 reflects depolarization of the left atrium, which is directed leftward,

inferior, and posterior. This all makes sense if you remember our discussion of anatomy in Chapter 2 where we learned that the right side of the heart is really an anterior structure and the left side posterior. The portion of the P wave loop between vectors 1 and 2 is a combination of both right and left atrial forces.

Using the vector loop helps us to visualize why the P wave is normally upright in leads I, aVF, and V6. It also explains why the P wave in lead VI can normally appear biphasic, with the first upright portion of the P wave representing the right atrium and the second inverted portion representing the left atrium. Enlargement of either the right or left atrium due to cardiac disease will cause changes in the magnitude and direction of the atrial vectors that will be evident on the ECG.

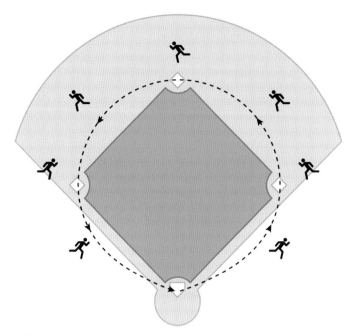

Figure 6-8. Connecting the tips of all the vectors creates a vector loop. The directional arrow indicates the sequence of the vectors over time and may be described here as a counterclockwise loop.

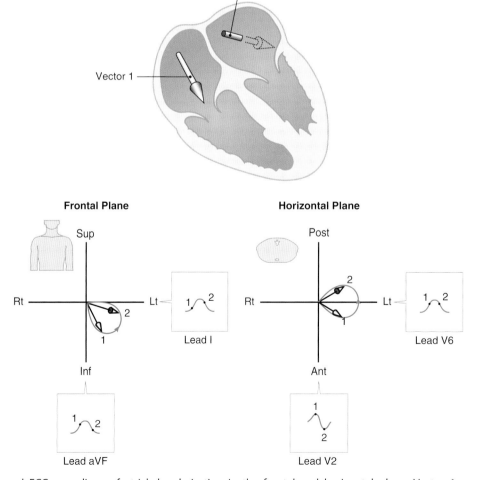

Figure 6-9. Vector and ECG recordings of atrial depolarization in the frontal and horizontal plane. Vector 1 represents right atrial depolarization, which is directed leftward, inferior, and anterior. Vector 2 reflects depolarization of the left atrium, which is directed leftward, inferior, and posterior. The P wave vector loop is usually small and is enlarged here for clarification.

Ventricular depolarization Activation of the ventricles can be divided arbitrarily into three vectors. Again, this is an oversimplification because the spread of the electrical current is continuous throughout the ventricular myocardium and is more complex than what will now be described. **Figure 6-10** illustrates the vectors, loops, and ECG patterns in the frontal and horizontal planes. Vector 1 represents depolarization of the left side of the interventricular septum, directed rightward, anterior, and (usually) superior. There is simultaneous right-to-left depolarization of the right side of the septum, but the greater left-sided forces predominate. Vector 2 represents simultaneous activation of the free walls of both ventricles beginning with the endocardium and spreading out toward the epicardium. The remaining right- and left-sided portions of the interventricular septum depolarize during this time, but the effects counterbalance one another. Both ventricles depolarize from apex to base, but again the greater mass of the left ventricle compared with the right ventricle predominates. Accordingly, vector 2 is oriented toward the left, inferiorly and posteriorly, reflecting the anatomical position of the left ventricle in the chest. Vector 3 represents the terminal activation of the posterobasal portions of both the left ventricle and interventricular septum. These structures lie rightward and posterior in relation to the other cardiac structures. Vector 3 can be variable, but is predominantly oriented to the right, somewhat superiorly and usually posteriorly.

Inspection of these vector loops helps us to understand the normal contour of the QRS complex. Let's summarize the key vector-QRS relationships.

- **Vector 1**. The left-to-right orientation of vector 1 explains why there is often a small initial Q wave in leads I, aVL, and V6. This reflects depolarization of the first portion of the interventricular septum, hence the term "septal Q wave." The anterior and rightward orientation explains the initial R wave in leads V1 and V2.
- **Vector 2**. This reflects the large mass of the left ventricle so this vector points leftward with large amplitude. Accordingly, we would expect to see tall R waves in leads that "look" from that direction, such as leads I, aVL, and V5-V6. Similarly, we expect to see deep S waves in leads that are oriented rightward, away from the direction of vector 2, such as leads V1 and aVR.

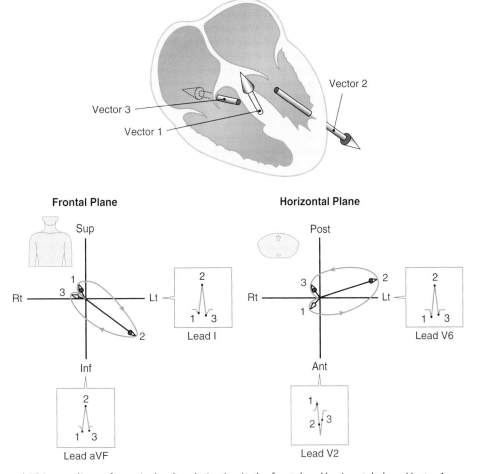

Figure 6-10. Vector and ECG recordings of ventricular depolarization in the frontal and horizontal plane. Vector 1 represents depolarization of the left side of the interventricular septum, directed rightward, anterior, and (usually) superior. Vector 2 represents activation of the free walls of both ventricles, oriented toward the left, inferiorly, and posteriorly. The greater mass of the left ventricle predominates. Vector 3 represents the terminal activation of the posterobasal portions of both the left ventricle and interventricular septum, and is oriented to the right, posteriorly and either superiorly or inferiorly.

- **Vector 3**. This vector is of small amplitude and variable in direction, so we would normally expect to see only small voltage waves at that point of the QRS complex. The orientation is mainly rightward, producing small S waves in leads I and V4-V6. In a small percentage of the population vector 3 is directed anteriorly, which would produce a small r´ in lead V1.

It is important to realize that the vector orientation described in the preceding discussion is only a generality. As we will learn shortly, the orientation of the cardiac vectors can vary considerably and is affected by age, body habitus, and the position of the heart in the chest.

Determining the Mean Frontal Plane QRS Axis

The *mean QRS vector* represents the average of *all* the instantaneous vectors occurring during ventricular depolarization. The orientation of this vector *in the frontal plane* is called the **mean QRS axis** (**Figure 6-11**). The normal mean QRS frontal plane axis is between −30 and +90 degrees. Note that these criteria are somewhat arbitrary and you will find some references that define the normal axis as between −30 and +110 degrees.

Left axis deviation is defined as an axis between −30 and −90 degrees. Causes of left axis deviation include left ventricular enlargement/hypertrophy, left anterior fascicular block, left bundle branch block, and inferior wall myocardial infarction. Some electrocardiographers further characterize left axis deviation as either moderate (between −30 and −45 degrees) or marked (between −45 and −90 degrees).

Right axis deviation is defined as an axis between +90 and +180 degrees. Causes of right axis deviation include right ventricular enlargement/hypertrophy, pulmonary embolism, and left posterior fascicular block. Some electrocardiographers further characterize right axis deviation as either moderate (between +90 and +120 degrees) or marked (between +120 and +180 degrees).

Extreme axis deviation is defined as an axis between −90 and ±180 degrees. This unusual finding may represent either extreme right or left axis deviation.

There are times where the mean QRS axis is directed out of the frontal plane, rendering the QRS equiphasic in multiple leads (see later). In this circumstance the mean frontal plane axis cannot be calculated and is characterized as **indeterminate**.

A variety of anatomical factors can cause the electrical axis to vary within the normal range (**Figure 6-12**). The term *horizontal heart* describes a mean QRS axis between 0 and −30 degrees, which may be related to obesity or alterations in abdominal pressure from pregnancy. A *vertical heart* describes a mean QRS axis close to +90 degrees, a finding that can be seen in lean, but otherwise healthy individuals.

 FOR BOOKWORMS: In infants and young children the normal QRS axis is rightward, greater than +90 degrees. With increasing age, the axis normally moves toward the left.

Every ECG interpretation includes a determination of the mean QRS axis and can be performed using a few simple steps. You do need to be familiar with the hexaxial system, so commit this to memory. You will need to inspect the QRS complex in each lead for **net amplitude**, which is determined by adding the amplitudes of the positive waves and subtracting them from the negative waves. Don't worry about making a lot of tedious measurements. In most cases you can just make an "eyeball" determination whether the net amplitude is either positive or negative. If the net amplitude is approximately equal, the complex is said to be **equiphasic** (isoelectric) in that lead. Modern computerized ECG machines can determine the mean QRS axis with extreme precision, but for practical purposes estimating a value within 15 degrees will suffice.

There are a number of different ways to determine the mean QRS axis. **Figure 6-13** shows the six limb leads of a typical ECG. Here is the method I recommend:

1. First look at the QRS complex in lead I. If the net amplitude of the QRS complex is positive (the amplitude of the R wave is greater than the S wave), then the mean QRS vector must be in the direction of lead I. If we use a globe analogy, the vector points toward the eastern hemisphere. Conversely, if the QRS complex is relatively negative in lead I, the mean vector points toward the western hemisphere. In the ECG tracing of Figure 6-13, the QRS in lead I is positive, so the mean vector must be between +90 and −90 degrees.

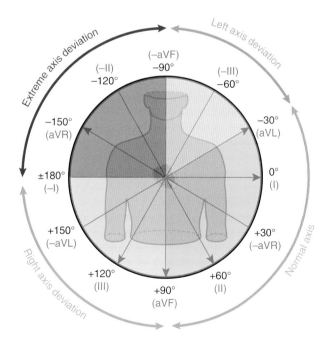

Figure 6-11. The normal mean QRS axis falls between −30 and +90 degrees. Left axis deviation is between −30 and −90 degrees. Right axis deviation is between +90 and +180 degrees. Extreme axis deviation is between −90 and ± 180 degrees.

Vertical heart

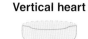

Horizontal heart

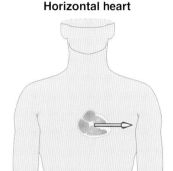

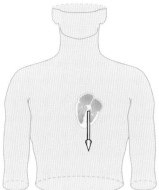

Figure 6-12. The mean QRS axis depends on the spatial orientation of the heart within the chest, which may be described as either a horizontal or vertical heart.

2. Next look at lead aVF. If the net QRS amplitude is positive, then the mean vector points toward lead aVF (ie, the southern hemisphere). Conversely, if the QRS is relatively negative in lead aVF, the mean vector points northward. In Figure 6-13, the QRS complex is positive in lead aVF, so the mean QRS vector must be between 0 and +180 degrees.

3. Combining steps one and two places the mean QRS vector between 0 and +90 degrees.

4. Finally search for a complex where the QRS is most equiphasic (isoelectric). An equiphasic complex places the mean QRS vector *perpendicular* to this lead, falling within the quadrant we previously determined. If the QRS is exactly equiphasic, then the mean vector is precisely perpendicular to that lead. If the net QRS amplitude is slightly positive in the equiphasic lead, find the perpendicular and adjust the mean vector approximately 15 degrees *toward* the equiphasic lead. Conversely, if the net QRS amplitude is slightly negative, find the perpendicular and adjust the mean vector approximately 15 degrees *away* from the equiphasic lead. In Figure 6-13, the most equiphasic lead is aVL, so the mean vector must be close to +60 degrees. But because the complex is more negative than positive in lead aVL, the vector is adjusted *away* from the direction of lead aVL, leaving us with a mean QRS vector of approximately +75 degrees.

There are other methods to analyze the mean QRS vector, but I prefer the systematic approach described in the preceding discussion. Here are some other methods you can use.

Equiphasic (zero net amplitude) method First look for an equiphasic lead and find a perpendicular using the method described earlier. You will then need to check that you are in the correct quadrant because if you're not careful you could place the axis in the wrong hemisphere. For example, if the QRS is equiphasic in lead II, the mean QRS vector could be either −30 degrees or +150 degrees.

Smallest QRS voltage method This is a variant of the equiphasic method and is used when there is no QRS complex that is truly equiphasic. Here you search for the smallest complex as the closest substitute for an equiphasic complex. Position the vector perpendicular to this complex, again making sure it is within the proper quadrant. Then make small corrections rightward or leftward as necessary.

Equal net amplitude method Here, you inspect the complexes in the frontal plane looking for two QRS complexes with equal net amplitudes. The mean QRS axis vector will lie exactly between the two leads. In our example, the net QRS amplitude is virtually identical in leads II and aVF, so the mean QRS vector must lie between these two leads at approximately +75 degrees. Again, you can make slight adjustments depending on which of the two complexes have slightly greater net QRS amplitude. The axis will be slightly closer to the lead with the higher amplitude of the two.

The fastest qualitative check for a normal QRS axis, without any further precision, is to look at leads I and II. If the net amplitude of the QRS is positive in those two leads, the axis is somewhere in the normal range, between +90 and −30 degrees.

Rotation of the Heart

The precordial leads are used to analyze the heart in the horizontal plane (**Figure 6-14**). The amplitude of the R waves normally increases from leads V1 to V6, reflecting the leftward and posterior direction of the dominant depolarization wave of the left ventricle. Leads V1 and V2 are right-sided, normally recording a QRS complex with small r waves and deep S waves. Leads V5 and V6 are left-sided, recording a QRS complex with tall R waves and small s waves. Leads V3 and V4 are transitional, with complexes relatively equiphasic. *R wave progression* is the term used to describe the normal increase in R waves across the precordial leads. The *transition zone* is the term for the lead where the QRS complex changes from one that is predominantly negative to one that is positive, usually occurring at lead V3.

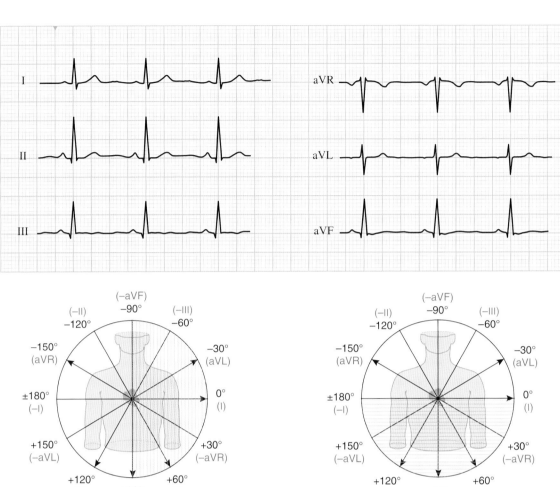

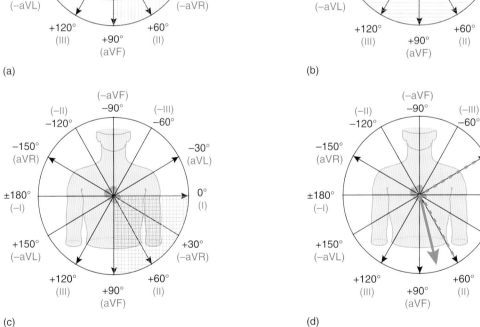

Figure 6-13. Determining the mean QRS axis in the frontal plane. Step 1 (a): Inspect lead I and assign the proper "hemisphere." Step 2 (b): Inspect lead aVF and assign the proper hemisphere. Step 3 (c): Combine steps 1 and 2 to determine the proper quadrant. Step 4 (d): Find the most equiphasic complex (aVL here) and follow the perpendicular. Make final adjustments as required (see text for details) as part of Step 4. The mean QRS axis of the tracing shown by the blue arrow in this example is +75 degrees.

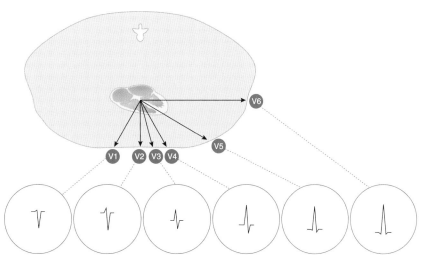

Figure 6-14. The transition zone of the precordial leads refers to the point where the amplitude of the R and S waves is approximately equal. Here the transition zone is at lead V3.

The heart can also rotate along its long axis, either clockwise or counterclockwise (**Figure 6-15**). The direction of rotation refers to the perspective from one looking up at the patient from below the diaphragm. It's the same type of view you see when you look at images from a chest CT scan, which is as if you were standing at the foot of the bed looking at a patient who is lying face up. The terms for cardiac rotation are somewhat antiquated and are a source of much confusion, but it's worthwhile to understand the terminology. Remember in Chapter 2 we described the axis of the heart and its football-like configuration. Imagine you are sitting in a chair in front of the patient placing a finger on the tip of the football. By spinning the football counterclockwise along its long axis, you swing the left ventricle more anterior and rightward. As you might expect, the R waves become taller in leads V3 and V4 and the transition zone is shifted rightward toward lead V2 (*early transition*). Clockwise rotation does the opposite, rotating the right ventricle more anterior and to the left, producing smaller R waves in leads V3-V4, moving the dominant R waves out of the recording field beyond V6, and shifting the transition zone leftward toward V4 (*delayed or late transition*).

Poor R wave progression is the term to describe when small R waves are present and there is an increase in voltage from leads V1-V3, but the R wave amplitude in V3 is ≤3 mm. This may be a normal variant or a reflection of cardiac rotation. Other, clinically important causes of poor R wave progression include anteroseptal wall myocardial infarction and chronic obstructive pulmonary disease. It may also be present with left anterior fascicular block. *Reverse R wave progression* is as discussed earlier, except that R wave voltage decreases from leads V1-V3.

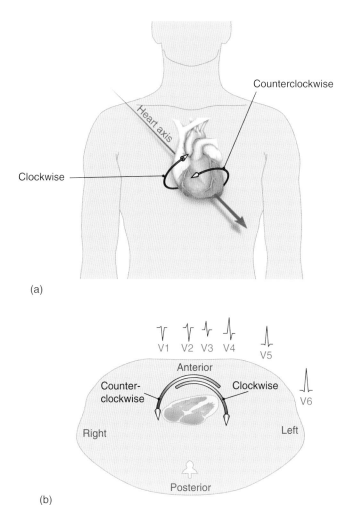

Figure 6-15. Rotation of the heart can be described in terms of rotation on its long axis (panel a). The terms refer to the rotation of the heart as viewed from below the diaphragm (panel b).

QUESTIONS

Chapter 6 • SELF-TEST

1. The magnitude and direction of an electrical wave traveling through the heart can be represented by what mathematical term?

2. When recorded by a cardiac lead, a wave of depolarization moving toward the positive electrode will inscribe a _____ deflection and a wave of depolarization moving away from the positive electrode will inscribe a _____ deflection.

3. The amplitude of a vector with respect to any given lead is obtained by drawing a line from the tip of the vector _____ to the lead of interest.

4. A diagrammatic representation of the sequence of vectors is called a _____.

5. Atrial depolarization begins with the _____ atrium and follows with the _____ atrium.

6. The three primary vectors of ventricular depolarization represent activation of which anatomical structures?

7. The term used to represent the average of all the instantaneous vectors that occur during ventricular depolarization is _____.

8. The normal mean QRS axis lies between _____ and _____ degrees.

9. Left axis deviation is defined as a mean QRS axis that lies between _____ and _____ degrees.

10. Right axis deviation is defined as a mean QRS axis that lies between _____ and _____ degrees.

11. A mean QRS axis that cannot be measured in the frontal plane is said to be _____.

12. Clockwise and counterclockwise rotation of the heart refers to rotation of the heart as viewed from _____.

ANSWERS

Chapter 6 • SELF-TEST

1. Instantaneous cardiac vector.

2. • Positive (upward).
   • Negative (downward).

3. Perpendicular.

4. Vector loop.

5. • Right.
   • Left.

6. • Vector 1: Left side of the interventricular septum.
   • Vector 2: Free walls of the left and right ventricles.
   • Vector 3: The posterobasal portions of the left ventricle and interventricular septum.

7. Mean QRS axis.

8. +90 and −30.

9. −30 and −90.

10. +90 and +180.

11. Indeterminate.

12. Below the diaphragm.

Further Reading

Hurst JW. Methods used to interpret the 12-lead electrocardiogram: Pattern memorization versus the use of vector concepts. *Clin Cardiol.* 2000:23;4-13.

Perez Riera AR, Uchida AH, Filho CF, et al. Significance of vectorcardiogram in the cardiological diagnosis of the 21st century. *Clin Cardiol.* 2007:30;319-323.

Surawicz B, Childers R, Deal BJ, Gettes LS. AHA/ACCF/HRS Recommendations for the standardization and interpretation of the electrocardiogram. Part III: Intraventricular conduction disturbances. *J Am Coll Cardiol.* 2009:53;976-981.

SECTION II
Chamber Enlargement, Bundle Branch Block, and Preexcitation

Chamber Enlargement

The electrocardiogram (ECG) provides vital clues to the size of the cardiac chambers, which may enlarge in response to a variety of cardiac disorders. Electrocardiographic evidence of chamber enlargement represents an abnormal increase in mass, which may be due to *hypertrophy* of the muscular walls, *dilation* of the internal cavity, or a combination of both processes (**Figure 7-1**). *Concentric hypertrophy* is a circumferential increase in the wall thickness relative to the internal dimension of the myocardial chamber. This is the characteristic response to *pressure overload*, where the heart is forced to pump against increased resistance. Cardiac enlargement may also result from *dilation*, which is an increase in the internal chamber dimension. *Eccentric hypertrophy* is the adaptive response of the heart to *volume overload*, where the heart needs to pump an added quantity of blood with each contraction. In this situation, wall thickness increases *proportional* to the degree of dilation. Cardiac disorders frequently involve both pressure and volume overload; therefore, enlargement of either the atria or ventricles may involve both hypertrophy and dilation.

 CLINICAL TIP: Aortic stenosis and hypertension are examples of pressure overload. Left ventricular hypertrophy (LVH) is the physiologic adaptation to the added workload of systolic contraction against the restricted aortic valve or elevated blood pressure. Examples of volume overload include aortic and mitral insufficiency. In this situation, the left ventricle dilates to accommodate the added quantity of blood flowing into the chamber during diastole.

▶ ATRIAL ENLARGEMENT: GENERAL CONCEPTS

The normal sinus P wave has two components representing depolarization of the right atrium followed by the left atrium (**Figure 7-2**). Remember that the right atrium is really an anterior structure and the left atrium is actually posterior. The initial right atrial vector is directed leftward, inferiorly, and anteriorly. The terminal left atrial vector follows, directed leftward, inferiorly, and posteriorly. In the frontal plane, the contour of the normal P wave is smooth, with an amplitude ≤2.5 mm, a duration ≤0.11 seconds, and an axis between 0 and +75 degrees. In the horizontal plane, the normal P wave may be upright, inverted, or biphasic (upright followed by inverted) in lead V1. The inverted terminal portion of a normal biphasic P wave is <0.1 second in duration and <1 mm in depth. Analysis of the P wave is best performed by first inspecting lead II in the frontal plane and lead V1 in the horizontal plane. The thin-walled atria dilate in response to both pressure and volume overload, so avoid using the term *hypertrophy* when referring to atrial enlargement (which will immediately identify you as an ECG rookie). Left and right *atrial abnormality* is the preferred term to describe the P wave findings related to

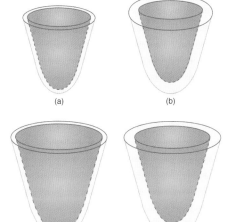

Figure 7-1. Forms of cardiac chamber enlargement. (a) Normal. (b) Concentric hypertrophy with increased wall thickness. (c) Dilation with increased internal dimension. (d) Eccentric hypertrophy with increased wall thickness proportional to chamber dilation.

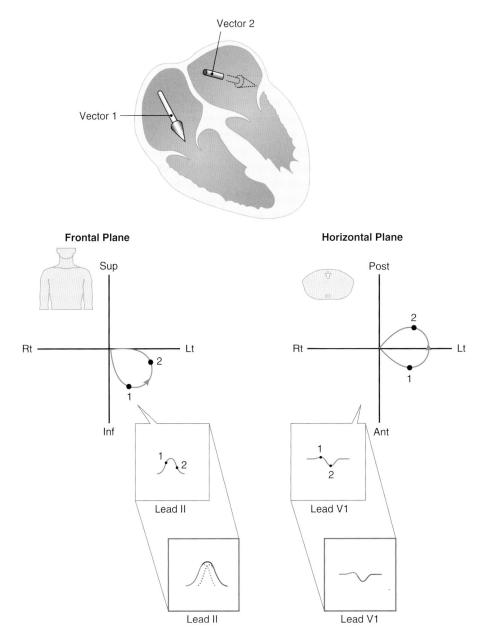

Figure 7-2. The normal P wave loop (enlarged for clarity). The P wave configuration has portions derived from vectors of the right atrium (blue), left atrium (red), and a combination of both atria (violet). The numbered dots represent the approximate ECG equivalents of the corresponding vectors.

increased chamber size, but it is also acceptable to use the term *atrial enlargement.*

 BE CAREFUL: The ECG criteria for left and right atrial abnormality/enlargement are neither sensitive nor specific. Echocardiographic techniques are preferred, with the *left and right atrial volume index* recognized as a more accurate and readily available measure of atrial size.

Right Atrial Abnormality/Enlargement

Enlargement of the right atrium causes the initial vector of the P wave to dominate (**Figure 7-3**). In the frontal plane, the P wave amplitude increases in leads II, III, and aVF with a

"peaked" configuration and a rightward axis shift. The duration of the P wave is unchanged because any prolongation of the initial right atrial portion merges within the left atrial contour. Findings of right atrial abnormality are less evident in the horizontal plane, but may increase the amplitude of the initial portion of the P wave in lead V1.

Criteria for Right Atrial Abnormality/Enlargement

- Increased P wave amplitude >2.5 mm in leads II, III, and aVF.
- Tall initial P wave amplitude >1.5 mm in lead V1.
- Normal P wave duration <0.12 seconds.
- Supporting criteria:
  - P wave axis shifted rightward (>+75 degrees).

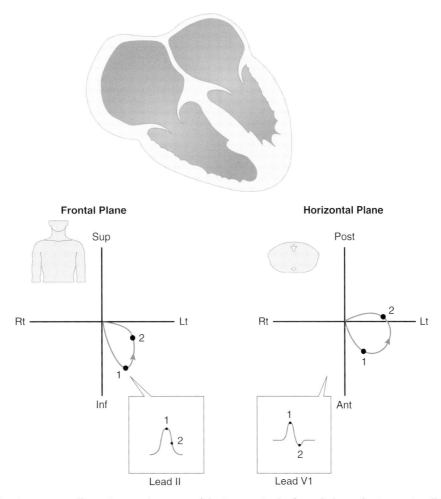

Figure 7-3. Right atrial enlargement affects the initial portion of the P wave. In the frontal plane, the P wave is tall in leads II, III, and aVF. In the horizontal plane, a tall initial P wave amplitude may be seen in lead V1.

 CLINICAL TIP: Right atrial enlargement may be seen in patients with chronic obstructive pulmonary disease, pulmonary hypertension, and congenital heart diseases that cause pressure or volume overload of the right heart. You may encounter the historical terms, *P pulmonale* and *P congenitale*, used to describe P wave abnormalities associated with these conditions.

Left Atrial Abnormality/Enlargement

Enlargement of the left atrium alters the terminal portion of the P wave with leftward and posterior forces now dominating (**Figure 7-4**). The P wave is notched and prolonged in the frontal plane with a leftward axis. The left and right atrial vectors separate and are distinguishable. In the horizontal plane, the inverted portion of the P wave in lead V1 is wide and deep. An *abnormal P terminal force* (Morris index) is a very specific clue to left atrial enlargement, which is defined as the product of the depth and duration of the inverted P wave in lead V1 of ≥0.04 mm-sec (at least one small box wide and one small box deep).

Criteria for Left Atrial Abnormality/Enlargement
• Prolonged and notched P wave with duration ≥0.12 seconds in leads I, II, aVF, V5, V6.

• Abnormal P terminal force ≥0.04 mm-sec in lead V1.
• Supporting criteria:
  ▪ P wave axis leftward of +15 degrees.

 CLINICAL TIP: Left atrial enlargement is frequently associated with disorders of left ventricular function, congestive heart failure, hypertension, and mitral valve disease. You may encounter the historical term, *P mitrale*, used to describe the P wave abnormalities associated with mitral stenosis. ECG findings of left atrial enlargement may also be found in the absence of cardiac disease.

 FOR BOOKWORMS: A prolonged, notched P wave of ≥0.12 seconds without other evidence of left atrial enlargement may be due to an abnormality of intra-atrial conduction. In this circumstance, you should use the terms *nonspecific atrial abnormality* or *intra-atrial conduction delay* to describe the findings.

Bi-atrial Abnormality/Enlargement

The presence of bi-atrial enlargement is identified when findings of both right and left atrial enlargement coexist

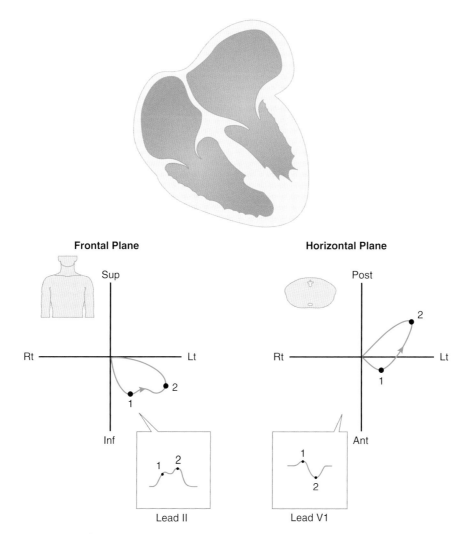

Figure 7-4. Left atrial enlargement affects the terminal portion of the P wave. The P wave is prolonged and notched in leads I and II. An abnormal P terminal force is seen in lead V1.

(**Figure 7-5**). Vectors of the two atria affect different portions of the P wave without canceling each other and remain distinguishable. The P wave of bi-atrial enlargement in the frontal plane is both tall and wide. In the horizontal plane, there is both a tall initial portion and abnormal P terminal force.

Criteria for Bi-atrial Abnormality/Enlargement
- In lead V1, a tall initial P wave amplitude >1.5 mm and an abnormal P terminal force ≥0.04 mm-sec.
- In the limb leads, a notched and prolonged P wave ≥0.12 seconds with an amplitude >2.5 mm.

 VENTRICULAR ENLARGEMENT: GENERAL CONCEPTS

Enlargement of the right, left, or both ventricles produces an array of ECG findings. These include (1) increase in QRS amplitude (voltage), (2) increase in QRS duration, (3) changes in QRS axis, and (4) repolarization abnormalities (ST segment and T wave).

The QRS complex reflects depolarization of both the right and left ventricles. But unlike the P wave, which has identifiable components of both atria, the normal QRS complex is dominated by the greater mass of the left ventricle. The QRS complex normally has a duration of 0.06 to 0.10 seconds, an axis of −30 to +90 degrees, and an R wave peak time (time to the intrinsicoid deflection or ventricular activation time) of <0.04 seconds in V1 and V2 and <0.05 seconds in leads V5 and V6. The ST segment is usually isoelectric, but may be slightly elevated or depressed (<1 mm) above or below the baseline. The T wave configuration is usually concordant with that of the QRS complex, meaning that it is upright in leads with a positive QRS and inverted in leads with negative QRS. All these items enter into the analysis of ventricular enlargement.

CLINICAL TIP: I prefer to use left and right ventricular *enlargement* (LVE, RVE) to describe the ECG findings of increased ventricular mass. However, the use of left and right ventricular *hypertrophy* (LVH, RVH) is embedded in the medical lexicon, so the terms may be used interchangeably in clinical practice.

Left Ventricular Enlargement/Hypertrophy

Analysis of the vector loop helps us to understand the findings we see on the scalar ECG. In Chapter 6 we described the normal sequence of ventricular activation, which we arbitrarily divided

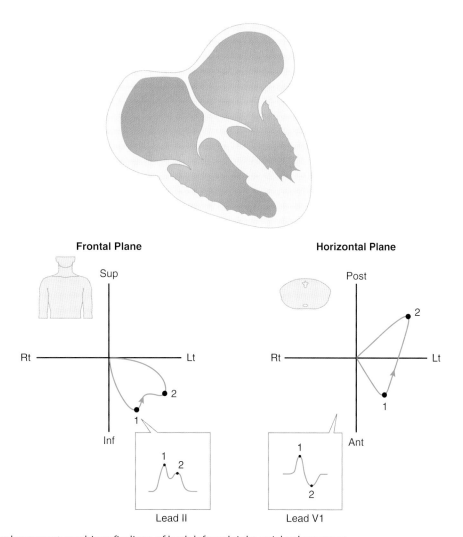

Figure 7-5. Bi-atrial enlargement combines findings of both left and right atrial enlargement.

into three vectors (**Figure 7-6**). Vector 1 represents depolarization of the left side of the interventricular septum. Vector 2 reflects activation of the free walls of both ventricles, with left ventricular forces predominating. Vector 3 denotes activation of the posterobasal portions of both the left ventricle and interventricular septum.

Left ventricular enlargement (LVE) amplifies the vector forces of the left ventricular free wall. An easy way to visualize the ECG findings of LVE is to imagine as if Hercules "the hypertropher" is pulling the vector loop by cables in a leftward and posterior direction (**Figure 7-7**). Hercules is strong enough to alter every part of the loop, including the initial, main, and terminal vectors, and can even change the loop's rotation (clockwise or counterclockwise). In the frontal plane, the initial forces are pulled leftward and inferiorly with the main portion of the enlarged loop following in a leftward and relatively superior direction (**Figure 7-8**). This results in a leftward axis shift, with tall R waves in leads I and aVL and deep S waves in lead III. In the horizontal plane, the enlarged vector loop is pulled leftward and posteriorly. This produces tall R waves in the left precordial leads (V5, V6) and deep S waves in the right precordial leads (V1, V2). The time delay required for depolarization of the increased left ventricular mass may result in widening of the QRS complex and an increase in the R wave peak time.

CLINICAL TIP: LVE provides important prognostic information in patients with hypertension. Overall cardiovascular morbidity and mortality is greater in subjects with increased left ventricular mass. Antihypertensive treatment that causes LVE regression improves prognosis independent of the degree of blood pressure lowering.

CLINICAL TIP: LVE does not always indicate pathology and may represent a physiologic adaptation to athletic training. Olympic athletes engaging in dynamic/aerobic events such as running or swimming characteristically have LV chamber dilation with little (or a proportional) increase in wall thickness. Those competing in static/power events such as weight lifting typically have increased wall thickness alone. The hearts of athletes competing in rowing and cycling demonstrate both increased chamber dimension and wall thickness, reflecting the combined dynamic and power demands of these sports. Hercules was said to have both legendary endurance and strength. We would expect his ECG to show LVE and his echocardiogram to demonstrate both chamber dilation and hypertrophy.

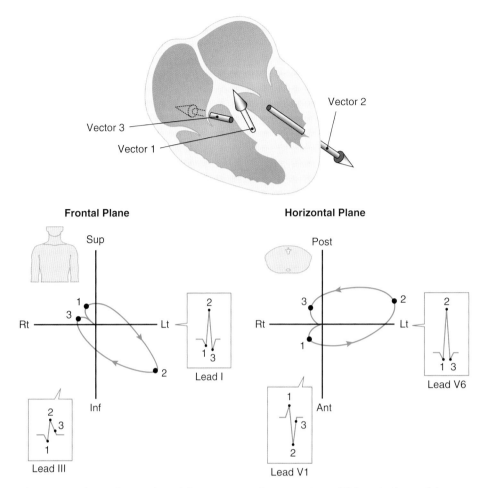

Figure 7-6. The normal QRS vector loop. The numbered dots represent the approximate ECG equivalents of the corresponding vectors.

Repolarization abnormalities are also found in LVE including ST segment depression and T wave inversion that is directed opposite to that of the QRS complex. Recall from Chapter 6 that depolarization of the left ventricle proceeds from endocardium to epicardium, but repolarization is in the opposite direction, epicardium to endocardium. That is why the direction of the normal T wave is concordant with the QRS complex, rather than the opposite we would normally expect (see Chapter 4). One theory to explain the ST segment and T wave findings of LVE is that depolarization of the thickened ventricle is so prolonged that

repolarization of the endocardium now occurs *before* the epicardium. The combination of an increased QRS voltage with deviation of the ST segment and T wave in an opposite direction to the QRS complex has been historically called the "*left ventricular strain*" pattern (**Figure 7-9**). It is preferable that this older term be replaced with the term "secondary ST segment and T wave abnormalities."

Criteria for Left Ventricular Enlargement/Left Ventricular Hypertrophy

A variety of criteria are available to diagnose LVE. All utilize measurements of QRS voltage and some include non-voltage-related items. Some of the more widely utilized criteria for LVE are as follows:

Sokolow-Lyon criteria (precordial lead-based)

- S wave in lead V1 + R wave in lead V5 or V6 is >35 mm (age >40).
- S wave in lead V1 + R wave in lead V5 or V6 is >40 mm (age 31-40).
- S wave in lead V1 + R wave in lead V5 or V6 is >60 mm (age 16-30).

Gubner-Ungerleider criteria (limb lead-based)

- R wave in lead I + S wave in lead III is >25 mm.

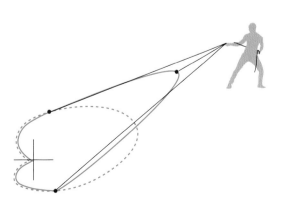

Figure 7-7. The vector loop of LVE in the horizontal plane is "pulled" in a leftward and posterior direction.

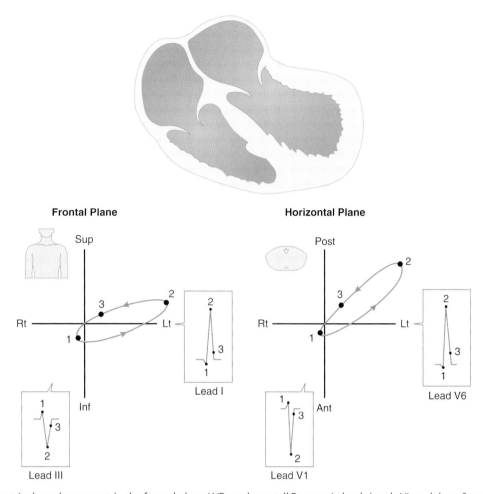

Figure 7-8. Left ventricular enlargement. In the frontal plane LVE produces tall R waves in leads I and aVL and deep S waves in lead III. In the horizontal plane, the findings include tall R waves in leads V5 and V6 and deep S waves in leads V1 and V2.

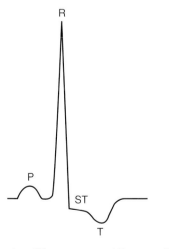

Figure 7-9. Secondary ST segment and T wave abnormalities in LVE. Also called the "left ventricular strain pattern," repolarization abnormalities associated with LVE include ST depression and T wave inversion in leads with a tall R wave.

Cornell criteria (combined precordial and limb lead-based)

- In men, R wave in lead aVL + S wave in lead V3 is >28 mm.
- In women, R wave in lead aVL + S wave in lead V3 is >20 mm.

Romhilt-Estes scoring system (4 = "probable" and ≥5 = "definite")

- R wave or S wave in any limb lead ≥20 mm (3 points).
- S wave in lead V1 or V2 ≥30 mm (3 points).
- R wave in lead V5 or V6 ≥30 mm (3 points).
- Left ventricular strain pattern.
  - Without digitalis (3 points).
  - With digitalis (1 point).
- Abnormal P terminal force lead V1 (3 points).
- Left axis deviation ≥−30 degrees (2 points).
- QRS duration ≥0.09 seconds (1 point).
- R wave peak time (time to the intrinsicoid deflection) in lead V5 or V6 ≥0.05 seconds (1 point).

These are but a few of the many published criteria for LVE. All have strengths and weaknesses and it is common that tracings that indicate LVE by one criterion fail to do so with another. When diagnosing LVE, always identify the criteria you are using to establish the diagnosis (**Figures 7-10 to 7-12**).

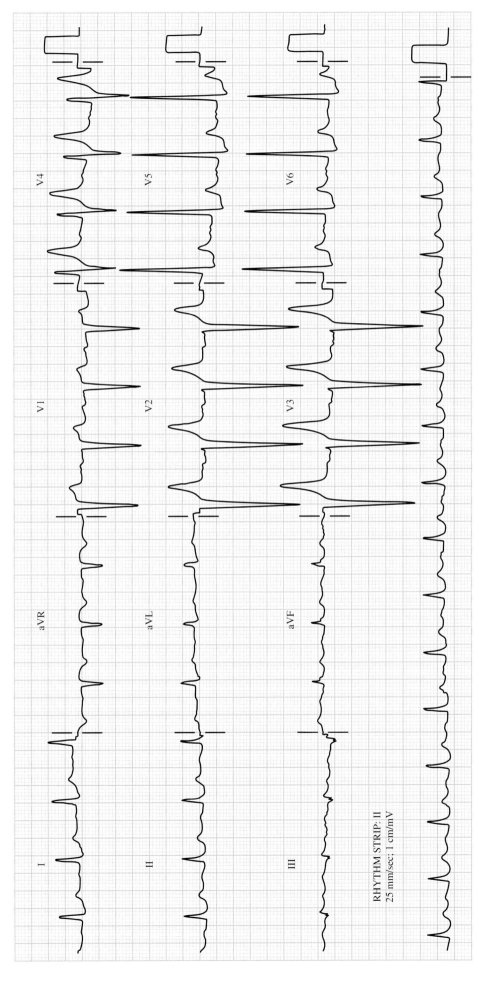

Figure 7-10. LVE is diagnosed based on both the precordial lead and Cornell criteria. The S wave in lead V1 + R wave in lead V5 or V6 is >35 mm and the R wave in lead aVL + S wave in lead V3 is >28 mm. Note also the secondary ST segment and T wave abnormalities (strain pattern) present in leads V5-V6.

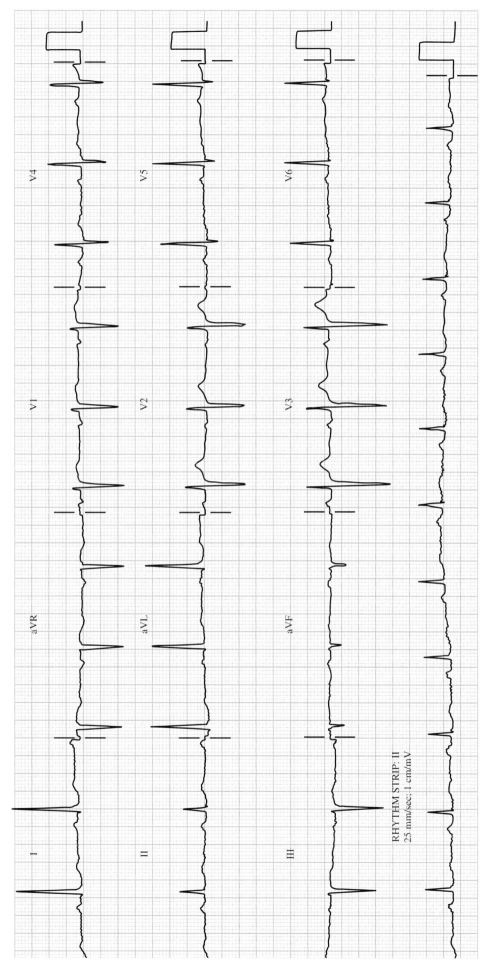

Figure 7-11. LVE is diagnosed based on both the limb lead and Cornell criteria. The R wave in lead III is >25 mm and the R wave in lead I + S wave in lead aVL + S wave in lead V3 is >28 mm.

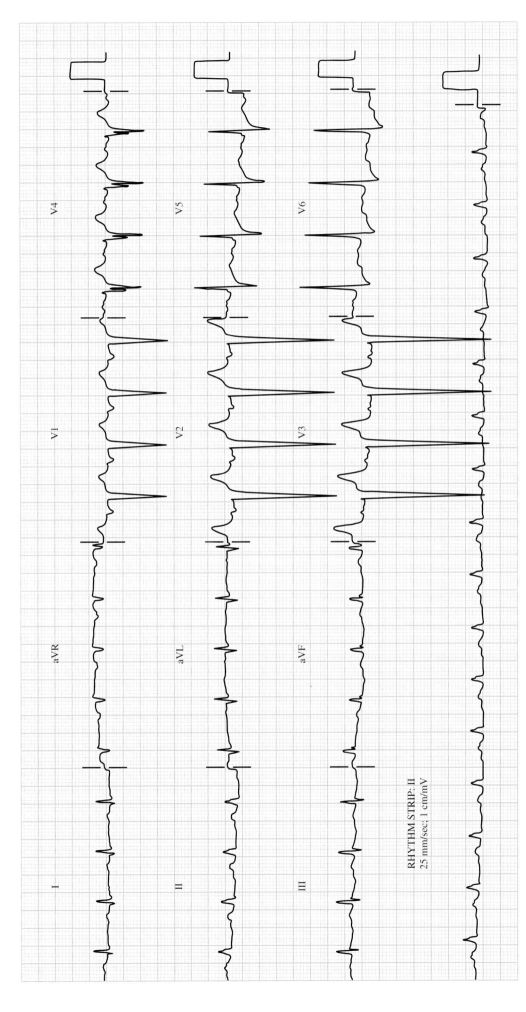

Figure 7-12. LVE is diagnosed based on the Cornell criteria. The R wave in lead aVL + S wave in lead V3 is >28 mm. Note also the secondary ST segment and T wave findings in leads V5-V6 and the left atrial abnormality in lead V1.

Problems and Pitfalls with Left Ventricular Enlargement

A number of factors unrelated to chamber size or mass impact the accuracy of QRS voltage criteria for ventricular enlargement. This is particularly true for the left ventricle, where QRS voltage may be affected by age, gender, race, and body habitus. The ECG of children and young adults normally exhibits a large QRS amplitude, therefore voltage criteria for LVE are applicable only for individuals 40 years of age or older. Men normally have a higher QRS amplitude in both the limb and precordial leads than women. Breast tissue impacts QRS voltage, which may be lower in women with large breasts and greater following mastectomy. Compared with values in Caucasians, the upper limit of normal QRS voltage is higher in individuals of African descent and lower in Hispanics. Precordial QRS voltage is less in obese individuals because the adipose tissue increases the distance between the electrode and the myocardium. Conversely, voltage may be increased in extremely lean individuals leading to an erroneous diagnosis of cardiac enlargement.

Disturbances of intraventricular conduction such as right bundle branch block, left bundle branch block, and left anterior fascicular block negatively impact the diagnostic accuracy of voltage criteria for LVE. Although criteria have been proposed, the diagnosis of LVE in the presence of conduction abnormalities must be considered tenuous.

 FOR BOOKWORMS: You may consider using the following voltage criteria for the diagnosis of LVE in the presence of conduction abnormalities.
- Left anterior fascicular block.
  - S wave in lead III + (sum of R + S voltage in the precordial lead with the greatest R + S amplitude) ≥30 mm.
- Right bundle branch block.
  - R wave in lead I + S wave lead III >25 mm.
  - R wave in lead V5 or V6 ≥25 mm.
  - R wave in lead aVL >12 mm.
- Left bundle branch block.
  - S wave in lead V2 + R wave lead V5 ≥45 mm.
- Incomplete left and right bundle branch block: Use standard criteria.

Right Ventricular Enlargement/Hypertrophy

The vector pattern of right ventricular enlargement is much more variable than that of LVE and is characteristically related to the underlying etiology, depending on whether the disorder is one of pressure or volume overload. In most circumstances, we can visualize Hercules as pulling the loop in an anterior and rightward direction, reflecting the position of the right ventricle in the chest (**Figure 7-13**). In some forms of RVE, posterior forces become evident. As with LVE, the change in forces may affect any portion of the vector loop and alter the direction of rotation.

Different patterns of RVE are broadly categorized as type A, B, or C based on the QRS morphology present in the right precordial leads. These general divisions can be useful, but there is considerable variability of the ECG and vector patterns

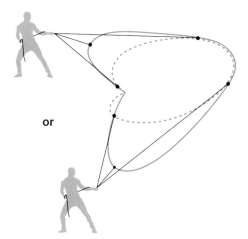

Figure 7-13. The vector loop of RVE in the horizontal plane is "pulled" rightward and either in an anterior or posterior direction.

within each category. I will review the different patterns later, but I recommend you use them to understand the subtleties of the diagnosis of RVE rather than worry about which type is present.

Type A (Tall R wave pattern) In the horizontal plane, increasing enlargement of the right ventricle pulls the vector loop in a rightward and anterior direction, changing the rotation clockwise. This produces very tall R waves in the right precordial leads and deep S waves in the left precordial leads (**Figure 7-14**). The frontal plane loop is pulled to the right and inferiorly, resulting in right axis deviation. This produces a small R wave and deep S wave in lead I. Tall R waves are found in leads II, III, and aVF.

 CLINICAL TIP: The type A pattern of RVE is characteristically found in patients with congenital pulmonic stenosis, tetralogy of Fallot, severe pulmonary hypertension (Eisenmenger syndrome) and other conditions in which pressure overload has caused the right ventricular mass to approach or exceed that of the left ventricle.

Type B (Rs pattern) Unlike pattern A, the vector loop in this form of RVE maintains its normal counterclockwise rotation in the horizontal plane (**Figure 7-15**). Pattern B also differs from pattern A in that the tall R wave in lead V1 is comparatively smaller and an S wave is present, hence the Rs pattern. S waves are found in the left precordial leads, but they are not as deep as those seen in type A RVE. In the frontal plane, the overall QRS pattern is fairly normal with the axis remaining either normal or directed to the right.

 CLINICAL TIP: The type B pattern of RVE is most often seen in patients with atrial septal defect or mitral stenosis that results in a more moderate degree of pulmonary hypertension.

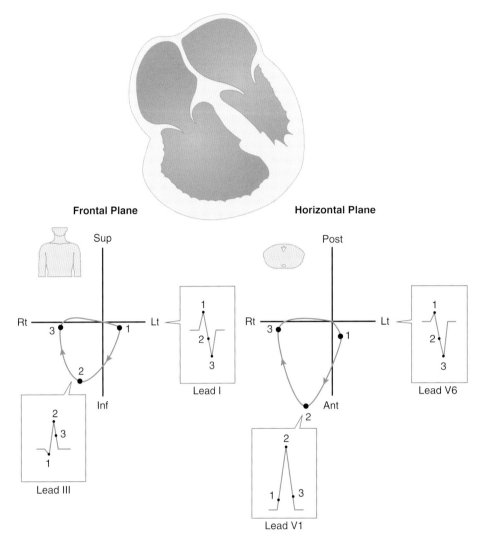

Figure 7-14. Type A (tall R wave) pattern of RVE. In the horizontal plane, the loop is turned clockwise and directed in a rightward and anterior direction.

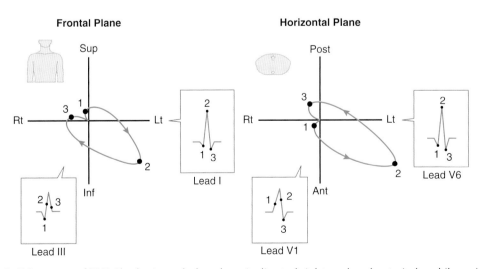

Figure 7-15. Type B (Rs) pattern of RVE. The horizontal plane loop is directed rightward and anteriorly, while maintaining its normal counterclockwise rotation.

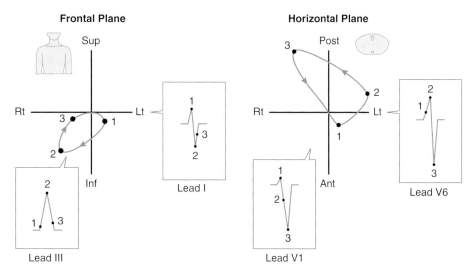

Figure 7-16. Type C (rS or rSr′) pattern of RVE. In the horizontal plane, the main portion of the counterclockwise loop is directed posteriorly.

Type C (rS or rSr′ pattern) The main feature of this form of RVE is the posterior position of the vector loop (**Figure 7-16**). In the horizontal plane the initial forces move anteriorly and either to the right or left, producing an initial r wave in lead V1. The main forces of the counterclockwise loop turn rightward and posteriorly, generating dominant S waves across the precordium (rS). In some cases, the terminal forces return anteriorly, producing a second r wave (rSr′). In the frontal plane, the forces are directed inferiorly and rightward, resulting in right axis deviation.

 CLINICAL TIP: Type C RVE is a pattern seen with *cor pulmonale* secondary to chronic obstructive pulmonary disease. Lung disease lowers the diaphragm, changing the position of the heart in the chest to a more vertical position with clockwise rotation along its vertical axis (see Chapter 6, Figures 6-12 and 6-15). The left ventricular free wall is now positioned more posteriorly, which is a reasonable explanation why a condition associated with enlargement of the *anterior* right ventricle produces the prominent *posterior* (LV) vector findings (deep precordial S waves) that we see in type C RVE.

Criteria for Right Ventricular Enlargement/Hypertrophy
There is no one group of criteria that sets the standard for the diagnosis of right ventricular enlargement. This is not surprising given the variety of vector and QRS patterns we just discussed. Clues to the diagnosis are that in virtually all cases, right axis deviation (>+110 degrees) and prominent R waves in the right precordial leads are present (**Figure 7-17**). ECG findings that suggest the presence of RVE are as follows:

- Right axis deviation (in the absence of other causes).
- R/S ratio in V1 >1.
- R/S ratio in lead V5 or V6 ≤1.

- R wave in lead V1 ≥7 mm.
- qR pattern in lead V1.
- rSR′ pattern in lead V1 with R′ wave ≥10 mm (normal QRS duration).
- Supporting criteria:
  - ST segment depression and T wave inversion in the right precordial leads.
  - Right atrial abnormality.
  - R wave peak time (time to the intrinsicoid deflection) in lead V1 ≥0.04 seconds.

Problems and Pitfalls with RVE

One of the problems with the ECG diagnosis of RVE is that the large mass of the left ventricle can mask the forces of even a substantially enlarged right ventricle. In addition, conditions that might predispose to RVE, such as COPD might actually reduce the diagnostic accuracy of the ECG because the hyperinflated lungs are poor electrical conductors, thereby lowering the QRS voltage.

Combined Right and Left Ventricular Enlargement/ Biventricular Hypertrophy

The ECG diagnosis of combined or biventricular enlargement is a tenuous proposition, particularly in adults. Vector examples are sparse and not well validated. The forces of the enlarged right and left ventricles may counterbalance each other producing a nearly normal QRS pattern. Alternatively, forces of either the right or left ventricle may predominate over the other. Nevertheless, there are clues to the diagnosis as follows:

- Precordial lead voltage criteria for LVE accompany a frontal plane QRS axis >+90 degrees.
- Tall, equiphasic complexes (R wave = S wave) in leads V2, V3, V4 (Katz-Wachtel pattern).

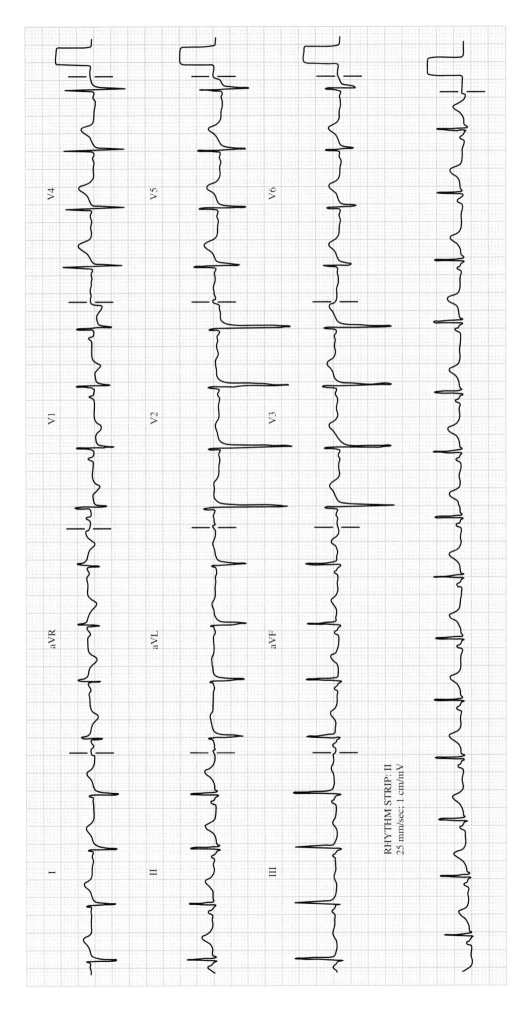

Figure 7-17. Typical findings of RVE. Note the right axis deviation, tall R wave voltage in lead V1 and R/S ratio in lead V5-V6 ≤1.

QUESTIONS

Chapter 7 • SELF-TEST

1. An increased chamber mass may be due to a change of which anatomical factors?
2. Name two clinical conditions that may result in pressure overload of the left ventricle.
3. Name two clinical conditions that may result in volume overload of the left ventricle.
4. The initial and terminal portions of the P wave represent depolarization of which chambers, respectively?
5. List the criteria for right atrial enlargement.
6. List the criteria for left atrial enlargement.
7. In the limb leads, how does left ventricular enlargement affect the voltage of the QRS complex?
8. In the precordial leads, how does left ventricular enlargement affect the voltage of the QRS complex?
9. List at least three different voltage criteria for LVE.
10. List two key ECG features that suggest right ventricular enlargement.

ANSWERS

Chapter 7 • SELF-TEST

1. Hypertrophy and dilation.
2. Aortic stenosis and hypertension.
3. Aortic insufficiency and mitral insufficiency.
4. The initial portion of the P wave represents depolarization of the right atrium. The terminal portion of the P wave represents depolarization of the left atrium.
5. • Increased P wave amplitude >2.5 mm in leads II, III, and aVF.
   • Tall initial P wave amplitude >1.5 mm in lead V1.
   • Normal P wave duration <0.12 seconds.
   • Supporting criteria:
     ▪ P wave axis shifted rightward of +75 degrees.
6. • Prolonged and notched P wave with duration ≥0.12 seconds leads I, II, aVF, V5, V6.
   • Abnormal P terminal force ≥0.04 mm-sec in lead V1.
   • Supporting criteria:
     ▪ P wave axis leftward of +15 degrees.
7. Produces tall R waves in leads I and aVL and deep S wave in lead III.
8. Produces tall R waves in leads V5 and V6 and deep S waves in leads V1 and V2.
9. • S wave in lead V1 + R wave in lead V5 or V6 is >35 mm (age >40).
   • R wave in lead aVL + S wave in lead V3 is >28 mm (men) or >20 mm (women).
   • R wave in lead I + S wave in lead III is >25 mm.
10. Right axis deviation and tall R waves in the right precordial leads (V1 and V2).

Further Reading

Alpert MA, Munuswamy K. Electrocardiographic diagnosis of left atrial enlargement. *Arch Intern Med*. 1989;149:1161-1165.

Bacharova L, Estes EH Jr. Left ventricular hypertrophy by the surface ECG. *J Electrocardiol*. 2017;50:906-908.

Casale PN, Devereux RB, Kligfield P, et al. Electrocardiographic detection of left ventricular hypertrophy: development and prospective validation of improved criteria. *J Am Coll Cardiol*. 1985;6:572-580.

Dorn GW, Robbins J, Sugden PH. Phenotyping hypertrophy: eschew obfuscation. *Circ Res*. 2003;92:1171-1175.

Estes EH Jr., Jackson KP. The electrocardiogram in left ventricular hypertrophy: past and future. *J Electrocardiol*. 2009;42:589-592.

Garg S, Drazner MH. Refining the classification of left ventricular hypertrophy to provide new insights into the progression from hypertension to heart failure. *Curr Opin Cardiol*. 2016;31:387-393.

Gubner R, Underleider HE. Electrocardiographic criteria of left ventricular hypertrophy. *Arch Intern Med*. 1943;72:196-209.

Hancock EW, Deal BJ, Mirvis DM, Okin P, Kliegfield P, Gettes LS. AHA/ACCF/HRS recommendations for the standardization and interpretation of the electrocardiogram. Part V: Electrocardiogram changes associated with cardiac chamber hypertrophy. *J Am Coll Cardiol*. 2009;53:982-1002.

Hazen MS, Marwick TH, Underwood DA. Diagnostic accuracy of the resting electrocardiogram in detection and estimation of left atrial enlargement: an echocardiographic correlation in 551 patients. *Am Heart J*. 1991;122:823-828.

Jain A, Chandna H, Silver EN, Clark WA, Denes P. Electrocardiographic patterns of patients with echocardiographically determined biventricular hypertrophy. *J Electrocardiol*. 1999;32:269-273.

Kannel WB, Dannenberg AL, Levy D. Population implications of electrocardiographic left ventricular hypertrophy. *Am J Cardiol*. 1987;60:85I-93I.

Lee KS, Applemton CP, Lester SJ, et al. Relation of electrocardiographic criteria for left atrial enlargement to two-dimensional echocardiographic left atrial volume measurements. *Am J Cardiol*. 2007;99:113-118.

Okin PM, Devereux RB, Fabsitz RR, Lee ET, Galloway JM, Howard BV. Quantitative assessment of electrocardiographic strain predicts increased left ventricular mass: the Strong Heart Study. *J Am Coll Cardiol*. 2002;40:1395-1400.

Romhilt DW, Bove KE, Norris RJ, et al. A critical appraisal of the electrocardiographic criteria for the diagnosis of left ventricular hypertrophy. *Circulation*. 1969;40:185-195.

Romhilt DW, Estes EH. A point-score system for the ECG diagnosis of left ventricular hypertrophy. *Am Heart J*. 1946;75:752-758.

Sokolow M, Lyon TP. The ventricular complex in left ventricular hypertrophy as obtained by unipolar precordial and limb leads. *Am Heart J*. 1949;37:161-185.

Surawicz B. Electrocardiographic diagnosis of chamber enlargement. *J Am Coll Cardiol*. 1986;8:711-724.

Bundle Branch Block and Related Conduction Abnormalities

▶ REVIEW OF ANATOMY AND CARDIAC CONDUCTION

Let's again review how the normal sinus impulse reaches the ventricles. The SA node depolarization first conducts through the atria, the AV node, and the bundle of His. Next, the stimulus proceeds through the right bundle branch and the left bundle branch and its divisions. The left common bundle branch divides into two major fascicles called the left anterior-superior fascicle and left posterior-inferior fascicle, as well as a smaller mid-septal fascicle (**Figure 8-1**). Remember that this is a simplified description of the left bundle branch because the two major divisions and one minor branch are arranged more like a fan-shaped array rather than distinct, isolated fibers. The right and left bundle branches arborize widely, dividing into an extensive network of Purkinje fibers that interconnects with the ventricular myocytes. Transmission of the sinus impulse through the atria and the remainder of the specialized conduction system (AV node and His-Purkinje system) is recorded on

the ECG as the PR interval. Electrical transmission through the His-Purkinje system is extremely rapid, with the majority of the duration of the PR interval representing conduction through the atria and AV node (**Figure 8-2**). The QRS complex records depolarization of the ventricular myocardium, a process that is normally completed within 0.10 seconds. Recall from Chapter 6 that we can simplify ventricular depolarization into three stages, each represented by a vector (**Figure 8-3**).

1. The left side of the interventricular septum.
2. The right and left ventricular free walls.
3. The posterobasal portions of the left ventricle and interventricular septum.

The first portion of the ventricle to be stimulated is the left side of the interventricular septum, which receives the electrical signal via a division of the left bundle branch (septal fascicle). This corresponds to vector 1, which is directed left-to-right, anterior, and (usually) superior. On the ECG it

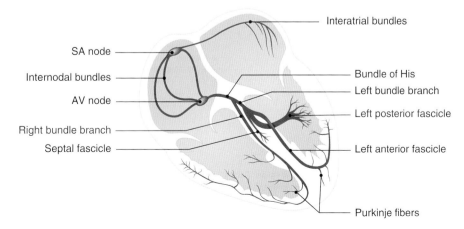

Figure 8-1. Conduction system of the heart (see text for details).

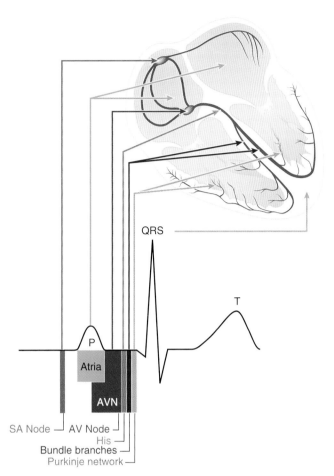

Figure 8-2. ECG timing relationship of transmission through the specialized conduction system.

produces an initial Q wave in leftward-looking leads (I, aVL, V5, V6) and an initial R wave in rightward-looking leads (V1, V2, aVR).

The next portions of the heart to depolarize are the free walls of the right and left ventricles, which correspond to vector 2. Remember that the much larger mass of the left ventricle predominates, resulting in a vector oriented toward the left, inferiorly and posteriorly. This produces the normal tall R wave in leftward-looking leads and deep S wave in rightward-looking leads.

Final activation of the interventricular septum and posterobasal portions of the left ventricle represent vector 3. This vector is of small amplitude and variable, oriented predominantly to the right, posteriorly and somewhat superiorly. This results in low voltage R waves in rightward-looking leads and small S waves in leftward-looking leads.

▶ DEFINITIONS AND TERMINOLOGY

Intraventricular conduction abnormalities are defined as either a delay of transmission or complete interruption of the electrical impulse in one or more of the conduction pathways located distal to the bundle of His (**Figure 8-4**). Disturbances within the main right or left bundle branches are termed **bundle branch**

blocks, which are further categorized as either complete or incomplete based on the duration of the QRS complex. A complete bundle branch block has a QRS duration of ≥0.12 seconds, whereas an incomplete bundle branch block is considered to have a QRS duration of >0.10 and <0.12 seconds. Intraventricular conduction abnormalities may also be localized to either of the divisions of the left bundle branch, which are termed **left anterior** or **left posterior fascicular blocks** (also called hemiblocks). The term *nonspecific intraventricular conduction delay* is used to describe findings that do not fit within a specific category of bundle branch block.

> **CLINICAL TIP:** The term *bundle branch block* is somewhat unfortunate because patients will often interpret this term as a "blockage" in their coronary arteries. A better term to use is to describe the findings as a bundle branch block *pattern*. I explain the term as a "slowing" of electricity through their heart rather than a "block." I also use an automobile analogy describing that the ECG pattern indicates the electrical impulse is traveling on a slow, winding route (conduction delay), rather than on the straight, high-speed highway (normal conduction).

▶ GENERAL CONCEPTS OF BUNDLE BRANCH BLOCK

Intraventricular conduction disturbances alter the normal sequence of ventricular activation and produce characteristic changes on the ECG. Two key electrocardiographic features of both left and right bundle branch blocks include (1) prolonged QRS duration and (2) terminal conduction delay. Additional findings typically include secondary ST segment and T wave changes. An important concept to understand is that the wide complexes seen with bundle branch blocks are the result of **asynchronous** activation of the left and right ventricles. It won't take you long to immediately recognize the characteristic features of the bundle branch blocks. But instead of asking you to memorize these patterns, I prefer that you understand the genesis of these ECG findings.

A narrow QRS complex is the result of both ventricles depolarizing in synchrony, concurrently receiving their impulses via the right and left bundle branches and the Purkinje fibers. In the presence of a bundle branch block, the electrical impulse cannot directly stimulate its corresponding portion of the myocardium, resulting in asynchronous ventricular depolarization. Electrical transmission occurs through the unblocked bundle branch in the normal fashion. But then the impulse must spread through the surrounding muscle to depolarize the myocardium below the block. This myocyte-to-myocyte transmission is less efficient than using the specialized conduction system, which causes the blocked ventricle to depolarize late, after the unblocked ventricle. To use our driving analogy, the electrical impulse first speeds down a highway to depolarize the unblocked ventricle, then lumbers off-road to activate the remaining myocardium. This two-part route explains the prolonged QRS duration and terminal conduction delay that are the characteristic ECG features of bundle branch blocks. In addition, the abnormal sequence

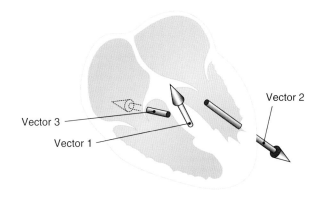

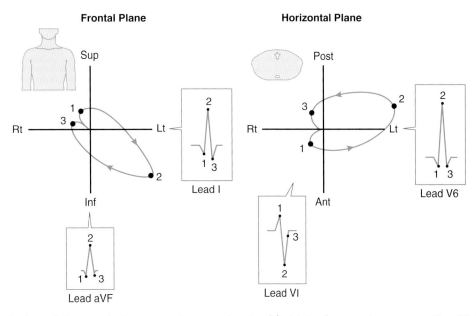

Figure 8-3. Depolarization of the ventricular myocardium can be simplified into three vectors representing (1) the left side of the interventricular septum, (2) the right and left ventricular free walls, and (3) the posterobasal portions of the left ventricle and interventricular septum. Normal vector loops are shown in the frontal and horizontal plane. Numbered points on the ECG correspond to the vector orientations.

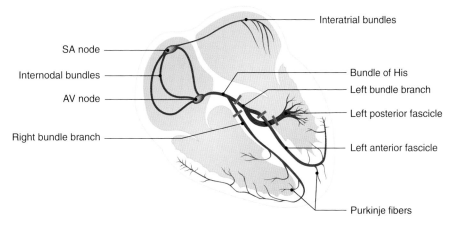

Figure 8-4. Common sites of block of the intraventricular conduction system (red bars).

of depolarization alters the course of repolarization, thereby producing secondary ST segment and T wave changes. OK, enough with the theory. Let's now discuss the various conduction abnormalities individually.

Right Bundle Branch Block

In right bundle branch block (RBBB), the primary abnormality is a delay in depolarization of the right ventricle (**Figure 8-5**). During normal conduction, the right ventricular forces are hidden, overwhelmed by the greater mass of the left ventricle. But in the presence of a RBBB, the conduction delay allows the now unopposed right-sided forces to become visible.

Depolarization of the interventricular septum is unaffected by RBBB and depolarizes via a division of the left bundle branch with normal speed in a normal left-to-right direction (vector 1). This preserves the initial Q waves in leftward-looking leads (I, aVL, V6). Transmission proceeds through the intact left bundle branch to activate the left ventricular free wall in a normal right-to-left direction (vector 2). Accordingly, leftward-looking leads show normal R waves and rightward-looking leads show normal S waves. As you can see, RBBB does little to alter vectors 1 and 2. The impulse now spreads via slow, myocyte-to-myocyte transmission to activate the right ventricle (vector 3). This final vector is directed rightward and anterior reflecting the anatomical position of the right ventricle in the chest.

The late, slowly transmitted impulse produces the characteristic large, wide terminal R′ wave in V1 and wide S wave in V6. You can visualize this pattern by holding up the second and third fingers of your right hand in front of you and making a "peace sign" (**Figure 8-6**). Another classic description of the pattern is to consider the rSR′ pattern in lead V1 as a set of "rabbit ears."

Secondary, discordant ST segment and T wave abnormalities are frequently present, opposite in the direction of the terminal portion of the QRS complex (**Figure 8-7**). For example, in lead V1, the ST segment is either isoelectric or depressed and the T wave is inverted, opposite in direction of the terminal R′.

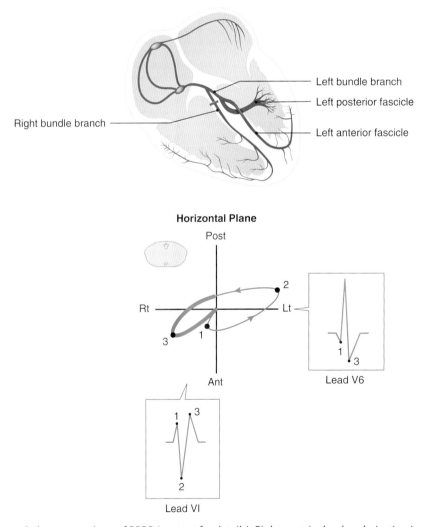

Figure 8-5. Typical horizontal plane vector loop of RBBB (see text for details). Right ventricular depolarization is delayed and slowed (wide portion of loop).

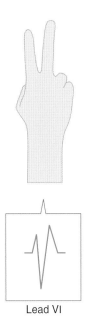

Lead VI

Figure 8-6. With RBBB, the QRS pattern resembles the right hand forming a "peace sign" in lead V1.

Criteria for Complete Right Bundle Branch block

- QRS duration ≥0.12 seconds.
- rsr´, rsR´, rSR´, or M-shaped pattern in leads V1 or V2.
- The secondary R´ wave is usually wider and of greater amplitude than the initial r wave.
- Secondary ST segment and T wave abnormalities in the right precordial leads directed opposite to that of the dominant R wave.
- Supporting criteria:
  - Prolonged R peak time (time to the intrinsicoid deflection) >0.05 seconds in lead V1.
  - Broad S waves in leads I, aVL, and V5-V6.

 CLINICAL TIP: Isolated RBBB may be clinically benign with no adverse prognosis. It may also be associated with any condition affecting the right heart including atrial septal defect, pulmonary embolism, and chronic obstructive pulmonary disease. RBBB may also be intermittent and rate related, appearing only with faster heart rates.

 FOR BOOKWORMS: In RBBB, the first 0.06 to 0.08 seconds of the QRS complex is unaffected by the conduction delay. Use this initial portion to measure the mean QRS axis. In addition, diagnostic Q waves of myocardial infarction are valid in the presence of RBBB.

 BE CAREFUL: An rSr´ pattern in lead V1 with a normal QRS duration is a normal variant in approximately 5% of the population. The absence of a prolonged QRS complex and secondary ST segment and T wave findings distinguishes this finding from an incomplete RBBB (see following discussion).

Left Bundle Branch Block

In left bundle branch block (LBBB) the primary abnormality is a delay in depolarization of the left ventricle. But unlike the case with RBBB, the entire sequence of ventricular activation is altered, affecting both the initial septal and subsequent ventricular forces (**Figure 8-8**).

The impulse conducts via the intact right bundle branch depolarizing the right side of the interventricular septum and free wall of the right ventricle. The initial forces are directed right-to-left, anteriorly, and inferiorly (vector 1). This produces either an rS or QS complex in lead V1 and V2. The leftward depolarization of the septum precludes the "septal q wave" that might be normally seen in left-oriented leads, I and V6. Indeed if you see a q wave in these leads, LBBB cannot be present. Although the direction is altered, this initial depolarization conducts at normal speed via the specialized conduction system. The impulse now spreads slowly via myocyte-to-myocyte transmission to depolarize the remainder of the left septal mass and adjacent free wall of the left ventricle (vector 2). These forces are directed to the left, posteriorly, and inferiorly. Delayed activation of the lateral wall of the left ventricle occurs last with the depolarization wave directed toward the left, posteriorly and either superiorly or inferiorly (vector 3).

The slow, delayed activation of the left ventricle produces the characteristic wide slurred or notched R waves in leads I, aVL, and V5-V6 along with slurred S waves in V1-V2. You can visualize how this pattern looks in leftward-looking leads by again making a peace sign, but this time use your left hand and place your fingers a little closer together (**Figure 8-9**). The relative amplitudes of the R waves can vary, resembling the fingers of either your right or left hand.

In LBBB, secondary, discordant ST segment and T wave abnormalities are directed opposite to the terminal portion of the QRS complex. In leads I, aVL, and V5-V6, the ST segment is typically isoelectric or depressed and the T wave is inverted, opposite to the orientation of the terminal R wave. ST elevation is typically seen in leads with a negative deflection, namely V1-V3 (**Figure 8-10**).

Criteria for Complete Left Bundle Branch block

- QRS duration ≥0.12 seconds.
- Broad, notched, or slurred R waves (rR´, RR´) in leads I, aVL, and V5-V6.
- Absent Q waves in leads I, V5-V6 (may be present in lead aVL).
- Secondary ST segment and T wave abnormalities in the left precordial leads directed opposite to that of the dominant R wave (also leads I and aVL).
- Supporting criteria:
  - Prolonged R peak time (time to the intrinsicoid deflection) >0.06 seconds in leads V5-V6.
  - Broad S waves in leads V1-V2 with rS or QS pattern.

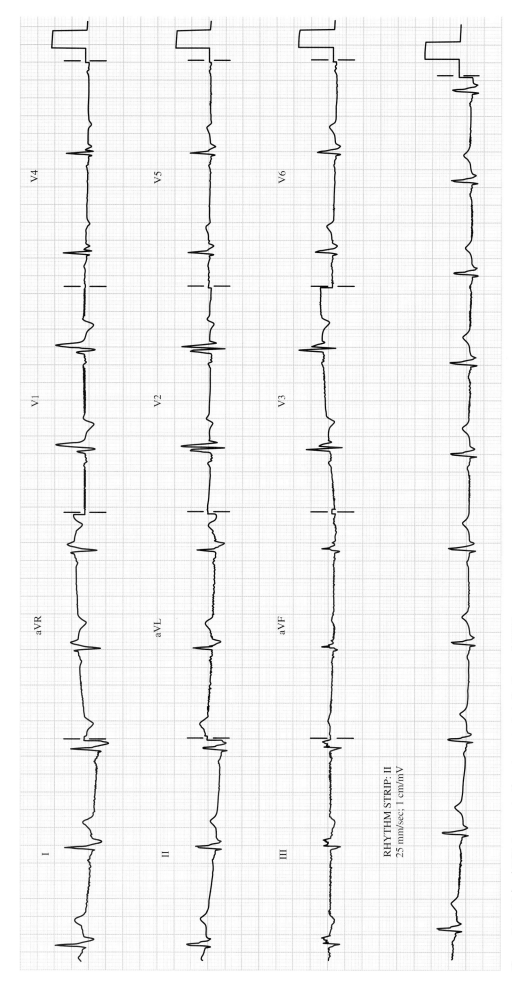

Figure 8-7. 12-lead ECG demonstrating characteristic findings of RBBB.

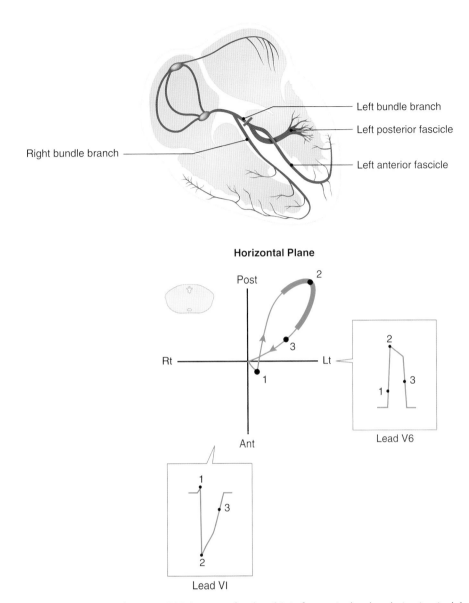

Figure 8-8. Typical horizontal plane vector loop or LBBB (see text for details). Left ventricular depolarization is delayed and slowed (wide portion of loop).

 CLINICAL TIP: LBBB usually has significant clinical implications. Most individuals with LBBB have left ventricular enlargement associated with either hypertensive or valvular heart disease. It is also frequently associated with coronary artery disease and congestive heart failure. The alteration of ventricular activation may cause loss of ventricular synchrony that worsens heart failure in patients with left ventricular dysfunction.

 CLINICAL TIP: In all cases of bundle branch block, take notice of T waves that are concordant in the direction of the terminal conduction delay (eg, an upright T wave in lead V1 with RBBB or an upright T wave in leads I, aVL, or V6 with LBBB). These may represent primary abnormalities of repolarization due to electrolyte abnormalities or myocardial ischemia.

Incomplete Right and Left Bundle Branch Block

Both RBBB and LBBB are characterized as incomplete if the QRS duration is between >0.10 and <0.12 seconds. Except for the shorter QRS duration, all of the findings described in the preceding discussion for complete bundle branch block are seen in their respective incomplete forms (**Figure 8-11**).

Nonspecific Intraventricular Conduction Delay

At times, the QRS is prolonged >0.10 seconds, but does not meet the criteria for either RBBB or LBBB (**Figure 8-12**). This may be present in patients with left ventricular enlargement, electrolyte abnormalities, and due to antiarrhythmic drug therapy. In these cases, it is appropriate to use the term *nonspecific intraventricular conduction delay*.

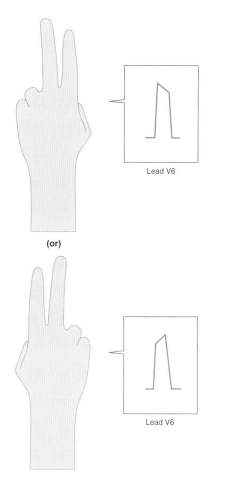

Figure 8-9. With LBBB, the QRS pattern resembles a "peace sign" in lead V6. Depending on the morphology, the complex may resemble the fingers of either the left or right hand.

▶ GENERAL CONCEPTS OF FASCICULAR BLOCKS (HEMIBLOCKS)

The simplified concept of the left bundle branch separates this structure into two major divisions, the left anterior fascicle and left posterior fascicle. The left anterior fascicle is oriented in an anterior and superior direction and the left posterior fascicle in a posterior and inferior direction. That's why I find it helpful to think of these two as the left anterior-*superior* fascicle and the left posterior-*inferior* fascicle. This makes it easier to understand the vector changes that result when conduction in each division is impaired. It's perfectly acceptable and customary to use the terms left anterior and left posterior fascicle, without my added hyphenation.

In both left anterior and posterior fascicular block, the initial depolarization of the ventricles is in the direction of the unblocked fascicle with the mid- and terminal-activation toward the blocked fascicle. This sequence produces a marked change of the QRS axis, which is the principle ECG effect of fascicular blocks. Left anterior fascicular block (LAFB) produces **left axis deviation** and left posterior fascicular block

(LPFB) causes **right axis deviation**. Unlike LBBB and RBBB, LAFB and LPFB do not appreciably prolong the QRS complex or cause ST segment and T wave findings. The reason is that the Purkinje fibers of the two fascicles intertwine, facilitating conduction from the unblocked to the blocked fascicle, which allows depolarization of the myocardium without appreciable delay.

Left Anterior Fascicular Block

In LAFB the primary abnormality is a delay in depolarization of the anterior and superior portions of the left ventricle (**Figure 8-13**). The loss of conduction in the left anterior fascicle removes the initial left, anterior, and superior forces. Conduction proceeds normally via the posterior fascicle with the initial forces directed inferiorly, posterior, and left-to-right. This usually preserves small Q waves in leads I and aVL, but now results in small R waves in the inferior leads, II, III, and aVF (vector 1). The forces then turn in a leftward and superior direction toward the blocked fascicle, producing a counterclockwise loop and left axis deviation (vector 2). In the frontal plane, the left axis deviation is characteristically more negative than −45 degrees. This produces prominent R waves in leads I and aVL and deep S waves in leads II, III, and aVF. As you can see from the pathway of the vector loop, the characteristic ECG findings of LAFB include an R wave voltage in lead aVL greater than lead I as well as an S wave voltage in lead III greater than lead II. The counterclockwise loop also indicates that the R wave in lead aVL should appear before an R wave in lead aVR (**Figure 8-14**). LAFB has little effect on the ECG in the precordial leads except that the loss of some anterior forces may lower the amplitude of the initial R waves in V1-V3, producing poor R wave progression.

 FOR HISTORY BUFFS: You will see some textbooks use left axis deviation of −30 degrees as a criterion for LAFB. However, the seminal textbook written on the subject by Mauricio Rosenbaum described LAFB with an axis leftward of −45 degrees. Indeed, left axis deviation is associated with, but is not synonymous with LAFB.

Criteria for Left Anterior Fascicular Block
- Left axis deviation between −45 and −90 degrees.
- QRS duration <0.12 seconds.
- A positive terminal deflection in aVL and aVR with the peak of the terminal R wave in aVR occurring later than in aVL (reflecting a counterclockwise vector loop).
- No other cause of left axis deviation (eg, left ventricular enlargement, inferior wall MI, congenital heart disease).
- Supporting criteria:
  - qR complex in leads I and aVL.
  - rS complex in leads II, III, aVF and an S wave in lead III, deeper than lead II.
  - Prolonged R peak time (time to the intrinsicoid deflection) ≥0.045 seconds in lead aVL.

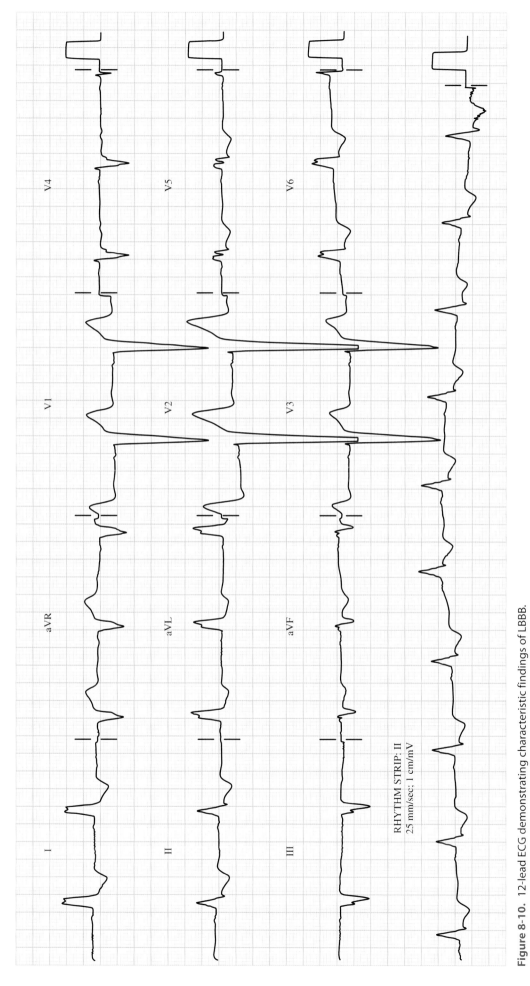

Figure 8-10. 12-lead ECG demonstrating characteristic findings of LBBB.

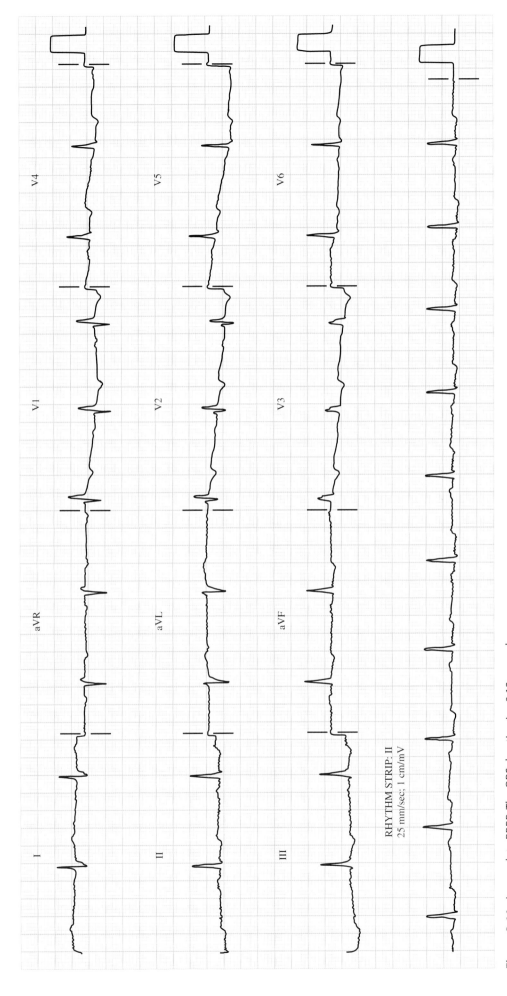

RHYTHM STRIP: II
25 mm/sec; 1 cm/mV

Figure 8-11. Incomplete RBBB. The QRS duration is <0.12 seconds.

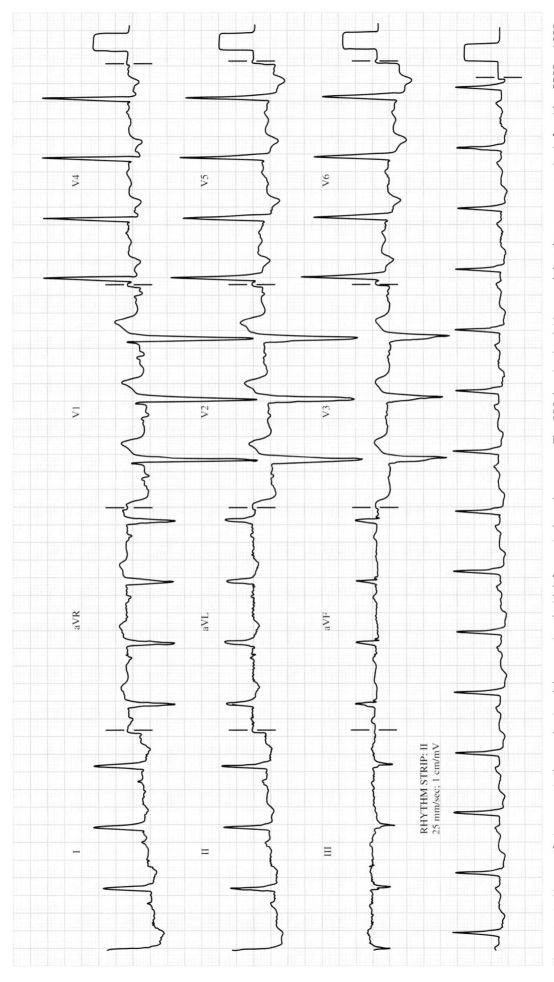

Figure 8-12. Nonspecific intraventricular conduction delay associated with left ventricular enlargement. The QRS duration is >0.10 seconds but does not meet criteria for either RBBB or LBBB.

I aVR V1 V4

II aVL V2 V5

III aVF V3 V6

RHYTHM STRIP: II
25 mm/sec; 1 cm/mV

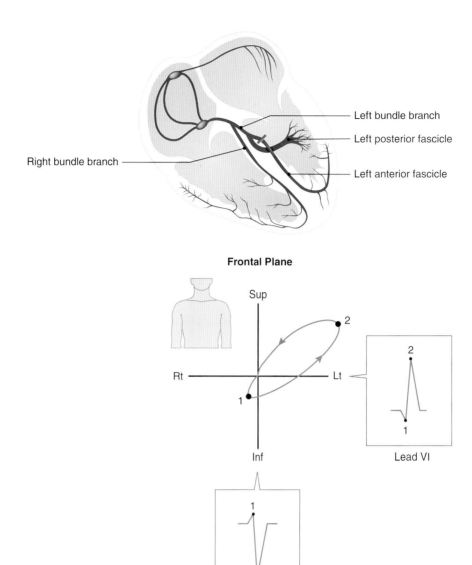

Figure 8-13. Typical frontal plane vector loop of LAFB. Initial forces are directed to the right and inferiorly. The loop then turns counterclockwise with left axis deviation.

 CLINICAL TIP: LAFB is the most common conduction abnormality, which may be seen either in the presence or absence of clinical cardiac disease. The left anterior fascicle is a long, thin structure located subendocardially in the left ventricular outflow tract and supplied by the left anterior descending coronary artery. Accordingly, clinical conditions that increase interventricular pressure as well as coronary artery disease can damage this structure, resulting in LAFB.

Left Posterior Fascicular Block

In left posterior fascicular block (LPFB) the primary abnormality is a delay in depolarization of the inferior and posterior portions of the left ventricle (**Figure 8-15**). Here the loss of conduction removes the initial inferior, posterior, and rightward forces. Conduction proceeds normally via the intact left anterior fascicle. The leftward direction of the activation wave gives rise to the initial R wave in leads I and aVL, whereas the superior forces produce initial q waves in leads II, III, and aVF (vector 1). The forces then turn inferiorly and rightward toward the blocked fascicle in a clockwise loop (vector 2). This gives rise to deep S waves in leads I and aVL and produces a qR pattern in leads II, III, and aVF. In the frontal plane, right axis deviation is present beyond +90 degrees (see Figure 8-15).

Criteria for Left Posterior Fascicular Block
- Right axis deviation between +90 and +180 degrees in adults
- QRS duration <0.12 seconds.
- rS pattern in leads I and aVL.
- qR pattern in leads II, III, and aVF (Q wave width <0.04 seconds).
- No other cause of right axis deviation (eg, extensive lateral wall MI, right ventricular enlargement, pulmonary disease).

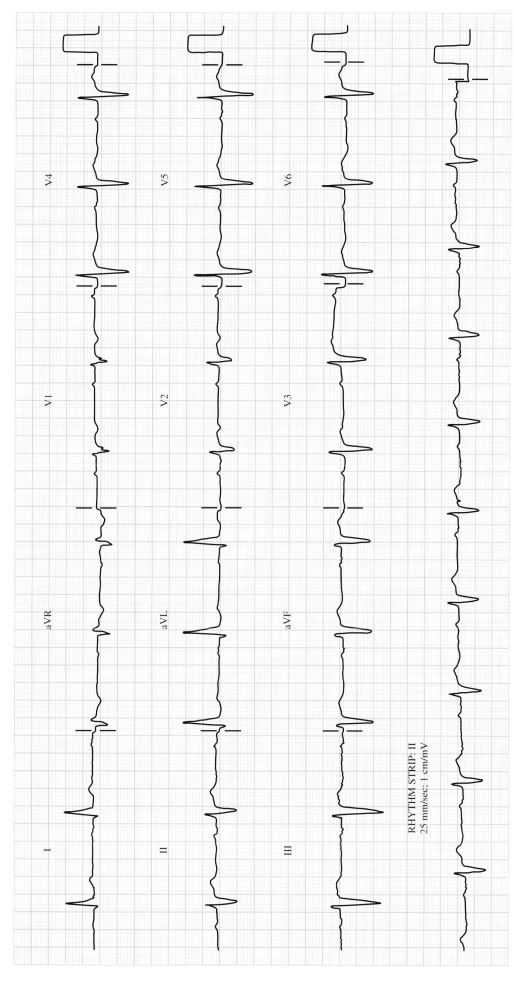

Figure 8-14. 12-lead ECG demonstrating characteristic findings of LAFB. There is left axis deviation of −45 degrees. The inferior leads show rS complexes. Also note that the R wave in aVL occurs prior to that in aVR, confirming a counterclockwise vector loop.

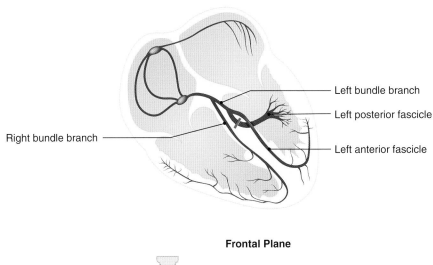

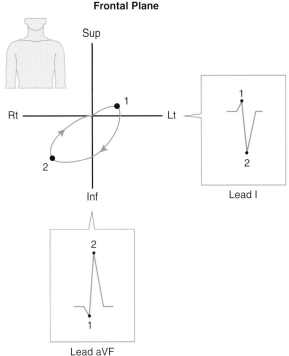

Figure 8-15. Typical frontal plane vector loop of LPFB. Initial forces are directed to the left and superiorly. The loop then turns clockwise with right axis deviation.

 CLINICAL TIP: Isolated LPFB is the least common intraventricular conduction disturbance. Unlike the left anterior fascicle, the left posterior fascicle has a dual coronary blood supply from both the left anterior descending and left posterior descending arteries. It is anatomically associated with the less turbulent left ventricular inflow tract and is thereby more protected than its anterior counterpart. LPFB is most often seen in conjunction with RBBB and reflects significant myocardial disease with associated impairment of intraventricular conduction (**Figure 8-16**).

▶ CONDUCTION CONUNDRUMS

You may encounter a number of additional terms related to intraventricular conduction disturbances on your electrocardiographic travels. I'm going to mention them for completeness, but my best advice is for you to concentrate on the basics reviewed in the preceding discussion, leaving it to us "old-timers" to debate their merit.

Bifascicular block refers to a conduction abnormality involving any two of the three fascicles. Examples include RBBB with LAFB or RBBB with LPFB.

Trifascicular block properly refers to disease in all of the fascicles below the bundle of His, namely, the right bundle branch, and both divisions of the left bundle branch. Note that such a total failure of conduction in all three fascicles would result in complete heart block as the supraventricular impulse has no pathway to the ventricles. Trifascicular block has been used *incorrectly* to describe the presence of first-degree AV block combined with any bifascicular block. The first-degree AV block most commonly reflects a conduction delay in the AV node and not a disorder of any third fascicle.

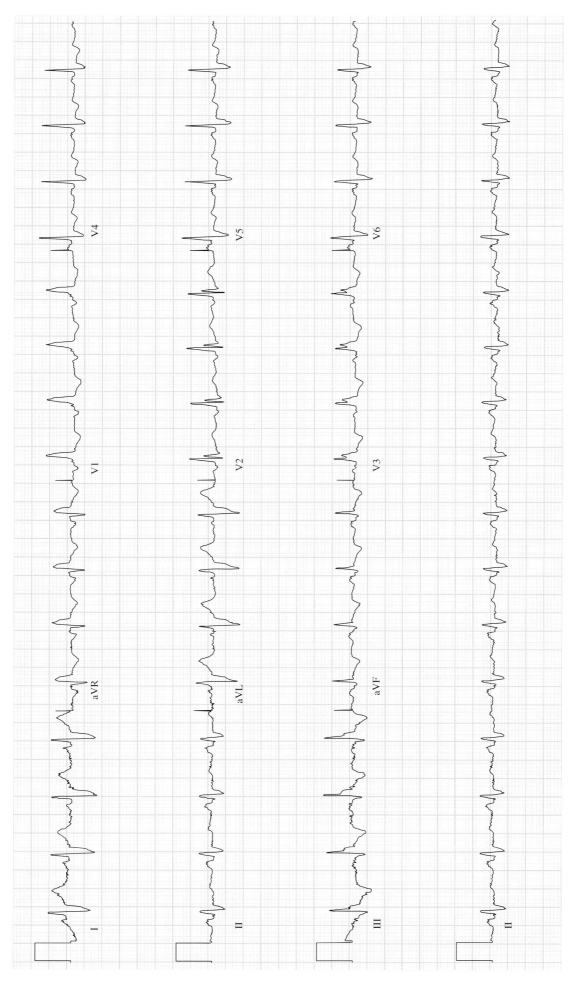

Figure 8-16. 12-lead ECG demonstrating characteristic findings of LPFB, here shown accompanying RBBB. There is right axis deviation of +120 degrees. Note the rS pattern in leads I and aVL and a qR pattern in the inferior leads. A RBBB pattern is evident in the precordial leads.

Septal fascicular block is an unlikely isolated finding. This controversial diagnosis may be considered when the ECG demonstrates isolated loss of Q waves in leftward-oriented leads, which would be expected to represent the normal left-to-right depolarization of the septum. The additional loss of the normal anterior septal vector may result in a QS pattern in leads V1-V2, which simulates anteroseptal myocardial infarction.

Chapter 8 • SELF-TEST

1. List the components of the specialized conduction system.
2. What ECG finding represents transmission of the electrical impulse through the atria and the remainder of the specialized conduction system?
3. What are the two major divisions of the left bundle branch?
4. Describe the three primary vectors of ventricular depolarization.
5. List the two key ECG features found in all complete bundle branch blocks.
6. What is the difference between complete and incomplete bundle branch block?
7. List the criteria for RBBB.
8. List the criteria for LBBB.
9. The hallmark of LAFB is what change in the QRS axis?
10. The hallmark of LPFB is what change in the QRS axis?

Chapter 8 • SELF-TEST

ANSWERS

1. SA node, interatrial and internodal bundles, AV node, bundle of His, left and right bundle branches, Purkinje fibers.

2. The PR interval.

3. Left anterior-superior fascicle and left posterior-inferior fascicle.

4. • Left side of the interventricular septum.
   • Right and left ventricular free walls.
   • Posterobasal portions of the left ventricle and interventricular septum.

5. Prolonged QRS duration ≥0.12 seconds and a terminal conduction delay.

6. The QRS duration for complete bundle branch is ≥0.12 seconds. Incomplete bundle branch block has a QRS duration of >0.10 and <0.12 seconds.

7. • QRS duration ≥0.12 sec.
   • rsr′, rsR′, rSR′, or M-shaped pattern in leads V1 or V2.
   • The secondary R′ wave is usually wider and of greater amplitude than the initial r wave.
   • Secondary ST segment and T wave abnormalities in the right precordial leads directed opposite to that of the dominant R wave.
   • Supporting criteria:
     ▪ Prolonged R peak time (time to the intrinsicoid deflection) >0.05 seconds in lead V1.
     ▪ Broad S waves in leads I, aVL, and V5-V6.

8. • QRS duration ≥0.12 seconds.
   • Broad, notched, or slurred R waves (rR′, RR′) in leads I, aVL, and V5-V6.
   • Absent Q waves in leads I, V5-V6 (may be present in lead aVL).
   • Secondary ST segment and T wave abnormalities in the left precordial leads directed opposite to that of the dominant R wave (also leads I and aVL).
   • Supporting criteria:
     ▪ Prolonged R peak time (time to the intrinsicoid deflection) >0.06 seconds in leads V5-V6.
     ▪ Broad S waves in leads V1-V2 with rS or QS pattern.

9. Left axis deviation between −45 and −90 degrees.

10. Right axis deviation between +90 and +180 degrees.

Further Reading

Baranchuk A, Enriquez A, Garcia-Neibla J, Bayes-Genis A, Villuendas R, Bayes de Luna A. Differential diagnosis of rSr′ pattern in leads V1-V2. Comprehensive review and proposed algorithm. *Ann Noninvasive Electrocardiol.* 2015;20:7-17.

Elizari MV, Acunzo RS, Ferreiro M. Hemiblocks revisited. *Circulation.* 2007;115:1154-1163.

Flowers NC. Left bundle branch block: a continuously evolving concept. *J Am Coll Cardiol.* 1987;9:684-697.

Francia P, Ball C, Paneni F, Volpe M. Left bundle branch block – pathophysiology, prognosis and clinical management. *Clin Cardiol.* 2007;30:110-115.

Leonelli FM, Bagliani G, DePonti R, Padeletti L. Intraventricular delay and blocks. *Card Electrophysiol Clin.* 2018;10:211-231.

MacAlpin RN. In search of left septal fascicular block. *Am Heart J.* 2002;144:948-956.

Milliken JA. Isolated and complicated left anterior fascicular block: a review of suggested electrocardiographic criteria. *J Electrocardiol.* 1983;16:199-212.

Perez-Riera AR, Barbosa-Barros R, Daminello-Raimundo R, de Abreu LC, Mendes JET, Nikus K. Left posterior fascicular block, state of the art review: a 2018 update. *Indian Pacing and Electrophysiol J.* 2018;28:217-230.

Perez-Riera AR, Barbosa-Barros R, de Rezende Barbosa MPC, Daminello-Raimundo R, de Abreu LC, Nikus K. Left bundle branch block: epidemiology, etiology, anatomic features, electrovectorcardiography, and classification proposal. *Ann Noninvasive Electrocardiol.* 2019;24:e112572.

Rosenbaum MB, Elizari MV, Lazzari JO. *The Hemiblocks.* Oldsmar, Florida: Tampa Tracings; 1970.

Schneider JF, Thomas HE, Kreger BE, McNamara PM, Kannel WB. Newly acquired left bundle branch block: the Framingham study. *Ann Intern Med.* 1979;90:303-310.

Schneider JF, Thomas HE, Kreger BE, McNamara PM, Sorlie P, Kannel WB. Newly acquired right bundle branch block: the Framingham study. *Ann Intern Med.* 1980;92:37-44.

Strauss DG, Selvester RH, Wagner GS. Defining left bundle branch block in the era of cardiac resynchronization therapy. *Am J Cardiol.* 2011;1087:927-934.

Surawicz B, Childers R, Dear BJ, Gettes LS. AHA/ACCF/ARS recommendations for the standardization and interpretation of the electrocardiogram. Part III. Intraventricular conduction disturbances. *J Am Coll Cardiol.* 2009;53:976-981.

Warner RA, Hill NE, Mookherjee S, Smulyan H. Improved electrocardiographic criteria for the diagnosis of left anterior hemiblock. *Am J Cardiol.* 1983;51:723-726.

Willems JL, Robles EO, Bernard R, et al. Criteria for intraventricular conduction disturbances and pre-excitation. *J Am Coll Cardiol.* 1985;5:1261-1275.

Accessory Pathways and Preexcitation

▶ BACKGROUND

In the normal heart a dense band of fibrous tissue forms early in embryogenesis to anatomically and electrically insulate the atria from the ventricles. The only natural electrical link between the atria and the ventricles is via the AV node and His-Purkinje system. Ventricular **preexcitation** is said to occur when all or part of the ventricular myocardium is activated by the atrial impulse *earlier* than would be expected if the stimulus were to reach the ventricles by way of the normal AV conduction system. This premature activation can occur only if there is an alternate route that allows the electrical stimulus to bypass the normal physiologic delay of the AV node. Atrioventricular bypass pathways are embryologic remnants of muscle bundles that bridge the heart's fibrous skeleton, providing the means for abnormal electrical conduction between the atrium and ventricle (**Figure 9-1**). Transmission of the electrical impulse over such an accessory pathway produces characteristic findings on the ECG and may provide a substrate for cardiac arrhythmias.

▶ PATHWAYS, CONNECTIONS, AND TRACTS, OH MY!

Accessory pathways are anomalous electrical conduits that are not part of the normal specialized conduction system. Although often used interchangeably, the terms *pathway*, *connection*, and *tract* should be used more precisely. In my experience, this ambiguity is a source of confusion for those trying to understand the anatomy and physiology behind preexcitation. We'll use "pathway" to describe *any* anomalous electrical route. A "connection" will describe an accessory conduction pathway that inserts into the working myocardium, regardless of its origin. A "tract" will define an atypical pathway of any origin that inserts into specialized conduction tissue. As we will see shortly, using these terms properly will help you understand how electrical transmission over these pathways affects their ECG appearance.

Types of Bypass Pathways

Accessory pathways between the atria and ventricles may take a number of anatomical forms. The most common and clinically

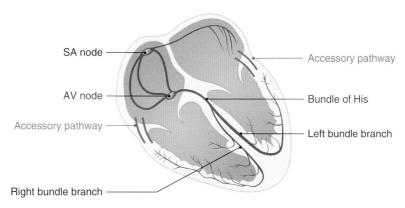

Figure 9-1. Conduction system of the heart showing accessory AV pathways in blue.

important of these are atrioventricular bypass connections, responsible for the classic Wolff-Parkinson-White pattern and syndrome (see following discussion). Rarely, preexcitation is due to accessory pathways that link the atria, AV node, bundle branches (fascicles), and the ventricles.

 FOR HISTORY BUFFS: You will encounter various eponyms to describe accessory pathways. Atrioventricular bypass connections are also called *bundles of Kent*. The unusual atriofascicular, nodofascicular, nodoventricular, and fasciculoventricular pathways are collectively known as *Mahaim fibers*. *James fibers* have been used to describe perinodal (also called atrionodal or intranodal) bypass tracts, but these pathways are disputed and of uncertain clinical significance. I discourage the use of these eponyms in favor of the more precise anatomical description.

▶ THE WPW PATTERN

Transmission of the normal sinus impulse over an atrioventricular type of accessory bypass connection produces distinctive findings on the ECG (**Figure 9-2**). These include (1) a **short PR interval**, typically <0.12 seconds, (2) slurring of the initial portion of the QRS called a **delta wave**, and (3) a **widened QRS** usually >0.12 seconds with **secondary ST segment and T wave changes**. In 1930, Louis Wolff, John Parkinson, and Paul Dudley White published their findings of 11 patients with paroxysmal tachycardia associated with this unique ECG pattern. Accordingly, this ECG morphology is termed the *Wolff-Parkinson-White* (WPW) pattern.

Genesis of the WPW Pattern (Atrioventricular Connection)

We can understand the unique appearance of the WPW pattern by examining the fate of the sinus impulse as it travels from the atria to the ventricles (**Figure 9-3**).

During sinus rhythm, the SA node depolarizes the atria in the usual fashion. The P wave, therefore, is normal.

The impulse splits into two simultaneous wavefronts, one conducting through the AV node, the other over the accessory bypass connection. The normally transmitted portion of the impulse encounters the physiologic delay of the AV node. The accessory pathway lacks this delay allowing the impulse to reach the ventricles early, producing a short PR interval. The *less delayed* transmission over the accessory pathway results in *early* activation of the ventricles, hence the terms, **accelerated conduction** or **preexcitation**. This is a bit of a misnomer because the shortened PR interval is not because of more rapid conduction over the accessory pathway, but results from the *absence* of the normal delay at the AV node. Let's use our automobile analogy to explain this further. Consider the AV node as a tollbooth, requiring the sinus impulse to delay and pay the toll before continuing down the His-Purkinje highway. The accessory pathway is like an old country road that bypasses the delay at the tollbooth. Your relatively greater speed through the alternate route is not because you accelerated, but because you avoided slowing down to pay the toll.

The split impulse proceeds to depolarize the ventricles via both the normal His-Purkinje system and the accessory bypass connection. The resulting QRS complex therefore represents the **fusion** of two portions of ventricular activation, one early and preexcited and the other with normal timing.

Although the impulse arrives early through the accessory connection, it depolarizes the ventricles utilizing less efficient, myocyte-to-myocyte transmission. As we learned with bundle branch blocks, this form of slow "off-road" conduction is recorded on the ECG as a wide QRS. But unlike bundle branch blocks where the ECG records a *terminal* conduction delay (r′or R′), preexcitation alters the *early* portion of the QRS (delta wave) (**Figure 9-4**).

The normally transmitted impulse delayed at the AV node follows after the preexcited portion, so the terminal portion

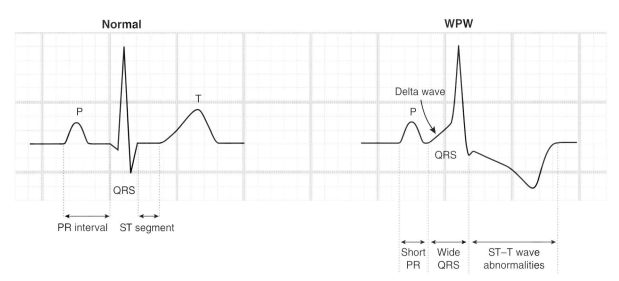

Figure 9-2. ECG demonstrating characteristic findings of the WPW pattern of preexcitation (right) compared with normal (left). Note the short PR interval, delta wave, wide QRS complex, and secondary ST segment and T wave abnormalities.

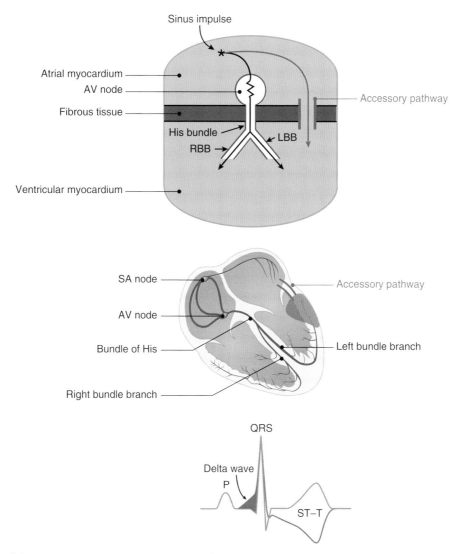

Figure 9-3. Genesis of the WPW pattern. (Top) Transmission of the electrical impulse to the ventricles occurs via both the normal His-Purkinje system and the accessory pathway (AP) shown in blue. (Middle) Ventricular muscle is depolarized by both the normal route and the AP. (Bottom) The ECG represents the fusion of both routes of transmission with the delta wave representing the preexcited portion of ventricular depolarization.

of the QRS complex is normal. Similar to bundle branch blocks, the abnormal depolarization of the preexcited ventricles also alters repolarization, producing ST segment and T wave findings typically opposite in direction to the QRS complex.

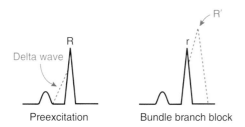

Figure 9-4. Preexcitation (WPW) affects the early portion of the QRS complex whereas bundle branch blocks produce a terminal conduction delay.

FOR BOOKWORMS: The size of the delta wave, the degree of PR interval shortening, and the amount of QRS complex prolongation, all depend on the relative amount of myocardium activated by the accessory pathway versus normal conduction. A larger delta wave is present if the normal sinus impulse encounters greater delay at the AV node as relatively more ventricular muscle is activated via the anomalous pathway. Conversely, more efficient AV conduction, such as might occur with enhanced sympathetic tone, results in a smaller delta wave as more ventricular tissue is activated by the normal His-Purkinje system. The location of the accessory pathway also affects the size of the delta wave. The SA node is located in the high right atrium; therefore it takes longer for the sinus impulse to reach a left-sided connection, versus one located nearby on the right. A right-sided pathway activates the ventricles comparatively earlier, so you would expect to see a more prominent delta wave than a left-sided location.

Localizing Atrioventricular Bypass Connections

Accessory atrioventricular bypass connections may occur anywhere around the AV ring, but may be broadly classified into left-sided and right-sided pathways (**Figure 9-5**). Left-sided connections provide a conduit within the mitral ring between the left atrium and the left ventricle. Right-sided connections traverse the tricuspid ring between the right atrium and the right ventricle. Detailed algorithms have been developed based on the 12-lead ECG that use the polarity of the QRS complex and delta wave to predict the location of the bypass connection. While generally useful, all have limitations and I prefer to leave it to our electrophysiology colleagues to debate their relative merits.

 FOR BOOKWORMS: The anatomical location of the accessory pathway can be described in greater detail, something important for electrophysiologists performing catheter ablation (**Figure 9-6**). For our purposes, it is reasonable to divide the AV ring into four regions with the distribution of AV bypass connections as follows: left ventricular free wall (46-60%), right ventricular free wall (13-21%), inferior paraseptal (left and right, 25%), and superior paraseptal (left and right, 2%). Even more precise localization is possible and you may encounter references that use different terminology to describe the regions of the AV ring. This reflects a change from an older nomenclature to the more anatomically correct terminology used earlier. Unfortunately old habits die hard, and you will likely encounter continuing descriptions of AV bypass tracts that are inconsistent. You can read more about this topic in the references provided at the end of this chapter.

 FOR HISTORY BUFFS: An older classification of WPW patterns described by Francis Rosenbaum and colleagues in 1945 separated bypass pathways into type A and type B according to the dominant QRS polarity in the right precordial leads. In the Rosenbaum classification, the type A pattern with positive QRS polarity in leads V1-V2 reflected a left-sided pathway. Type B with negative polarity in lead V1 (+/− lead V2) suggested a right-sided pathway. The modern recognition of the multitude and complexity of accessory pathways renders this classification obsolete.

Terminology Old and New

You will encounter a number of terms related to preexcitation. Some like the Kent, Mahaim, and James eponyms noted earlier are best considered of historical interest. Others are more clinically useful.

The **WPW pattern** refers to the classic ECG findings reviewed earlier. The **WPW syndrome** applies to the clinical diagnosis of patients with paroxysmal tachyarrhythmias associated with an atrioventricular bypass connection.

Conduction of the electrical impulse over any accessory pathway may be either **anterograde** (conducting from atria to ventricles), or **retrograde** (conducting from ventricles to atria). The pathway may have the ability to conduct in only anterograde, only retrograde, or in both directions. Most AV connections exhibit rapid and **nondecremental** conduction. This means that transmission of the impulses does not slow with a rise in heart rate. Contrast this with the **decremental** conduction exhibited by the AV node where conduction will slow as the heart rate increases.

The bypass pathway may be considered **manifest** or **overt**, meaning it transmits the normal sinus impulse anterograde from atrium to ventricle and demonstrates the classic WPW pattern on the ECG. A **concealed** pathway is one that is only capable of conducting retrograde from ventricle to atrium and is not apparent on the ECG during normal sinus rhythm. The presence of a concealed pathway becomes evident only when

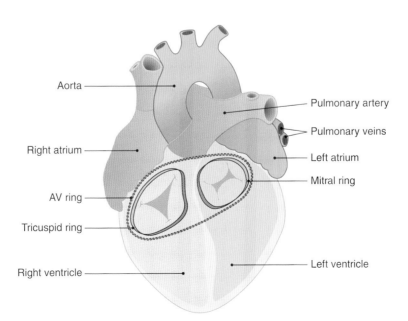

Figure 9-5. Left anterior oblique (LAO) view of the heart viewed from the apex showing internal and external cardiac structures. Accessory pathways can occur in multiple locations around the tricuspid and mitral rings.

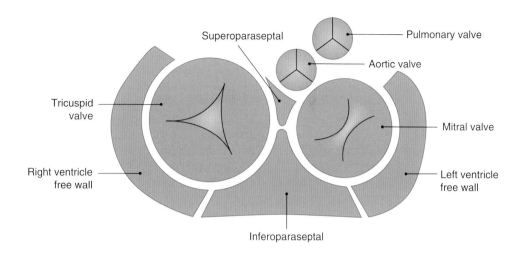

Traditional and Anatomically Correct AV Ring Nomenclature

REGION	TRADITIONAL	ANATOMICALLY CORRECT
Right Ventricular Free Wall	Anterior Anterolateral Posterior	Superior Superolateral Inferior
Left Ventricular Free Wall	Anterior Anterolateral Lateral Posterolateral Posterior	Superior Superoposterior Posterior Inferoposterior Inferior
Septal-Paraseptal	Anteroseptal Posteroseptal Midseptal	Superoparaseptal Inferoparaseptal Septal

Figure 9-6. Schematic LAO view of the heart as viewed from the apex. Accessory pathways are broadly classified into four regions surrounding the AV rings: left ventricular free wall, right ventricular free wall, inferoparaseptal, and superoparaseptal. The table below describes the differences between the traditional and anatomically correct nomenclature of these regions.

it participates in the genesis of a tachyarrhythmia or when revealed during electrophysiologic testing.

The degree of preexcitation, reflected in the prominence of the delta wave, may fluctuate from beat to beat in a cyclical pattern, a phenomenon known as the *concertina effect*. This is due to variable AV node conduction associated with respiratory alteration in vagal tone.

Preexcitation may be *intermittent*, defined as the variable presence and absence of preexcitation on the same tracing. This might result from transient alteration in the refractory period of the accessory pathway that affects antegrade conduction. *Inapparent or latent preexcitation* is defined as preexcitation that is absent during sinus rhythm but evident during atrial arrhythmias or with atrial stimulation. Inapparent preexcitation is a result of the sinus depolarization reaching the ventricles via the AV node and His-Purkinje system faster than the accelerated conduction over the accessory pathway. This may be due to a combination of factors, including sympathetic enhanced AV nodal conduction, delayed conduction via the bypass connection, and a longer distance of the accessory pathway relative to the depolarizing stimulus.

Clinical Significance

The WPW pattern is estimated to be present in 0.15 to 0.25% of the population and is typically discovered on a routine ECG. The clinical importance of the WPW pattern is primarily related to its association with cardiac arrhythmias (WPW syndrome). Note that the exact percentage of the population with an accessory bypass pathway is unknown because the pathway may be concealed or is not evident on the surface ECG due to its location or conduction characteristics.

Depending on the population studied, only 1 to 2% of individuals with the WPW pattern have clinical arrhythmias. Of those patients with arrhythmias, approximately 80% have supraventricular tachycardia, with the remainder atrial fibrillation and atrial flutter. The two distinct conduction pathways provide the substrate for a specific type of supraventricular arrhythmia called **atrioventricular reentrant tachycardia** (AVRT), where the accessory pathway and the normal His-Purkinje system each provide one limb of an electrical circuit. Typically, a premature impulse travels down one limb of the circuit and proceeds retrograde through the other, returning to rapidly stimulate the original chamber again and repeat the process. This is an example of **reentry**, a process we will review in greater detail in later chapters.

Atrial fibrillation is found in 10 to 20% of individuals with the WPW syndrome. This may be life-threatening because transmission over the accessory bypass connection avoids the "blocking" function of the AV node, which may result in extremely rapid conduction to the ventricles that degenerates into ventricular fibrillation.

The Great Imitator

It is important for you to recognize the WPW pattern because it may be easily mistaken for a variety of other ECG diagnoses (**Figures 9-7** and **9-8**). Examples include:

- The wide QRS may be mistaken for a bundle branch block.
- The anomalous conduction may increase QRS voltage leading to an erroneous diagnosis of left ventricular enlargement.
- A negative delta wave and change in QRS polarity may simulate Q or QS waves leading to an incorrect diagnosis of myocardial infarction.
- The positive delta wave and tall R waves in the right precordial leads may wrongly suggest either right ventricular enlargement or posterior wall myocardial infarction.

▶ ATYPICAL PREEXCITATION PATHWAYS

Atypical accessory pathways are a rare group of tracts and connections that bypass all or part of the normal conduction system. It is unlikely that you will encounter many patients with atypical accessory pathways and I recommend you concentrate on learning about the classic WPW pattern and related arrhythmias. But this can be a confusing and difficult topic and I felt compelled to spend some time here to clarify the subject. **Table 9-1** should serve as a valuable resource should the need arise.

The various atypical accessory pathways include atriofascicular and nodofascicular tracts, as well as nodoventricular and fasciculoventricular connections. Perinodal bypass tracts are of uncertain clinical significance. Atrio-Hisian bypass tracts are rare. Unlike the muscular AV connections of WPW, these pathways may form fibers containing cells with properties resembling those of the normal AV node or specialized conduction system. This is an important consideration because the degree of preexcitation on the resting ECG depends on the relative rate of transmission through both the AV node and the accessory pathway. This relationship also impacts whether a delta wave is evident for those pathways that insert directly into ventricular myocardium. Atypical tracts and connections comprise only 3 to 5% of all accessory pathways and not all are associated with cardiac arrhythmias.

The most common of the atypical accessory pathways are atriofascicular tracts. These tracts originate in the right atrial free wall and terminate in a distal fascicle of the right bundle branch. Recall that the term "tract" is used because the fiber inserts into the specialized conduction system. Although the AV node is bypassed, atriofascicular tracts exhibit properties similar to the AV node; hence the PR interval will be nearly normal. The tract inserts into specialized conduction tissue, therefore a delta wave is absent. The QRS complex at rest is usually normal. During an arrhythmia with maximal preexcitation, the QRS exhibits a left bundle branch pattern with left axis deviation.

Atypical pathways may rarely arise from the AV node and exhibit similar conduction properties. A nodoventricular connection originates in the AV node, bypassing some of that structure to insert directly into the right ventricular myocardium in the region of the AV junction. Depending on the site of exit, the PR interval will be either normal or slightly short. The QRS complex may either be normal or relatively prolonged with a small delta wave. Maximal preexcitation over this pathway exhibits a left bundle branch block configuration. A nodofascicular tract has similar properties to a nodoventricular connection but inserts into the right bundle branch instead of ventricular myocardium. Accordingly, the resting ECG does not exhibit a delta wave.

Fasciculoventricular connections are the most rare form of preexcitation. They link the His bundle or bundle branches with the ventricular myocardium. Normal conduction occurs through the AV node followed by slow myocardial transmission. The result is a normal PR interval and a small delta wave with either a normal or slightly prolonged QRS complex. This form of preexcitation is not associated with cardiac arrhythmias.

The Short PR Pattern

Some patients with an otherwise normal QRS complex have a short PR interval of <0.12 seconds (**Figure 9-9**). This may result from a variety of causes including enhanced AV nodal conduction, increased sympathetic tone, an anatomically small AV node, or a variant of normal. Rarely, a short PR interval is due to preexcitation from an atrio-Hisian tract that links the atrium with the His bundle, bypassing the normal physiologic delay at the AV node.

 FOR HISTORY BUFFS: In 1952, Bernard Lown, William F. Ganong Jr., and Samuel Levine described a series of patients with a short PR interval, narrow complex QRS, and recurrent supraventricular tachycardia; hence the term, Lown-Ganong-Levine (LGL) syndrome. The perinodal (atrionodal or intranodal) fibers described by James were hypothesized as the anatomical substrate to explain the short PR interval. They arise from internodal pathways that normally connect the SA and AV nodes. These fibers insert into the lower AV node or bundle of His, thereby circumventing the main body of the AV node. Conduction via this pathway would theoretically explain the short PR interval. The concept was called into question with the recognition that atrial tracts that skirt the AV node are present in all normal hearts. Electrophysiologists currently doubt the physiologic significance of these perinodal fibers and no longer recognize the LGL syndrome as a single clinical entity.

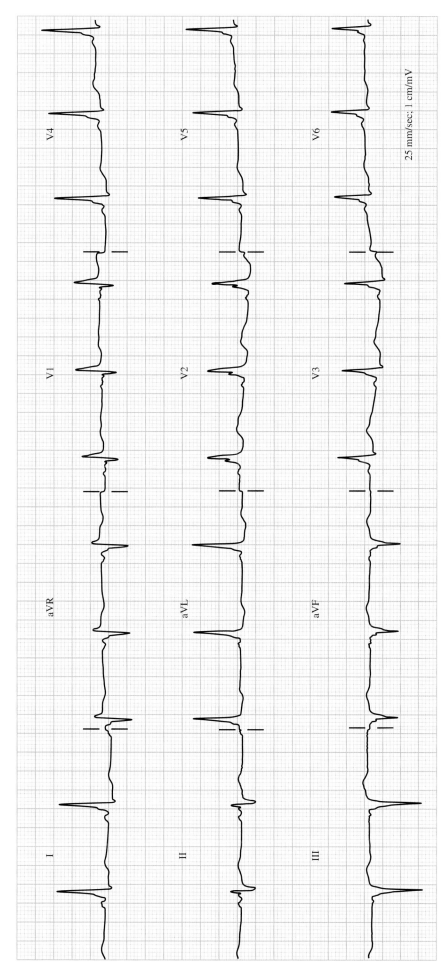

25 mm/sec; 1 cm/mV

Figure 9-7. WPW pattern. A short PR interval, delta waves, and ST segment and T wave abnormalities are evident throughout the tracing. Also note the negative delta waves in leads III and aVF with deep S waves that might be mistaken for inferior wall MI. The QRS configuration in leads V1 and V2 might also be confused with RBBB.

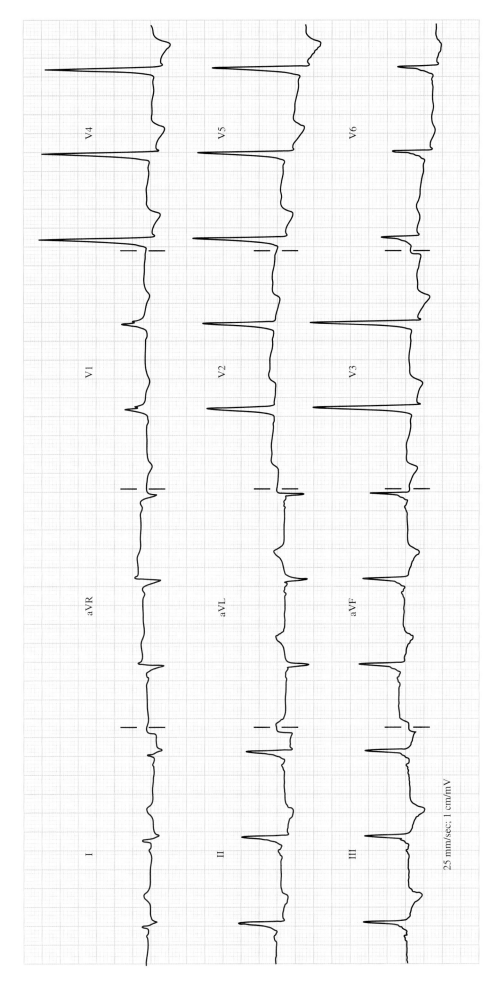

Figure 9-8. WPW pattern. Abnormal R wave voltage with ST segment and T wave abnormalities characteristic of preexcitation might be mistaken for ventricular enlargement.

25 mm/sec; 1 cm/mV

TABLE 9-1 Characteristics of Typical and Atypical Accessory Bypass Pathways

Name	Anatomical Link	Diagram	PR	Delta	QRS	Eponym	Comment
Atrioventricular connection	Atrium to ventricle		Short	Yes	Wide	Bundle of Kent	Responsible for typical WPW pattern and syndrome
Atriofascicular tract	Atrium to right bundle branch		Normal or slightly short	No	Normal	Mahaim fiber	Most common atypical pathway. LBBB pattern during maximal preexcitation
Atrio-Hisian tract	Atrium to His bundle		Short	No	Normal	None	Very rare
Nodoventricular connection	AV node to right ventricle		Normal or slightly short	No or minimal	Normal or mildly wide	Mahaim fiber	LBBB pattern during maximal preexcitation
Nodofascicular tract	AV node to right bundle branch		Normal or slightly short	No	Normal	Mahaim fiber	LBBB pattern during maximal preexcitation
Fasciculoventricular connection	His bundle or bundle branch to ventricle		Normal	Minimal	Normal or mildly wide	Mahaim fiber	Rarest form of preexcitation. May resemble WPW pattern, but not associated with arrhythmias
Perinodal tract	Perinodal pathways (SA-AV node) to the lower AV node or His bundle		Short	No	Normal	James fiber	Once suggested to explain "LGL syndrome," but now considered normal variant and not clinically significant

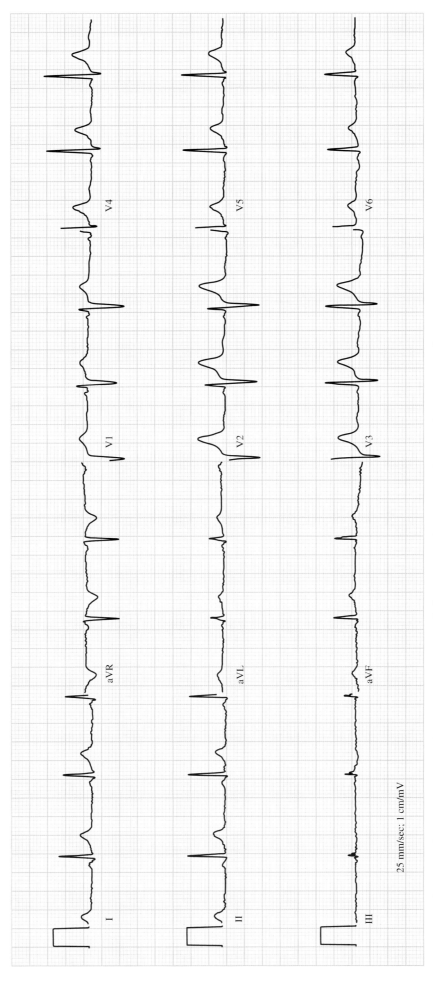

Figure 9-9. Short PR without preexcitation. There is a short PR interval of approximately 0.10 seconds in an otherwise normal ECG.

Chapter 9 • SELF-TEST

QUESTIONS

1. What is the only natural electrical link between the atria and the ventricles?
2. Define preexcitation.
3. Identify the characteristic ECG findings of preexcitation from an atrioventricular bypass connection (WPW pattern).
4. How does AV node conduction affect preexcitation?
5. What is the difference between "WPW pattern" and WPW syndrome?
6. What is the difference between anterograde and retrograde conduction?
7. What is a "concealed" bypass pathway?
8. The WPW pattern can be mistaken for what other ECG diagnoses (name at least three)?
9. What is the most common arrhythmia associated with WPW?
10. What is the danger of atrial fibrillation associated with preexcitation?

Chapter 9 • SELF-TEST

ANSWERS

1. The AV node and His-Purkinje system.
2. Preexcitation is said to occur if all or part of the ventricular myocardium is activated by the normal atrial impulse earlier than would be expected by way of the normal His-Purkinje system.
3. • Short PR interval of <0.12 seconds.
   • Slurring of the upstroke of the initial portion of the QRS (delta wave).
   • Widened QRS of >0.12 seconds.
   • Secondary ST segment and T wave changes.
4. The greater the AV delay, the more opportunity for preexcitation via the accessory bypass pathway.
5. The "WPW pattern" represents the visible ECG findings associated with an overt atrioventricular bypass pathway. The "WPW syndrome" refers to patients with arrhythmias associated with this pathway.
6. Anterograde conduction indicates the pathway conducts the impulse from atrium to ventricle. Retrograde conduction reflects conduction from ventricle to atrium.
7. A concealed pathway is one capable only of retrograde conduction and is not evident on the surface ECG.
8. The WPW pattern can be mistaken for (1) bundle branch block, (2) left ventricular enlargement, (3) right ventricular enlargement, (4) myocardial infarction patterns.
9. Supraventricular tachycardia (atrioventricular reentrant tachycardia).
10. Conduction over an accessory bypass connection avoids the normal "blocking" function of the AV node. This may lead to extremely rapid conduction of the atrial impulse to the ventricles that can degenerate into ventricular fibrillation.

Further Reading

Anderson RH, Becker AE, Tranum-Jensen J, Janse MJ. Anatomico-electrophysiological correlations in the conduction system – a review. *Br Heart J.* 1981;45:67-82.

Anderson RH, Becker AE, Brechenmacher C, Davies MJ, Rossi L. Ventricular preexcitation: a proposed nomenclature for its substrates. *Eur J Cardiol.* 1975;3:27-36.

Arruda MS, McClelland JH, Wang X, et al. Development and validation of an ECG algorithm for identifying accessory pathway ablation site in Wolff-Parkinson-White syndrome. *J Cardiovasc Electrophysiol.* 1998;9:2-12.

Bagliani G, DePonti R, Notaristefano F, Cavallini C, Padeletti M, Leonelli FM. Ventricular preexcitation: an anomalous wave interfering with the ordered ventricular activation. *Card Electrophysiol Clin.* 2020;12:447-464.

Cosio FG, Anderson RH, Kuck KH, et al. Living anatomy of the atrioventricular junctions. A guide to electrophysiologic mapping. *Circulation.* 1999;100:e31-e37.

Fitzpatrick AP, Gonzales RP, Lesh MD, Modin GW, Lee RJ, Scheinman MM. New algorithm for the localization of accessory atrioventricular connections using a baseline electrocardiogram. *J Am Coll Cardiol.* 1994;23:107-116.

Issa ZF, Miller JM, Zipes DP. Variants of preexcitation. In: Issa ZF, Miller JM, Zipes DP, eds. *Clinical Arrhythmology and Electrophysiology.* Philadelphia, PA: Elsevier; 2012.

Prystowsky EN, Miles WM, Heger JJ, Zipes DP. Preexcitation syndromes: mechanisms and management. *Med Clin North Am.* 1984;68:831-893.

Sternick EB, Gerken LM. The 12-lead ECG in patients with Mahaim fibers. *Ann Noninvasive Electrocardiol.* 2006;11:63-83.

Myocardial Ischemia, Infarction, and Pericarditis

Myocardial Ischemia, Injury, and Infarction

▶ INTRODUCTION

This chapter will focus on the recognition of myocardial ischemia and infarction, one of the most important aspects of electrocardiography. It's absolutely vital that you master the ECG manifestations of acute and chronic coronary syndromes because you are going to use these skills to make urgent clinical decisions. Let's start our discussion with a review of anatomy.

Coronary Artery Anatomy

We learned in Chapter 2 that the heart muscle derives its supply of oxygen from the coronary arteries. The two coronary openings (ostia) give rise to the right coronary (RCA) and left main (LM) coronary arteries (**Figure 10-1**).

The RCA circles around the right (anterior) surface of the heart, coursing in the plane of the AV groove that divides the atria and the ventricles. This vessel normally supplies the right atrium and the right ventricular free wall. In 85% of individuals, the RCA gives rise to the posterior descending artery (PDA) that supplies the inferior surface of the left ventricle; a pattern termed a *right dominant* circulation. Septal branches from the PDA supply the inferior portion of the interventricular septum.

The LM coronary artery divides into the left anterior descending (LAD) and left circumflex (LCx) coronary arteries. The LAD

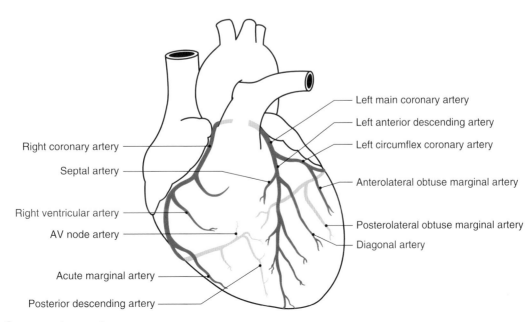

Left main coronary artery
Left anterior descending artery
Left circumflex coronary artery
Anterolateral obtuse marginal artery
Posterolateral obtuse marginal artery
Diagonal artery

Right coronary artery
Septal artery
Right ventricular artery
AV node artery
Acute marginal artery
Posterior descending artery

Figure 10-1. Coronary artery anatomy.

courses in the plane of the interventricular septum and supplies the anterior wall of the left ventricle. Septal branches supply the majority of the interventricular septum and diagonal branches supply portions of the anterolateral wall. The LCx circles leftward in the plane of the AV groove, typically supplying the posterior and lateral portions of the left ventricle. Anterolateral and posterolateral obtuse marginal branches supply their corresponding segments of the left ventricle. In 15% of individuals, the PDA arises from the LCx and is called a *left dominant* circulation.

It is important to note that the coronary anatomy depicted in Figure 10-1 is only a generality because there is wide variability from person to person. In some individuals, the left main trifurcates into three branches, the LAD, LCx, and a diagonal-type vessel termed the *ramus intermedius*. In most individuals the first branch of the LAD is the first diagonal artery, but in others it is the first septal artery. The size and distribution of the LCx and marginal vessels also vary widely. All these variations impact the ECG patterns of myocardial infarction.

Circulation to the Cardiac Conduction System

The coronary arteries provide circulation to the specialized conduction system. Accordingly, cardiac conduction abnormalities may be present in acute coronary syndromes. The SA node is supplied by the RCA in 60% of individuals and the LCx in 40%. The circulation to the AV node follows the coronary dominance as determined by the vessel that gives rise to the PDA; therefore, the AV nodal artery is a branch of the RCA in 85% and the LCx in 15% of individuals. The His bundle is supplied by the AV nodal branch of the RCA with a contribution from LAD septal branches. The right bundle branch derives its primary blood supply from septal branches of the LAD. The left anterior fascicle of the left bundle branch is supplied by LAD septals and is more prone to ischemic damage than the posterior fascicle, which receives a dual blood supply from septal branches of both the LAD and PDA.

The Layers of the Heart

Recall from Chapter 2 that the heart muscle is comprised of three layers, an inner *endocardium*, middle *myocardium,* and outer *epicardium*. The myocardium is further subdivided into an inner, *subendocardial,* and outer *subepicardial* layer.

The epicardium contains the coronary arteries, which then branch and penetrate the more inner layers to provide oxygen and other nutrients. The myocardium is the thick muscular layer responsible for cardiac contraction. The subendocardium has a high metabolic demand and is fed by the most distal branches of the coronary arteries; therefore, it has the greatest risk of injury from diminished coronary blood flow.

The endocardium is the thin layer lining the innermost surface of the cardiac chambers and derives a secondary source of oxygen from intracavitary blood.

Coronary Ischemia, Injury, and Infarction

Myocardial cells require an adequate supply of oxygen-containing blood from the coronary arteries. A deficiency between the degree of coronary blood flow and the demands of the heart muscle is called **myocardial ischemia**. This imbalance produces clinical symptoms and interferes with the normal contractile and electrical functions of cardiac muscle.

Cardiac ischemia most often results from **coronary stenosis** (narrowing) that reduces coronary blood flow. The most common cause of coronary stenosis is from **atherosclerosis,** which is a buildup of fatty, inflammatory, and fibrous material called **plaque**. The limitation of blood flow can produce myocardial ischemia during exercise, or any other process that increases metabolic demand. There are conditions where cardiac ischemia can occur in the absence of coronary obstruction. Examples include patients with severe aortic stenosis or those with profound anemia, both of which may cause a mismatch of oxygen supply and demand. **Angina** refers to clinical manifestations of coronary ischemia such as chest discomfort and related symptoms.

 CLINICAL TIP: You should avoid asking patients with suspected ischemic symptoms whether they have "chest pain." Instead, I recommend you use the term "discomfort." Patients with angina typically describe symptoms of "pressure," "heaviness," "tightness," or even "burning." These symptoms are uncomfortable, but not necessarily painful. The location may be the chest, neck, jaw, or either arm. Anginal symptoms are most often dull rather than sharp, last minutes rather than seconds, and are associated with either physical or emotional stress. Coronary ischemia can manifest only as shortness of breath or exercise intolerance. If you drop this book on your little toe, you're likely to experience sudden intense pain. Anginal symptoms are typically more subtle.

If rapidly reversed, coronary ischemia produces only temporary clinical symptoms or cardiac dysfunction without permanent damage to the heart muscle. But if the ischemic episode is prolonged, cellular damage occurs that results in **myocardial injury**.

Myocardial infarction occurs when the interruption of blood flow is sustained as to cause cell death, termed *myocardial necrosis*. Acute myocardial infarction is typically caused by the sudden rupture of an atherosclerotic plaque that triggers **coronary thrombosis** (clot) with either partial or complete occlusion of a coronary artery. Unless adequate circulation is restored, myocardial infarction and cell death will result. The infarction may be either *transmural*, reflecting full-thickness necrosis of a segment of the heart muscle or *nontransmural*, representing partial thickness damage confined to the subendocardium (**Figure 10-2**). Rarely, myocardial infarction is limited to the subepicardial layer. Biochemical evidence of myocardial cell death is confirmed by measuring serum levels of the myocardial contractile protein **troponin**, which become elevated with myocardial necrosis.

You can think of the coronary syndromes described in the preceding discussion as a continuum of a single process. Myocardial ischemia reflects an imbalance between supply and demand, which may be either transient or prolonged. Myocardial injury is the result of continuing ischemia with some degree of cellular death. Myocardial infarction involves varying

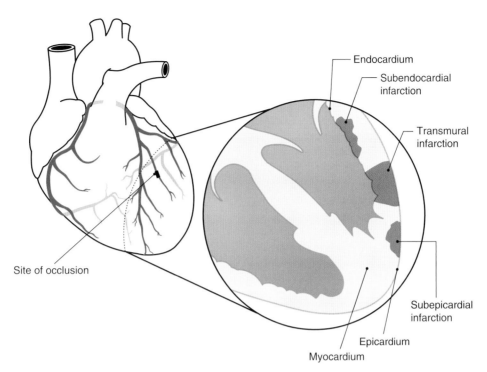

Figure 10-2. The heart muscle is divided into an inner endocardium, middle myocardium, and outer epicardium. Occlusion of a coronary artery may result in full thickness, transmural infarction. Partial thickness, nontransmural infarction may be limited to either the subendocardial or subepicardial region.

degrees of necrosis with potentially irreversible damage to the myocardium.

Myocardial ischemia, injury, and infarction each produce characteristic patterns on the electrocardiogram. These syndromes alter the Q wave, R wave, ST segment, T wave, QT interval, and sometimes the U wave. The findings you observe will depend both on the unique pathophysiologic process and when the ECG is obtained. Before we discuss each of these abnormalities, let's review the pertinent components of the normal electrocardiogram (**Figure 10-3**).

Review of the Normal ECG

Small, narrow Q waves ≤0.03 seconds related to septal depolarization may be normally found in leads I, II, III, aVL, aVF, and V4-V6. A wider Q wave ≥0.04 seconds may be a normal finding in lead III, as is a QS complex in leads aVR and V1. The ST segment

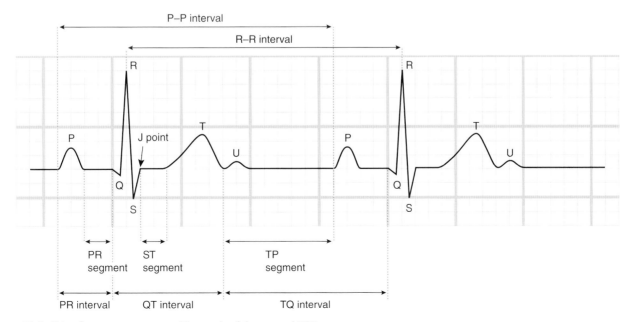

Figure 10-3. Waveforms, segments, and intervals of the normal ECG.

is normally isoelectric, but may be slightly elevated or depressed by <1 mm relative to the baseline. Somewhat greater ST elevation may be a normal finding in leads V2 and V3 (<1.5 mm in women and <2 mm in men younger than 40 years). The point where the QRS complex and ST segment meet is called the J point or J junction. The normal T wave configuration is rounded, smooth, and slightly asymmetric, with the terminal portion exhibiting a steeper downslope. The direction of the T wave usually parallels that of the normal QRS complex in that lead. Accordingly, leads that contain a tall, positive R wave will also have an upright T wave. The amplitude of the T wave should not exceed 6 mm in the limb leads or 10 mm in the precordial leads. As we learned in Chapter 4, the normal QT interval is affected by heart rate and gender. A clue for an abnormally prolonged QT interval is when it is more than half of the R-R interval. The amplitude of the U wave (if visible) should be <25% that of the T wave in that lead and normally follows in the same direction.

OK, so now you think you're ready to see the dramatic ECG findings of acute myocardial ischemia and infarction. Not so fast! Our goal is not to memorize patterns, but to understand their genesis. And for that we need a quick refresher on vectors.

Review of Cardiac Vectors

In Chapter 6 we arbitrarily divided ventricular depolarization into three basic vectors. But remember, this is a gross simplification. Each of the three vectors is not a single measurement, but represents the mathematical resultant of all the electrical forces moving in every direction at that moment (**Figure 10-4, top**). The electrocardiogram records the movements of these

vectors over time, with a vector oriented toward the positive electrode inscribed as a positive deflection and one pointed away as a negative deflection. By combining all the sequential cardiac vectors as a loop, we derive the corresponding vector-cardiogram (**Figure 10-4, bottom**).

- Vector 1 represents depolarization of the left side of the interventricular septum, directed rightward, anterior, and (usually) superior. There is simultaneous right-to-left depolarization of the right side of the septum, but the greater left-sided forces predominate. The net left-to-right orientation of vector 1 explains why there is often a small initial Q wave in leads I, aVL, and V6. This reflects depolarization of the first portion of the interventricular septum, hence the term "septal Q wave." A slight superior orientation of this vector may also allow for small Q waves in the inferior leads.
- Vector 2 represents simultaneous activation of the free walls of both ventricles with the predominant force reflecting the greater mass of the left ventricle. The remaining right and left-sided portions of the interventricular septum also depolarize during this time, but the effects counterbalance one another. The net effect is that vector 2 is of large amplitude and oriented toward the left, inferiorly and posteriorly, reflecting the anatomical position of the left ventricle. We, therefore, expect to see tall R waves in leads that "look" from that direction, such as leads I, aVL, and V5-V6. Similarly, we expect to see deep S waves in leads that are oriented rightward, looking away from the direction of vector 2, such as leads V1 and aVR.
- Vector 3 represents the terminal activation of the posterobasal portions of both the left ventricle and interventricular

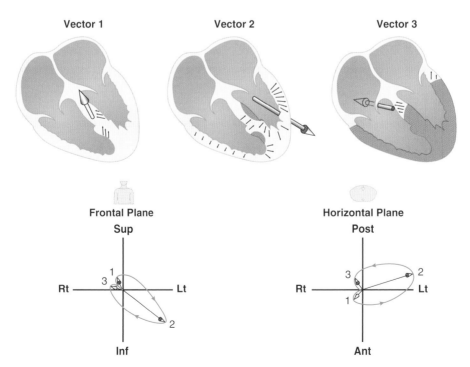

Figure 10-4. Sequence of left ventricular depolarization (top) and vector loops (bottom). Interventricular septum (vector 1), left and right ventricular free walls (vector 2), posterobasal left ventricle (vector 3). The large arrows represent the mathematical resultant of multiple simultaneous vectors. See text for details.

septum. These structures lie rightward and posterior in relation to the other cardiac structures. This vector is of small amplitude and variable, but is predominantly oriented to the right, somewhat superiorly and usually posteriorly. Accordingly, we normally expect to see small S waves in leads I and V4-V6.

Leading the Way with Contiguous Leads

The ECG allows us to record the heart's electrical events from different perspectives, with each of the 12 leads providing a different "view" of the same electrical sequence. Electrodes that face the same anatomical region from closely related perspectives are called **contiguous leads** (**Figure 10-5**).

We can use the concept of contiguous leads to identify an area of cardiac injury and the potential site of coronary obstruction. In the frontal plane, leads II, III, and aVF all face the inferior surface of the heart muscle, while leads I and aVL view the lateral wall. In the horizontal plane, contiguous leads are defined as any two numerically consecutive chest leads, V1-V6. Leads V1 and V2 view the interventricular septum, leads V2-V4 the anterior wall, and leads V4-V6 the lateral wall. Note that some contiguous leads overlap each other. By analyzing the abnormalities in these groupings we can predict the probable site of myocardial infarction. To optimize diagnostic accuracy, all the findings we are about to discuss should be present in **at least two contiguous leads** of a grouping.

Reciprocal changes are mirror image findings in leads oriented *opposite* to those facing the primary abnormalities. For example, a vector pointed in an anterior-superior direction will be recorded as positive in leads V1, V2, and aVL, but appear negative in leads II, III, and aVF. To use a baseball analogy, a ball thrown from the mound to the plate is moving toward the catcher and away from the pitcher. The identical

pitch would be graphically recorded as a positive vector from the catcher's perspective, but a negative vector as viewed by the pitcher.

OK, now that we've reviewed the basics, let's discuss the specific findings of the acute coronary syndromes.

▶ ACUTE ST ELEVATION MYOCARDIAL INFARCTION (STEMI)

Sudden, complete occlusion of a coronary artery is the principal cause of acute transmural myocardial infarction. This event produces dramatic evolutionary findings on the ECG characterized by ST segment elevation in the leads facing the myocardial infarction, hence the acronym STEMI. Let's now review each of these changes in the order that they occur (**Figure 10-6**).

Peaked (hyperacute) T waves are the earliest signs of sudden coronary occlusion. Within minutes of the cessation of blood flow, the T wave becomes tall and symmetric. Although

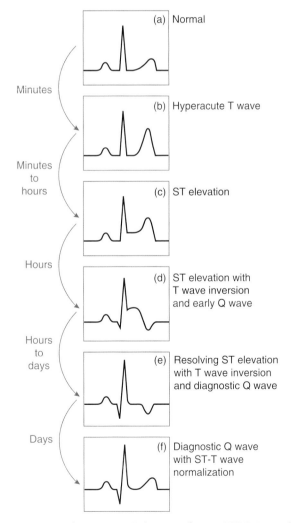

Figure 10-6. Evolutionary ECG changes of acute STEMI. Normal (a), hyperacute T wave (b), ST segment elevation with evolving T wave inversion (c-d), resolving ST segment elevation with developing Q wave (e), normalized ST segment and T wave with diagnostic Q wave (f).

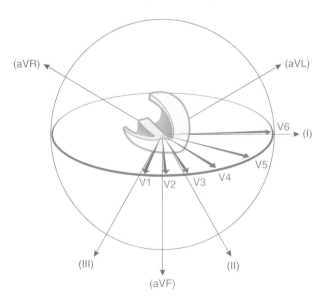

Figure 10-5. Contiguous limb leads (blue) and precordial leads (orange) are used to identify areas of cardiac injury and infarction. The regions are defined as: inferior (II, III, aVF), septal (V1, V2), anterior (V2, V3, V4), lateral (I, aVL, V4, V5, V6), and posterior (mirror image, reciprocal findings in leads V1, V2).

nonspecific, a clue to the presence of hyperacute T waves is a T wave amplitude more than two-thirds of the R wave in that lead. This initial T wave finding may be so brief as to not be evident when the patient presents for evaluation.

ST segment elevation is the defining abnormality of acute STEMI. Within minutes to hours, the ST segment rises at the J point above the baseline to merge with the T wave in a variety of patterns. In general, abnormal ST segment elevation is defined as ≥1 mm in two contiguous leads. In leads V2 and V3 the criteria for abnormal ST segment elevation is ≥2 mm in men and ≥1.5 mm in women. The ST segment elevation is initially horizontal to upsloping, which becomes more concave down ("domed" or "coved") over time. ST segment elevation is also called the *current of injury*, reflecting full thickness, transmural injury that reaches the epicardium. Marked ST segment elevation that reaches the level of the R wave is called a *tombstone pattern*, which is apropos because of the poor prognosis of untreated patients with this ECG finding. Reciprocal ST segment depression may be seen in leads opposite to those recording ST segment elevation. Over hours to days, the ST segment returns to baseline. The initial T wave peaking and ST segment elevation define the *acute* period of STEMI.

BE CAREFUL: ST segment elevation is not always due to acute myocardial infarction. Slight upsloping ST segment elevation is often normally seen in leads V2 and V3, which is why the criteria for abnormal ST segment elevation are more restrictive in these leads. A high J-point takeoff for the ST segment may reflect either a normal variant or a pattern of *early repolarization*. A particularly important clinical decision is distinguishing patients who have *pericarditis*, who may present with chest discomfort and ST segment abnormalities. A helpful ECG clue is that the ST segment elevation of acute myocardial infarction is typically concave down like a dome (frowning), whereas the ST segment elevation in the other conditions is upsloping (smiling) (**Figure 10-7**). We will review these and other imitators of acute coronary syndromes in the next chapter.

CLINICAL TIP: Transient, reversible ST segment elevation may also be due to *coronary spasm* (*Prinzmetal or variant angina*). In this syndrome, intense coronary spasm produces marked ST segment elevation indistinguishable from acute STEMI due to coronary thrombosis. What differentiates this syndrome from acute MI is the rapid

resolution of symptoms and ECG findings after relief of the ischemia with nitroglycerin. If the spasm does not resolve however, myocardial infarction may occur in the absence of coronary atherosclerosis. *Takotsubo syndrome* (stress cardiomyopathy) is another clinical syndrome that has transient ECG findings indistinguishable from acute STEMI, but is unrelated to atherosclerotic coronary artery disease.

Over the next few hours to days, the ST segments return to baseline, usually accompanied by **T wave inversion**. These changes typify the *evolving* phase of the infarction. In the absence of ongoing ischemia, the inverted T waves usually return to baseline over hours to days.

Pathological Q waves will develop in most patients with ST elevation MI. As the infarction evolves and completes, Q or QS waves will form. This process usually occurs within hours to days, reflecting necrotic tissue that is *electrically silent*. As a result, the ECG records the depolarization from the *unopposed* electrical forces of the viable tissue. Therefore, the negative deflection of the Q wave represents the "infarction vector" that points *away* from the area of necrosis (**Figure 10-8**).

There are a number of definitions for pathological Q waves. A classic criterion is a Q wave ≥0.04 seconds wide with an amplitude ≥1 mm deep. Specificity is increased when the Q wave has an amplitude that exceeds 25% of the corresponding R wave. These characteristics help to distinguish the pathological Q wave of myocardial infarction from one resulting from normal septal depolarization or other normal variants. Remember that whatever criterion is used, the diagnosis of myocardial infarction requires evidence of pathological Q waves in **at least two contiguous leads of a regional group**. One abnormal Q wave is not enough!

More detailed consensus criteria for pathological Q waves used for the universal definition of myocardial infarction are published as follows:

- Any Q wave ≥0.02 seconds or a QS complex in leads V2 and V3.
- Any Q wave ≥0.03 seconds and ≥1 mm deep or QS complex in ≥2 leads of a contiguous lead grouping (II, III, aVF), (I, aVL, V6), (V4-V6).
- R wave ≥0.04 seconds in V1-V2 and R/S ≥1 with a concordant positive T wave in the absence of a conduction defect. This R wave criterion is used for posterior wall MI as a mirror image "Q wave equivalent" (see following discussion).

Additional findings that may be seen associated with acute STEMI include QT prolongation and rarely, U wave inversion. ST segment elevation that persists for 2 weeks or more after Q wave myocardial infarction suggests the formation of a **ventricular aneurysm**.

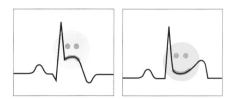

Figure 10-7. The ST segment of an acute STEMI (left) is characteristically domed (frowning), whereas it is usually concave upward (smiling) in noncoronary syndromes such as pericarditis or early repolarization (right).

CLINICAL TIP: Prompt recognition of the ECG findings of acute STEMI will help you to determine if your patient is a candidate for reperfusion therapy, either with thrombolytic agents or catheter-based coronary intervention. But remember that each tracing represents only one

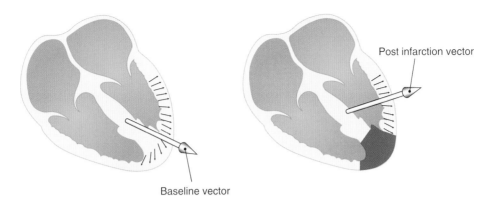

Figure 10-8. An instantaneous cardiac vector represents the sum of multiple, simultaneous wavefronts (left). Myocardial infarction renders the necrotic tissue electrically silent, shifting the vector toward the unopposed viable muscle and away from the injury (right). Contiguous leads facing the region of the infarction will now record the negative deflection of the infarction vector as a Q wave.

snapshot of an ongoing process. Compare each ECG with available prior recordings and analyze serial tracings over time. Subtle findings may become clearer when you make the comparison and never hesitate to order a repeat ECG to take a fresh look.

To Q or Not to Q, That is the Question

Most, but not all patients with STEMI will develop pathological Q waves. Conversely, Q waves may be present in the absence of STEMI. Ultimately the presence or absence of pathological Q waves depends on the extent of myocardial necrosis, which may be either transmural (full thickness) or nontransmural (subendocardial). This tells us that Q waves alone cannot be used to differentiate transmural from nontransmural infarction. Pathological studies show that some patients without Q waves have transmural infarction and some with Q waves have only subendocardial infarction. Yet another factor is that pathological Q waves may regress or even disappear entirely in up to 25% of patients with myocardial infarction.

Some patients with completed STEMI will only show loss of R waves, without developing Q waves. This is particularly true with anteroseptal wall MI. *Poor R wave progression* is the term used to describe R wave voltage ≤3 mm in leads V1-V3. *Reverse R wave progression* is as above, except that R wave voltage decreases instead of increases in leads V1-V3.

There are no leads in the standard 12-lead ECG that face the posterior wall of the left ventricle. Accordingly the ECG is unable to record ST segment elevation or Q waves in patients with myocardial infarction in this location. We solve this problem by examining the mirror image findings in the contiguous reciprocal leads of V1-V2. These leads will record **ST segment depression** and **T wave elevation** in place of the ST segment elevation and T wave inversion that we would have seen if we had examining leads facing the infarction. Similarly, leads V1-V2 will record **tall, broad R waves** that are the mirror image equivalents of posteriorly recorded Q waves.

In some patients with myocardial infarction the only ECG finding will be a **fragmented QRS**. This is believed to represent myocardial scar that results in nonhomogeneous depolarization. A fragmented QRS (fQRS) is a *narrow* complex: (<0.12 sec) that contains an additional R wave (R′) or notching of the R or S wave to create a "splintered" QRS. A variety of patterns may be seen, which like diagnostic Q waves should be present in ≥2 contiguous leads (**Figure 10-9**).

Exceptions, Confounders, and Diagnostic Dilemmas

We reviewed in the preceding discussion that small septal Q waves may be normally found in leads I, II, III, aVL, and V4-V6. The position of the heart in the chest also influences normal Q wave findings. Individuals with a more vertical heart position may show a wide and deep Q wave in lead aVL. Similarly, those with a horizontal heart position may have a more prominent Q wave in lead III that is ≥0.04 seconds and >25% of the amplitude of the corresponding R wave. And as noted earlier, a QS pattern may be normally found in leads aVR and V1.

In addition to these variations of the normal septal Q wave, a number of clinical conditions may produce apparently pathological Q waves in one or more leads that do not represent myocardial infarction. These include:

- Left ventricular enlargement.
- Right ventricular enlargement.
- Left bundle branch block.
- Left anterior fascicular block.
- Left posterior fascicular block.
- Preexcitation (WPW).
- Acute cor pulmonale due to pulmonary embolism.
- Emphysema.
- Hypertrophic cardiomyopathy.
- Cardiac amyloidosis.
- Pacemaker complexes.

 BE CAREFUL: Incorrect lead placement is a not uncommon confounder of the diagnosis of myocardial infarction. Typical scenarios are when the precordial leads are positioned incorrectly high on the chest or misplaced due to breast tissue. You need reliable data to make the correct diagnosis!

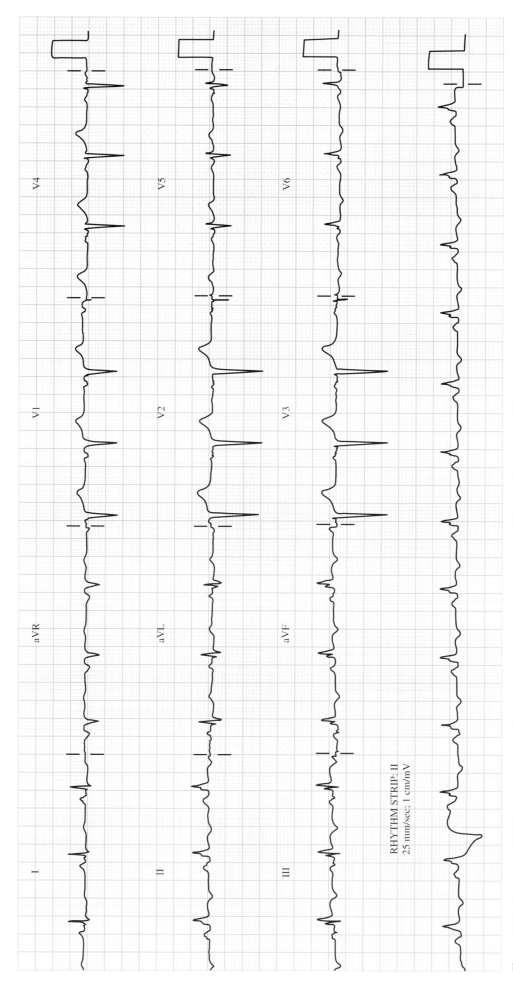

Figure 10-9. Fragmented QRS. Some patients with documented myocardial infarction will have a fragmented QRS as the only clue. Note the narrow complex QRS with prominent notching in leads II, III, aVF, V5, and V6. Additional findings supporting coronary disease in this example include small or absent R waves in leads V1-V5 as well as ST segment and T wave abnormalities in leads I, II, III, aVF, and V6.

RHYTHM STRIP: II
25 mm/sec; 1 cm/mV

TABLE 10–1	ECG Localization of Myocardial Infarction (MI)		
Site of Infarction	Diagnostic Leads[a]	Culprit Coronary Artery[b]	Comment
Anteroseptal	V1-V2 ± V3	LAD (variable location that involves both septal and diagonal branches)	Normal small septal Q waves are lost. Healed infarction may manifest only with diminution of R waves (poor R wave progression).
Anterior	V3-V4 ± V2	LAD (mid to distal portion) or Diagonal vessel	Initial septal forces are preserved.
Anterolateral	V4-V6 ± I, aVL	Diagonal branch of the LAD or Anterolateral marginal branch of the LCx	May show reciprocal ST depression in leads II, III, aVF. May involve only leads I, aVL, termed a "high lateral" MI.
Extensive anterior	V1-V5 ± V6	Proximal LAD involving multiple septal and diagonal branches	May show reciprocal ST depression in leads II, III, aVF.
Inferior	II, III, aVF	RCA-PDA branch or less commonly LCx-PDA branch	May show reciprocal ST depression in leads I, aVL. Also called diaphragmatic MI.
Posterior	V1-V2	LCx (mid to distal) or RCA (distal)	Healed infarction demonstrates tall R waves ≥0.04 sec with R>S. More proximal LCx obstruction results in postero-lateral MI.
Right ventricular	V3R-V6R ± V1	Proximal RCA involving the RV branches	Associated with inferior wall MI.

Left anterior descending (LAD), left circumflex (LCx), right coronary (RCA), posterior descending (PDA), right ventricular (RV).
[a]*Acute or recent infarction demonstrates ST elevation for all regions except posterior MI, which results in mirror image ST depression. MI that is old or of indeterminate age exhibits diagnostic Q waves for all regions except posterior MI, which demonstrates diagnostic R waves.*
[b]*Coronary anatomy exhibits marked variability.*

Location, Location, Location: Identifying the Site of Myocardial Infarction

It's time we put our understanding of the findings of acute STEMI, pathological Q waves, and cardiac anatomy to good use. By analyzing the ECG findings present in contiguous leads, we can determine the approximate anatomical location of the myocardial infarction. We can also use our knowledge of coronary anatomy to predict the likely culprit vessel involved. In addition, the evolutionary ST segment, T wave, and Q wave findings discussed earlier allow us to determine the likely age of the infarction. If we see early peaked T wave abnormalities and particularly ST segment elevation, then we can characterize the infarction as **acute or recent**. The presence of diagnostic Q waves with either normal or nonspecific ST segments and T waves classifies the infarction as **old or of indeterminate age**.

We can categorize the potential sites of myocardial infarction into several major regions (**Table 10-1**). These are the anteroseptal, anterior, anterolateral, extensive anterior, inferior (diaphragmatic), posterior, and right ventricular. There are other classifications and combinations of locations, but these categories have remained in common usage. Occlusion of one or more coronary arteries corresponds to the infarcted segments. In general, inferior and right ventricular infarctions correlate with

obstruction of the RCA, anterior infarctions with the LAD, and posterior infarctions with the LCx. Let's now review the findings of each myocardial infarction location in more detail.

BE CAREFUL: Description of the region of myocardial infarction is made more difficult because of differences in terminology used by electrocardiographers, anatomists, pathologists, imaging specialists, and clinicians. Accordingly, international societies have made an effort to standardize terminology for describing left ventricular anatomy. Advances in cardiac magnetic resonance imaging have allowed for precise correlation of anatomy with ECG findings. Using this updated classification, the left ventricle is divided into four walls: septal, anterior, lateral, and inferior, each with further subdivisions. Note the elimination of the term "posterior," which is now included within the lateral region. Until there is universal consensus and widespread usage of the new classification, I will opt to continue using the classical terminology familiar to most clinicians.

Anteroseptal myocardial infarction typically results from occlusion of the LAD in the mid to distal portion (**Figure 10-10**). Interruption of the blood supply through the septal and diagonal branches injures portions of the interventricular septum

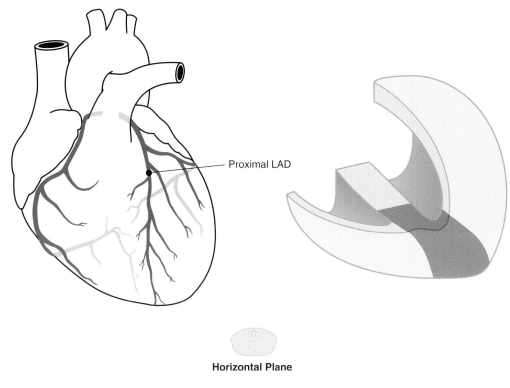

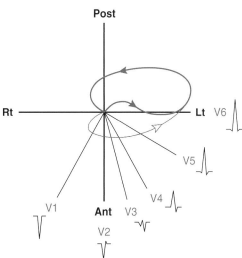

Figure 10-10. Anteroseptal MI. Typical location of coronary occlusion, myocardial segment, and vector loop (blue). The normal vector loop appears in shade.

and anterior wall. This results in loss of the initial rightward and anterior forces, displacing them posteriorly and to the left. Accordingly, we see Q or QS waves in leads V1, V2, and sometimes V3 (**Figure 10-11**). The septal Q wave normally seen in leftward-facing leads is usually lost. If some anterior forces in the frontal plane are preserved, smaller than normal R waves rather than Q waves are present in leads V1-V3, described as poor or reverse R wave progression (**Figure 10-12**).

Anterior wall myocardial infarction results from occlusion of either the mid to distal LAD or a diagonal vessel (**Figure 10-13**). This damages a localized area of the anterior wall, largely sparing the interventricular septum. Acute ST segment and T wave findings are typical in leads V2-V4 (**Figure 10-14**). Myocardial necrosis results in the loss of anterior forces, shifting the vector posteriorly. This produces Q waves in leads V3-V4, and sometimes lead V2. The initial septal depolarization remains intact, preserving the normal R wave in lead V1 and the natural septal Q wave in leftward-facing leads (**Figure 10-15**).

Apical myocardial infarction is a term used to describe an anterior infarction pattern that also includes findings in leads II, III, and aVF, in addition to those seen in leads V3 and V4. This may be seen when the LAD occlusion occurs in a vessel that "wraps around" the left ventricular apex to supply part of the inferior wall.

Anterolateral wall myocardial infarction is caused either by occlusion of a large diagonal branch of the LAD or an anterolateral obtuse marginal branch of the LCx (**Figure 10-16**). In either case, portions of the anterior and lateral segments of the left ventricle are injured. The normal leftward forces are shifted to the right, resulting in Q waves in leads V4-V6, ± leads I and aVL. Septal forces are preserved, which combine with the subsequent rightward forces to reverse the normal direction of the vector loop in both the frontal and horizontal planes.

The typical ECG findings of anterolateral infarction are recorded in the lateral precordial leads, with or without limb lead findings (**Figure 10-17**). Less frequently, patients with lateral infarction will demonstrate ECG findings only in leads I and aVL, without affecting the precordial leads. This pattern has been termed a *high lateral* myocardial infarction. The typical culprit artery of a high lateral MI is a diagonal branch of the LAD.

Extensive anterior myocardial infarction combines the features of an anteroseptal, anterior, and anterolateral wall MI and is due to occlusion of the proximal LAD (**Figure 10-18**). Dramatic ECG findings in acute MI are the norm (**Figure 10-19**). The extensive area of necrosis shifts vector forces posteriorly and to the right, resulting in diagnostic Q waves in leads I, aVL, V1 through V6 (**Figure 10-20**).

Inferior wall myocardial infarction results from occlusion of the PDA (**Figure 10-21**). As noted previously, this vessel arises from the RCA in 85% of individuals. In patients with a left dominant circulation, the LCx gives rise to the PDA and

this system contains the culprit vessel. Inferior MI injures the portion of the left ventricle that rests on the diaphragm, hence you may encounter the term *diaphragmatic MI* to describe this type of infarction. The vector forces are shifted superiorly in the frontal plane, producing Q waves in leads II, III, and aVF. There is little effect of isolated inferior infarction in the horizontal plane; therefore the precordial leads are unchanged (**Figure 10-22**).

Posterior (posterolateral) wall myocardial infarction is usually caused by occlusion of the mid to distal LCx or a posterolateral obtuse marginal artery (**Figure 10-23**). At times, distal occlusion of a large RCA can also produce this infarction pattern. The ECG recording of posterior MI is unique because there are no standard leads that face the infarction; therefore, we must rely on "mirror image" findings to make the diagnosis. With posterior MI, the initial rightward and anterior septal forces remain intact. The late depolarization of the injured posterobasal portion of the left ventricle (vector 3) is compromised, shifting this vector anteriorly. This results in tall (R>S), broad (≥0.04 seconds) R waves in leads V1 and V2 that may be considered "Q wave equivalents." Similarly, acute posterior wall MI will produce mirror image ST segment depression in the anterior precordial leads instead of the ST segment elevation we are accustomed to seeing in all other forms of acute MI (**Figure 10-24**).

Posterior wall MI patterns often occur in conjunction with other infarcted regions. Examples include the inferior wall (inferoposterior MI) and lateral wall (posterolateral MI).

 FOR BOOKWORMS: The diagnosis of acute posterior wall MI can be facilitated by the use of special posterior chest leads that are placed on the patient's back in the fifth intercostal space (V7 at the left posterior axillary line, V8 at the left mid-scapular line, and V9 at the left paraspinal border). ST segment elevation ≥1 mm in these special leads suggests acute posterior wall STEMI.

Right ventricular MI (RVMI) is caused by proximal occlusion of the RCA, involving the branches supplying the right ventricle. Accordingly, RVMI is typically accompanied by inferior wall MI. The diagnosis of RVMI is made by analyzing right ventricular leads V3R-V6R, which are obtained by placing electrodes over the corresponding mirror image interspaces on the right chest instead of their usual left-sided locations (**Figure 10-25**). (Note that recording leads V1 and V2 in a mirror image location provides no new information, so it is acceptable to leave these leads in their usual position.) The limb leads remain in their proper location. RVMI may be diagnosed if there is any ST segment elevation ≥1 mm in any right ventricular lead, with lead V4R being both the most sensitive and specific (**Figure 10-26**).

Atrial infarction may accompany proximal occlusion of the RCA. The diagnosis may be suspected when the PQ segment is either markedly elevated or depressed, particularly if accompanied by a notched P wave. These findings, however, are neither sensitive nor specific.

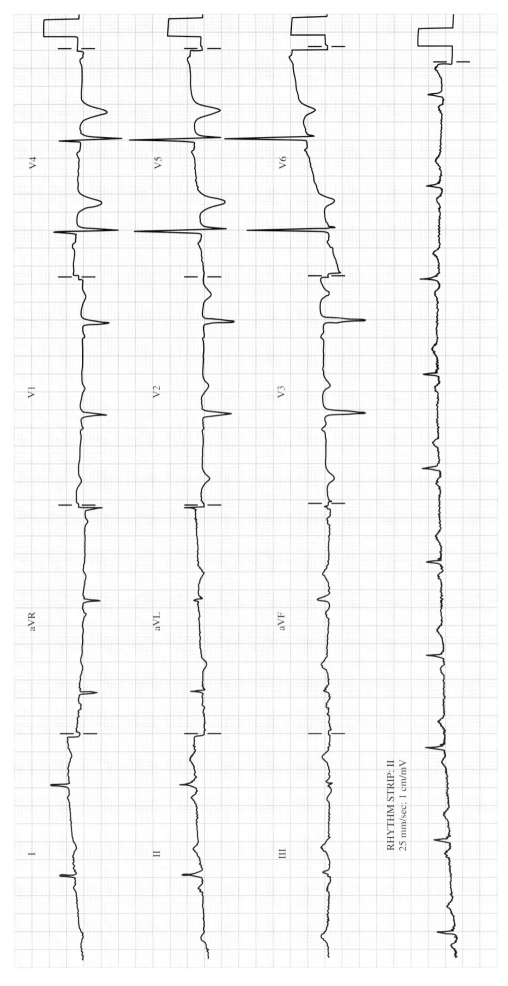

Figure 10-11. Anteroseptal MI, possibly recent. QS waves are present in leads V1-V3. There is diffuse T wave inversion, but not diagnostic acute ST segment elevation. Accordingly, it is best to categorize the MI as recent. Comparison with prior tracings is necessary to determine whether the MI should be described as old or of indeterminate age.

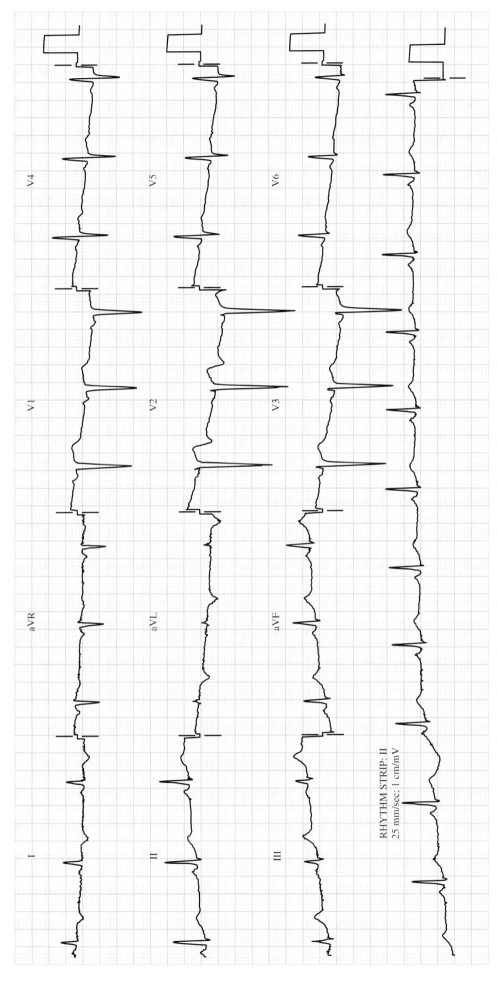

Figure 10-12. Poor R wave progression may be the only manifestation of anteroseptal MI. The abnormal ST segment and T wave findings here indicate a recent or evolving MI.

RHYTHM STRIP: II
25 mm/sec; 1 cm/mV

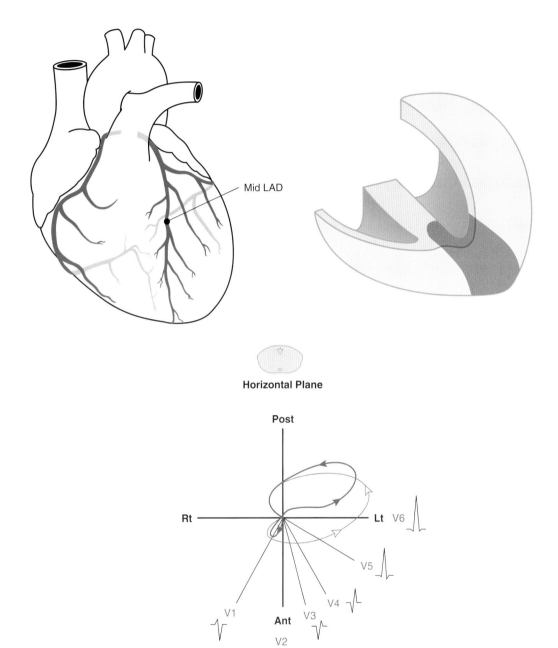

Horizontal Plane

Figure 10-13. Anterior MI. Typical location of coronary occlusion, myocardial segment, and vector loop (blue). The normal vector loop appears in shade.

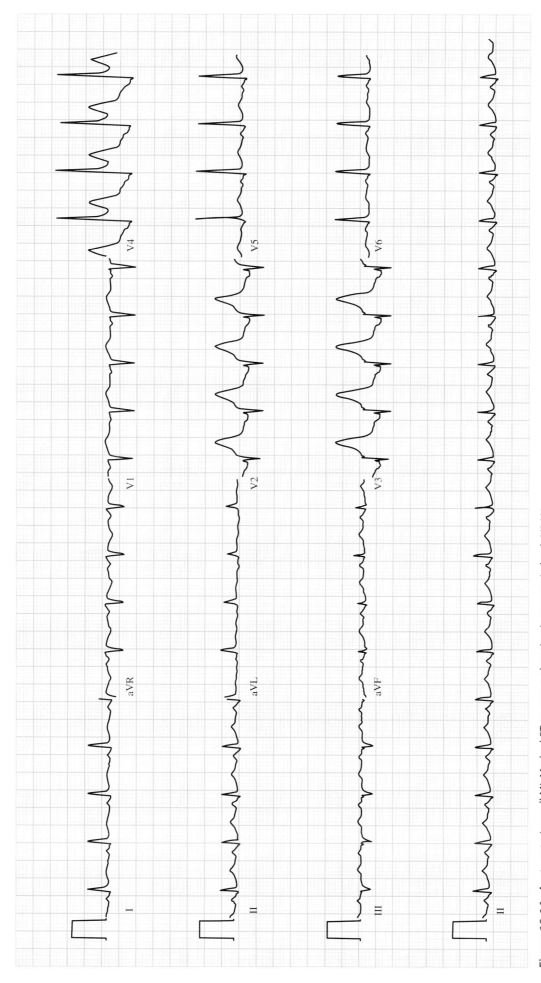

Figure 10-14. Acute anterior wall MI. Marked ST segment elevation is present in leads V2-V4.

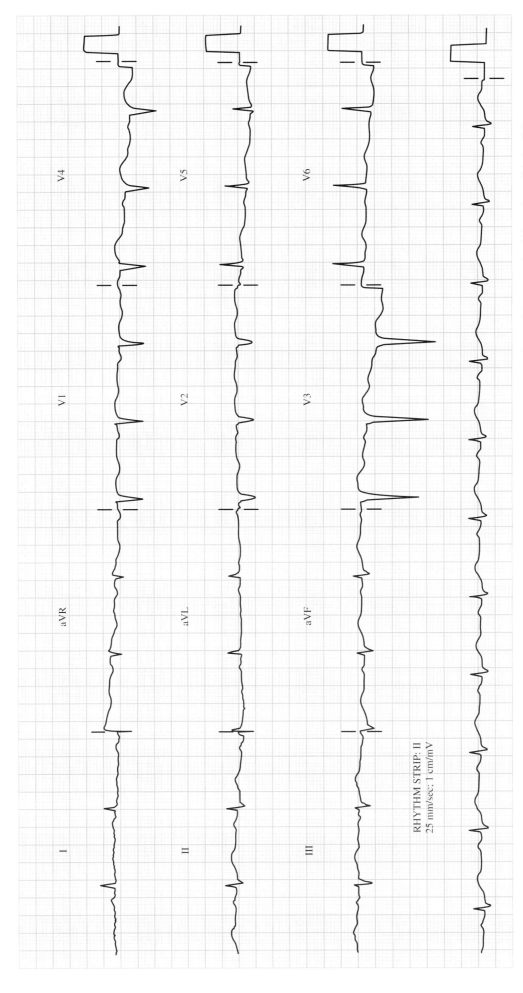

Figure 10-15. Anterior MI, old or age indeterminate. Diagnostic Q waves are present in leads V3 and V4 with preservation of a small R wave in lead V1 and possibly lead V2.

RHYTHM STRIP: II
25 mm/sec; 1 cm/mV

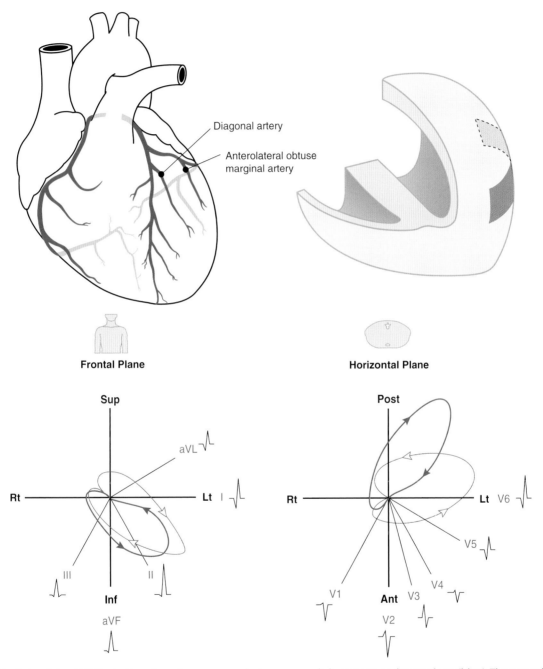

Figure 10-16. Anterolateral MI. Typical location of coronary occlusion, myocardial segment, and vector loop (blue). The normal vector loop appears in shade.

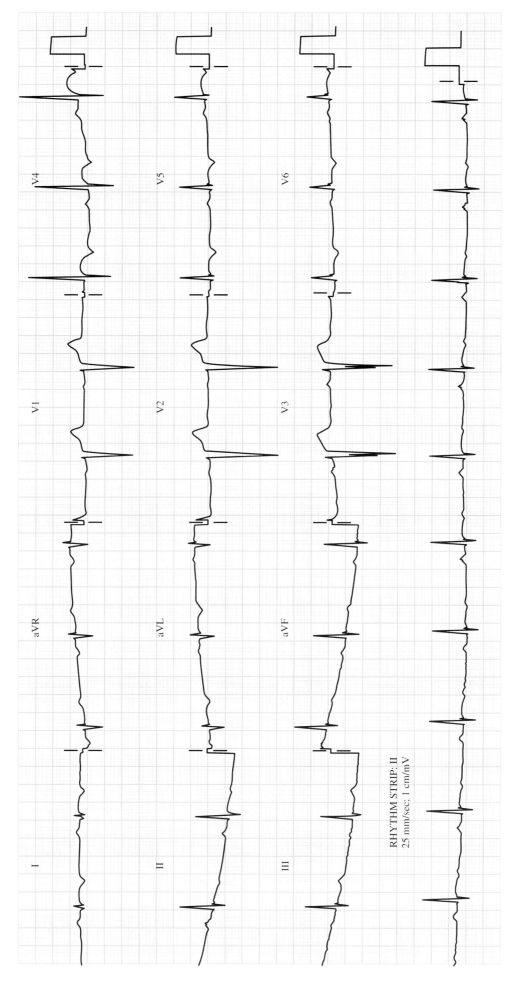

Figure 10-17. Acute or evolving anterolateral MI. ST segment elevation and T wave inversion are most prominent in leads V4-V6, I, and aVL.

RHYTHM STRIP: II
25 mm/sec; 1 cm/mV

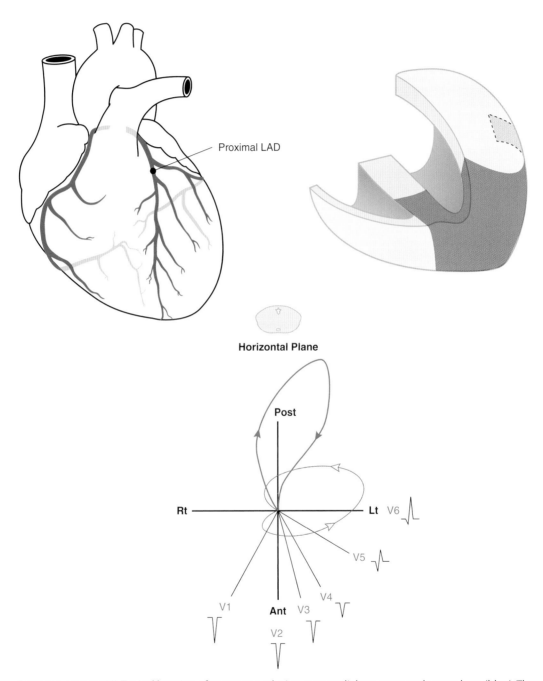

Figure 10-18. Extensive anterior MI. Typical location of coronary occlusion, myocardial segment, and vector loop (blue). The normal vector loop appears in shade.

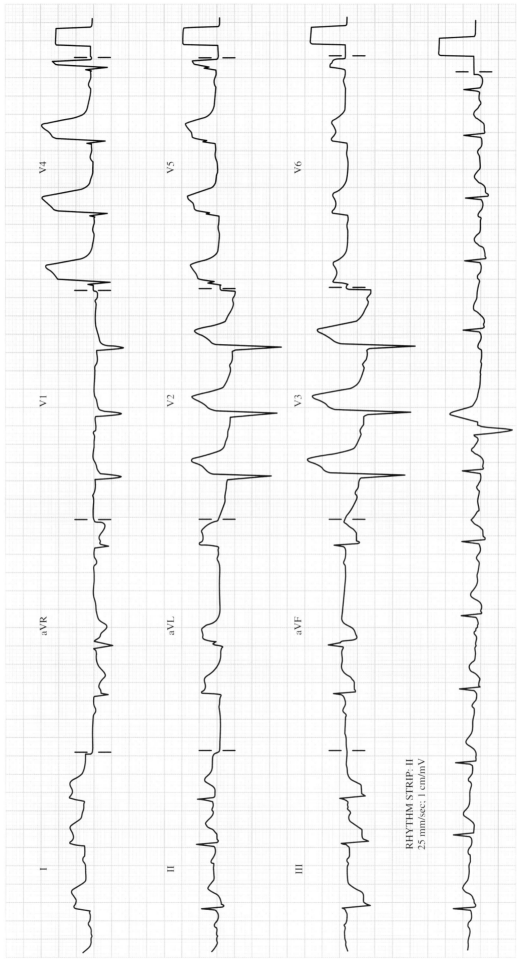

Figure 10-19. Acute extensive anterior MI. Diffuse ST segment elevation with "tombstoning" in leads I, aVL, V2–V6. Reciprocal ST depression is present in leads II, III, and aVF.

RHYTHM STRIP: II
25 mm/sec; 1 cm/mV

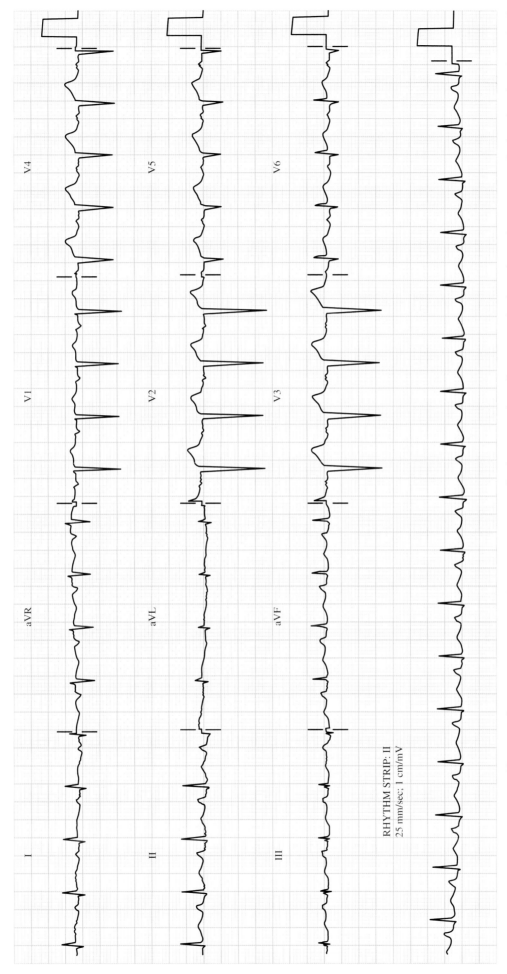

Figure 10-20. Extensive anterior MI, old or age indeterminate. Diagnostic Q waves are present in leads V2–V6 with small Q waves in leads I and aVL. The ST segment findings have largely resolved.

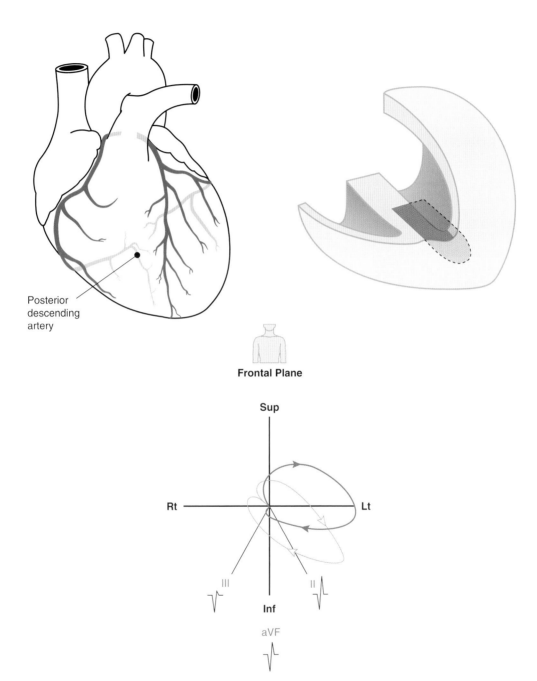

Figure 10-21. Inferior MI. Typical location of coronary occlusion, myocardial segment, and vector loop (blue). The normal vector loop appears in shade.

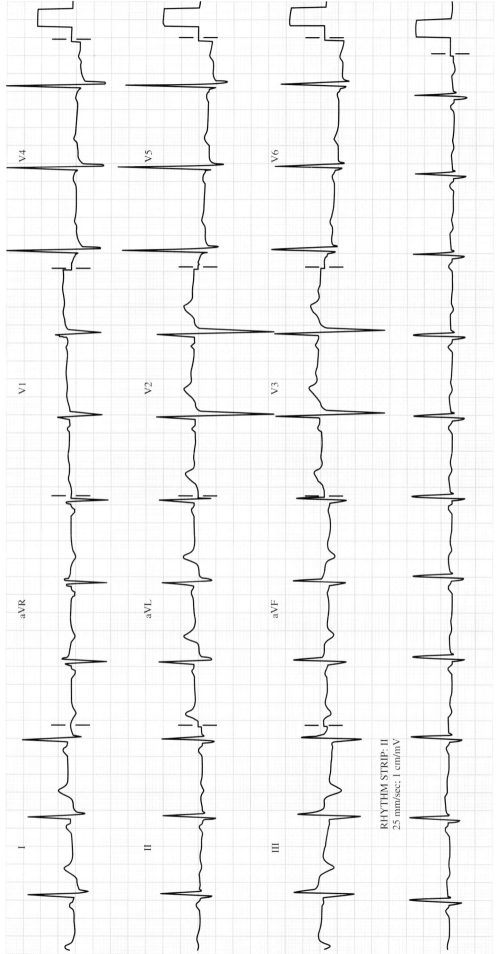

Figure 10-22. Acute inferior MI. Diagnostic Q waves are present with evolving ST elevation and T wave inversion in leads II, III, and aVF. Reciprocal ST segment depression is present in leads I and aVL.

RHYTHM STRIP: II
25 mm/sec; 1 cm/mV

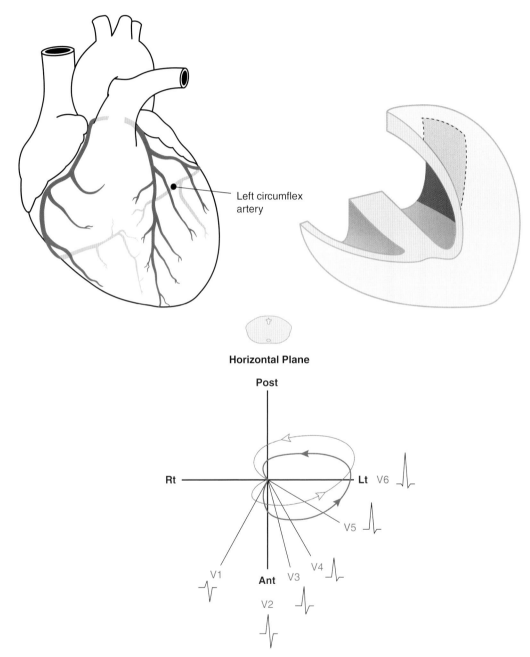

Horizontal Plane

Figure 10-23. Posterior MI. Typical location of coronary occlusion, myocardial segment, and vector loop (blue). The normal vector loop appears in shade.

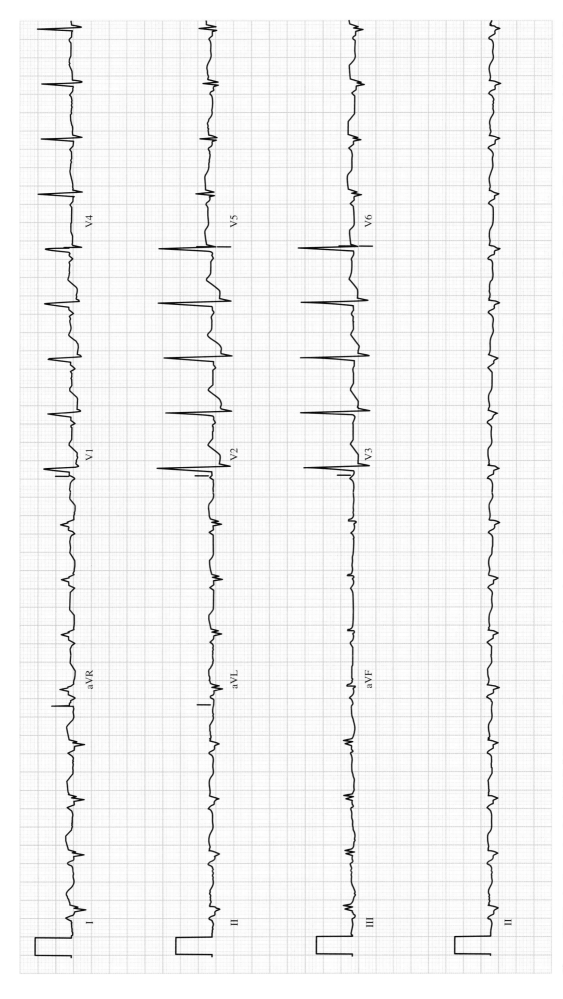

Figure 10-24. Acute posterolateral MI. Tall R waves with ST segment depression and an upright T wave are noted in leads V1-V2. Also note the Q waves with ST segment elevation in leads I, II, aVL, V5, and V6 indicating lateral (and likely inferior) involvement. This pattern typically results from proximal occlusion of a large, dominant LCx artery.

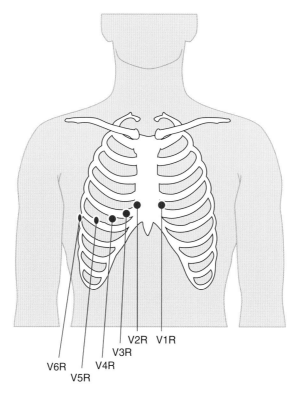

Figure 10-25. Right ventricular leads are typically obtained by placing leads V1-V6 in a mirror image position on the right chest. (It is acceptable to transfer only leads V3-V6 to the right side, leaving leads V1 and V2 in their usual positions.)

▶ **MYOCARDIAL ISCHEMIA AND ACUTE NON-ST ELEVATION MYOCARDIAL INFARCTION**

Acute and chronic myocardial ischemia may be limited to the subendocardium, resulting in alterations of the ST segment and T wave. In these syndromes, which may or may not involve actual myocardial necrosis, ST elevation and diagnostic Q waves are absent.

ST segment depression is the characteristic finding of myocardial ischemia. Whereas the normal ST segment is either flat or slightly upsloping, myocardial ischemia produces ≥1 mm horizontal or downsloping ST segment depression (**Figure 10-27**). Physiological, upsloping ST segment depression may be noted with rapid heart rates in the absence of myocardial ischemia. ST segment depression may be present either as a chronic finding or occur only transiently during an episode of myocardial ischemia (**Figure 10-28**). The presence of an elevated serum troponin indicates that myocardial necrosis (eg, subendocardial infarction) has occurred.

 CLINICAL TIP: ST segment depression may be recorded during an episode of angina. It also may be present in the absence of clinical symptoms, a reflection of *silent ischemia*. The ST segment findings of silent and symptomatic ischemia are the basis for the evaluation of coronary artery disease with exercise or pharmacologic stress testing.

Other clinical conditions and ECG diagnoses alter the ST segment in the absence of myocardial ischemia. As reviewed in previous chapters, these include left ventricular enlargement, intraventricular conduction delays (RBBB, LBBB), as well as preexcitation (WPW pattern). Unlike the *primary* ECG alterations due to coronary syndromes, these are *secondary* ST segment changes of repolarization. Hypokalemia and digitalis treatment are other examples that cause ST segment depression unrelated to coronary obstruction.

T wave inversion is another manifestation of either myocardial ischemia or non-Q wave infarction. Recall that the normal T wave is upright, asymmetric, and generally follows the direction of the R wave in that lead. The abnormal T wave is symmetrical and is either flat or inverted in a direction typically opposite to that of the R wave (**Figures 10-29** and **10-30**). Ischemic T wave inversion may occur alone or along with ST depression.

 CLINICAL TIP: In patients presenting with angina, the presence of marked T wave inversion in the anterior precordial leads, V2-V3 (often V1-V6) is a clue for a severe stenosis of the proximal LAD called the *Wellen syndrome*.

Like the ST segment, left ventricular enlargement, intraventricular conduction delays, and preexcitation produce secondary repolarization alterations of the T wave. Cerebrovascular events, particularly subarachnoid hemorrhage may result in dramatic T wave inversion in the absence of myocardial

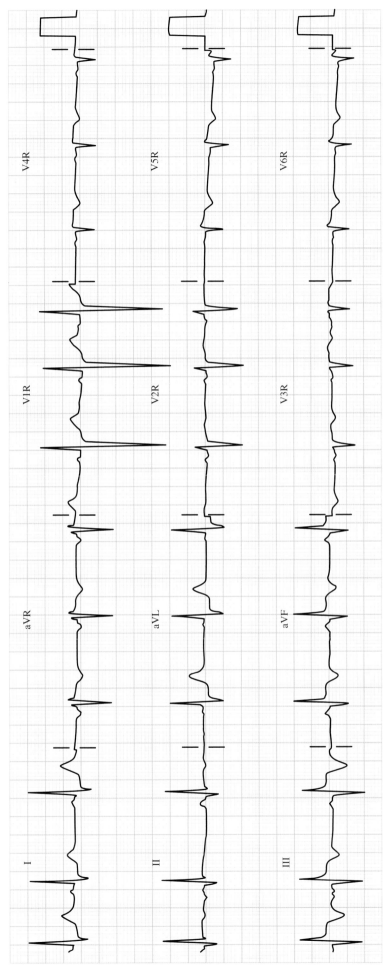

Figure 10-26. Right ventricular infarction. RV leads from the patient of **Figure 10-22.** Note the ST segment elevation in leads V3R-V6R. In this example, all the precordial electrodes (V1-V6) are placed in a mirror image position over their corresponding interspaces on the right chest. The limb leads remain in their proper locations.

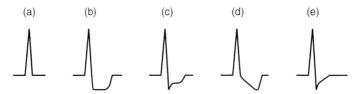

Figure 10-27. The normal ST segment is isoelectric (a), but may be slightly elevated or depressed by <1 mm relative to the baseline. Ischemic ST segment depression is ≥1 mm and is horizontal (b, c) or downsloping (d). Physiological ST segment depression is upsloping (e).

ischemia. Other noncardiac conditions that may produce T wave inversion include hypokalemia, acute cholecystitis, perforated ulcer, and pancreatitis. An inverted T wave with otherwise normal configuration in leads V1 through V3 may be a normal finding in some individuals, termed the *persistent juvenile pattern*.

MI in the Presence of Bundle Branch Block

The findings of myocardial infarction may be evident despite the presence of right bundle branch block. In RBBB, the QRS vectors during the first 0.04 to 0.06 seconds remain normal. Therefore, anterior and inferior wall MI patterns with ST segment elevation and Q waves appear as expected (**Figure 10-31**). The exception is a posterior wall MI where it may be difficult to differentiate the late, mirror image anteriorly directed forces in leads V1-V2 from the RBBB-related terminal conduction delay.

The ECG diagnosis of myocardial infarction in the presence of left bundle branch block is difficult if not impossible. LBBB affects both the early and late portions of the QRS complex, eliminating the normal left-to-right depolarization of the septum and producing secondary ST segment and T wave changes that resemble those of acute MI (**Figure 10-32**). Accordingly, there are no indisputable criteria to diagnose either an acute or chronic infarction. In the proper clinical setting, a clue to an acute coronary syndrome in patients with LBBB is the presence of *new*, primary ST segment changes that are *different* from a baseline tracing, particularly ST segment elevation that is concordant with the main QRS axis. Even so, these findings should be considered as suggestive, but not diagnostic evidence of MI.

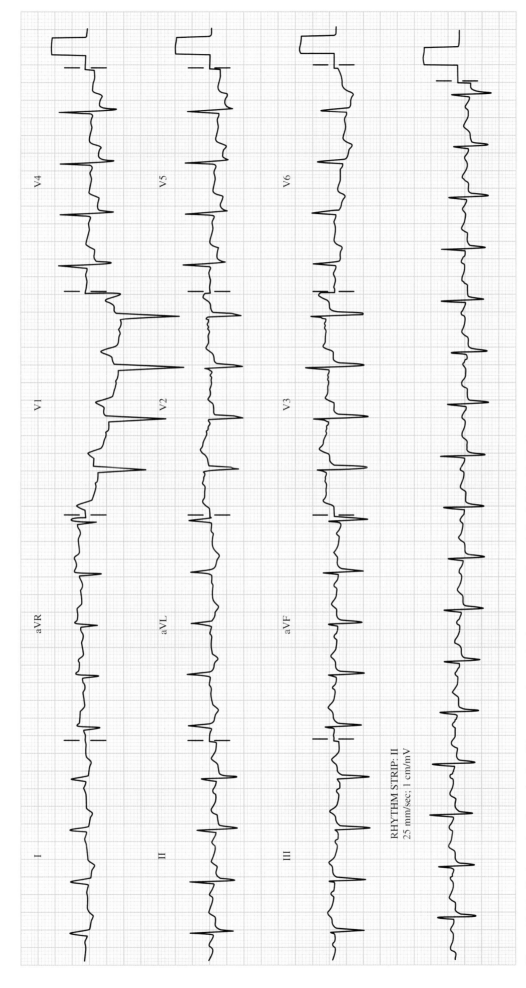

Figure 10-28. Horizontal or downsloping ST segment depression is most prominent in leads I, II, aVL, V2-V6.

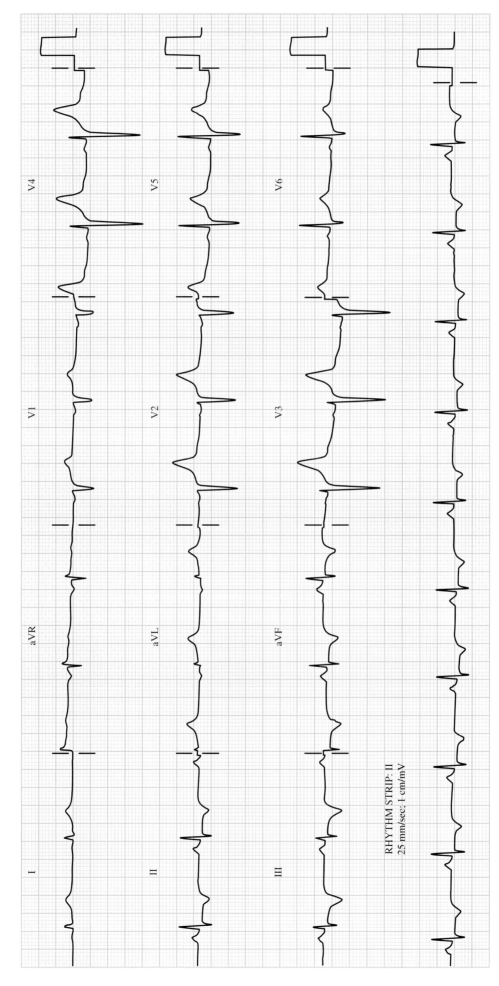

Figure 10-29. Abnormal T wave inversion is present in leads II, III, and aVF.

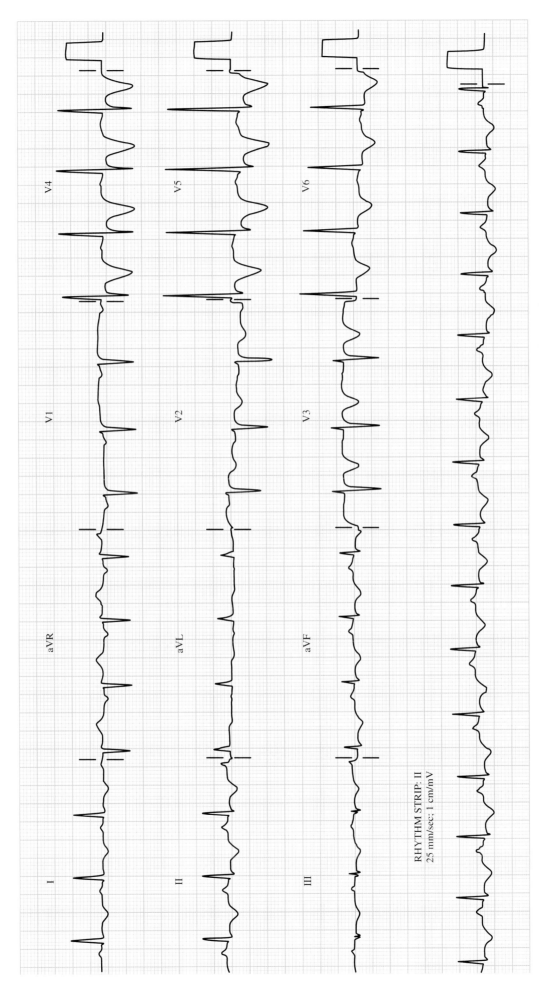

Figure 10-30. Diffuse T wave inversion involving multiple leads. ST segment depression accompanies T wave inversion in leads V5 and V6.

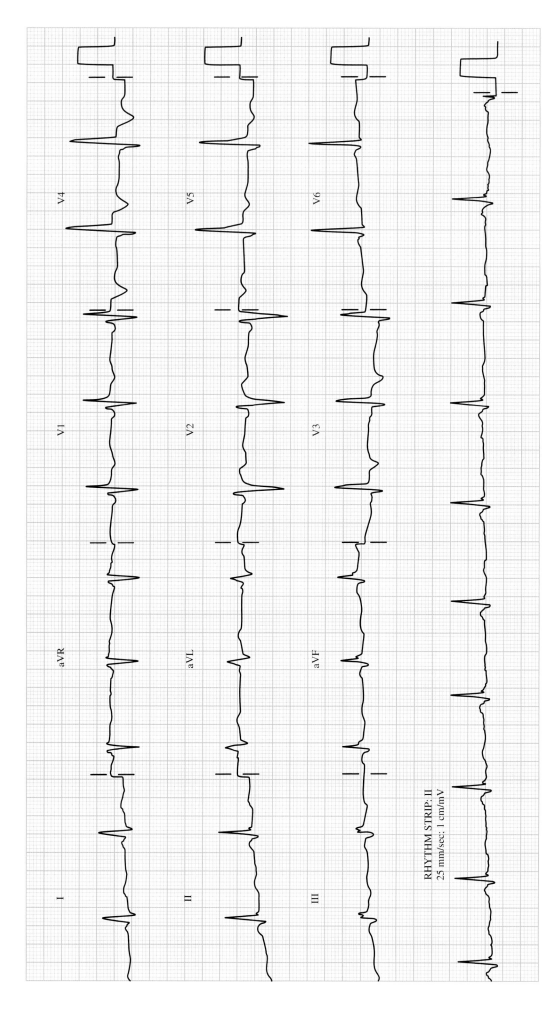

Figure 10-31. MI in the presence of RBBB. Diagnostic Q waves in leads II, III and aVF are identified that reflect old, or indeterminate inferior wall MI. ST segment elevation with early Q waves in leads V3-V5 are present that indicate acute anterior injury.

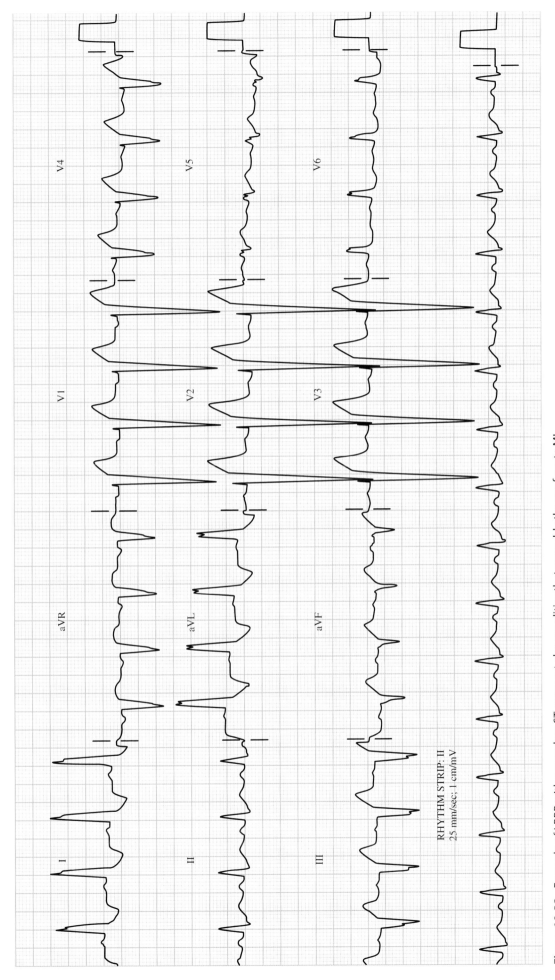

Figure 10-32. Example of LBBB with secondary ST segment abnormalities that resemble those of acute MI.

RHYTHM STRIP: II
25 mm/sec; 1 cm/mV

Chapter 10 • SELF-TEST

QUESTIONS

1. What part of the myocardium is supplied by each of the following arteries?
   - RCA.
   - LAD.
   - LCx.

2. What terms are used to describe the following?
   - An imbalance between myocardial supply and demand.
   - Myocardial cell death.

3. List the classic criteria for an abnormal (pathological) Q wave.

4. Describe the evolutionary findings of an acute ST elevation MI.

5. List the six basic regions of myocardial infarction, the groups of contiguous leads used for analysis, and the likely vessel occluded.

6. What special leads are used to diagnose a right ventricular MI?

7. What are the criteria used to diagnose acute posterior MI?

8. List at least five ECG diagnoses that may produce ST segment and T wave abnormalities unrelated to MI.

9. ST segment elevation that persists for >14 days post-MI suggests what diagnosis?

10. Myocardial ischemia without infarction typically results in what ECG finding?

ANSWERS

Chapter 10 • SELF-TEST

1. • The RCA supplies the right atrium and right ventricular free wall.
   • The LAD supplies the majority of the interventricular septum, anterior and anterolateral walls of the left ventricle.
   • The LCx supplies the posterior and lateral walls of the left ventricle.

2. • Myocardial ischemia.
   • Myocardial necrosis or infarction.

3. A Q wave that is ≥0.04 seconds wide and ≥1 mm deep.

4. The evolutionary ECG findings of acute STEMI are:
   • Hyperacute T waves.
   • ST segment elevation.
   • T wave inversion.
   • Early formation of pathological Q waves.
   • Development of pathological Q waves with resolution of ST segment elevation and T wave inversion.

5. The six basic regions of myocardial infarction, the groups of contiguous leads used for analysis, and the likely culprit vessel are:
   • Anteroseptal (V1, V2 ± V3). LAD, midportion.
   • Anterior (V2, V3, V4). LAD, mid to distal segment or diagonal vessel.
   • Anterolateral (V4, V5, V6 ± I, aVL). LAD, diagonal branch or LCx, anterolateral branch.
   • Extensive anterior (V1, V2, V3, V4, V5, V6, ± I, aVL). LAD, proximal.
   • Inferior (II, III, aVF). PDA, which is usually a branch of the RCA.
   • Posterior (V1, V2). LCx.

6. Right ventricular leads (V3R-V6R), which are precordial leads that are placed on the right chest in a mirror image pattern to their usual left-sided location.

7. Tall, broad (≥0.04 seconds) R waves with ST depression and upright T wave in leads V1 and V2.

8. ST segment and T wave abnormalities unrelated to MI are typically seen with (see text for complete list):
   • Left ventricular enlargement.
   • Bundle branch block.
   • Preexcitation (WPW).
   • Pacemaker complexes.
   • Hypertrophic cardiomyopathy.

9. Left ventricular aneurysm.

10. ST segment depression that is either flat or downsloping.

Further Reading

Bar FW, Brugada P, Dassen WR, van der Werf T, Wellens HJJ. Prognostic value of Q waves, R/S ratio, loss of R wave voltage, ST-T segment abnormalities, electrical axis, low voltage and notching: correlation of electrocardiogram and left ventriculogram. *J Am Coll Cardiol*. 1984;4:17-27.

Bayes de Luna A, Wagner G, Birnbaum Y, et al. A new terminology for left ventricular walls and location of myocardial infarcts that present Q wave based on the standard of cardiac magnetic resonance imaging: a statement for healthcare professionals from a committee by the international society for holter and noninvasive electrocardiography. *Circulation*. 2006;114:1755-1760.

Das MK, Khan B, Jacob S, Kumar A, Mahenthiran J. Significance of a fragmented QRS complex versus a Q wave in patients with coronary artery disease. *Circulation*. 2006;113:2495-2501.

Engelen DJ, Gorgels AP, Cheriex EC, et al. Value of the electrocardiogram in localizing the occlusion site in the left anterior descending coronary artery in acute anterior myocardial infarction. *J Am Coll Cardiol*. 1999;34:389-395.

France RJ, Formolo JM, Penney DG. Value of notching and slurring of the resting QRS complex in the detection of ischemic heart disease. *Clin Cardiol*. 1990;132:190-196.

Fuchs RM, Aschuff SC, Grunwald L, Yin FCP, Griffith LSC. Electrocardiographic localization of coronary artery narrowings: studies during myocardial ischemia and infarction in patients with one-vessel disease. *Circulation*. 1982;66:1168-1176.

Goldberger AL. ECG simulators of myocardial infarction. Part I: Pathophysiology and differential diagnosis of pseudo-infarct Q wave patterns. *PACE*. 1982;5:106-119.

Haji SA, Movahed A. Right ventricular infarction diagnosis and treatment. *Clin Cardiol*. 2000;23:473-482.

Michael MA, El Masry H, Khan BR, Das MK. Electrocardiographic signs of remote myocardial infarction. *Prog Cardiovasc Dis*. 2007;50:198-208.

Moon JDD, Perez de Arenza D, Elkington AG, et al. The pathological basis of Q-wave and non-Q-wave myocardial infarction. *J Am Coll Cardiol*. 2004;44:554-560.

Phibbs B, Marcus F, Marriott HJC, Moss A, Spodick DH. Q-wave versus non-Q wave myocardial infarction: a meaningless distinction. *J Am Coll Cardiol*. 1999;33:576-582.

Robalino BD, whitlow PL, Underwood DA, Salcedo EE. Electrocardiographic manifestations of right ventricular infarction. *Am Heart J*. 1989;118:138-143.

Schweitzer P. The electrocardiographic diagnosis of acute myocardial infarction in the thrombolytic era. *Am Heart J*. 1990;119:642-654.

Selvester RH. The Selvester QRS scoring system for estimating myocardial infarct size. *Arch Intern Med*. 1985;145:1877-1881.

Sgarbossa E. Value of the ECG in suspected acute myocardial infarction with left bundle branch block. *J Electrocardiol*. 2000;33:87-92.

Tabas JA, Rodriguez RM, Seligman HK, Goldschlager NF. Electrocardiographic criteria for detecting acute myocardial infarction in patients with left bundle branch block: a met-analysis. *Ann Emerg Med*. 2008;52:329-336.

Thygesen K, Alpert JS, Jaffe AS, Simoons ML, Chaitman BR, White HD: the writing group on behalf of the joint ESC/ACCF/AHA/WHF task force for the universal definition of myocardial infarction. Third universal definition of myocardial infarction. *Circulation*. 2012;126:2020-2035.

Thygsesen K, Alpert JS, White HD; on behalf of the ESC/ACCF/AHA/WHF task force for the universal redefinition of myocardial infarction. Universal definition of myocardial infarction. *Circulation*. 2007;116:2634-2653.

Wagner GS, Macfarlane P, Wellens, H, et al. AHA/ACCF/HRS recommendations for the standardization and interpretation of the electrocardiogram. Part IV: Acute ischemia/infarction. *J Am Coll Cardiol*. 2009;53:1003-1011.

Zema MJ. ECG poor R wave progression. *Arch Intern Med*. 1982;142:1145-1148.

Zimetbam PJ, Josephson ME. Use of the electrocardiogram in acute myocardial infarction. *N Engl J Med*. 2003;348:933-940.

Pericarditis and Other Infarction Imitators

▶ INTRODUCTION

In the last chapter we learned about the dramatic ECG findings of acute ST elevation myocardial infarction (STEMI). We also reviewed other ischemic syndromes that produce alterations of the ST segment and T wave. But not every case of ST segment elevation represents an acute myocardial infarction. In this chapter, we'll examine the many important conditions that can affect the ST segment, first focusing on items that produce ST segment elevation, imitating the findings of acute MI. At the end of the chapter, we'll describe some infarction imitators that do not involve ST segment elevation.

▶ THE NORMAL AND ABNORMAL ST SEGMENT

You know by now that the ST segment is the interval between the end of the QRS complex and the beginning of the T wave (**Figure 11-1**). Recall that the ST segment is normally isoelectric, but may be slightly elevated or depressed by <1 mm relative to the baseline. The ST segment should be measured at the J point compared to a baseline of either the PR segment or TP segment, using whichever appears the most stable and accurate.

Clinically important abnormalities of the ST segment include displacement from the baseline and changes in morphology. Abnormal ST segment displacement is defined as elevation or depression of ≥1 mm from the baseline in at least two contiguous leads. In leads V2 and V3 the criteria for abnormal ST segment elevation is ≥2 mm in men and ≥1.5 mm in women. Displacement of the ST segment may take different morphologies that may be described as horizontal, upsloping, downsloping, or with more complex patterns.

Thinking back to Chapter 3 you will recall that ST segment changes ultimately reflect alterations of repolarization.

The J point represents the end of early repolarization (phase 1) and the ST segment corresponds to the plateau (phase 2) of the ventricular action potential (**Figure 11-2**).

▶ ST ELEVATION INFARCTION IMITATORS

Abnormal ST segment elevation unrelated to MI may be either a primary or secondary phenomenon. Primary ST segment elevation is caused by clinical conditions that directly affect repolarization, whereas secondary ST segment elevation results as a consequence of alterations of depolarization.

Primary ST segment elevation unrelated to acute STEMI and other ischemic syndromes is characteristically seen with the following:

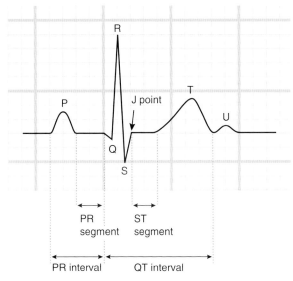

Figure 11-1. ECG segments and intervals.

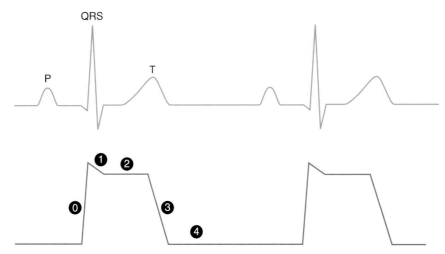

Figure 11-2. Electrocardiogram matched with phases of the ventricular action potential. Phase 0: Rapid depolarization. Phase 1: Early repolarization. Phase 2: Plateau phase (delayed repolarization). Phase 3: Terminal rapid repolarization. Phase 4: Resting phase.

- Pericarditis.
- Early repolarization.
- Brugada syndrome.
- Arrhythmogenic right ventricular cardiomyopathy.
- Hypothermia.
- Acute pulmonary embolus.
- Hyperkalemia.
- Hypercalcemia.

Secondary ST segment elevation unrelated to acute STEMI is characteristically seen with the following:

- Left bundle branch block.
- Pacemaker depolarization.
- Ectopic ventricular complexes.
- Preexcitation.
- Left ventricular enlargement/hypertrophy.

Pericarditis

Acute pericarditis is an inflammation of the pericardium. Causes include infections (viral, bacterial, mycobacterial, fungal), neoplasia (commonly metastatic), connective tissue diseases (lupus, rheumatoid arthritis), trauma, acute myocardial infarction, post cardiac surgery, and idiopathic. The process directly involves the epicardium and surrounding tissue, resulting in the deposition of inflammatory cells and fluids within the pericardial sac. Both pericarditis and acute myocardial infarction may cause clinical symptoms of chest discomfort and ECG findings of ST segment elevation. This often presents the clinician with a difficult diagnostic dilemma.

The characteristic ECG finding of acute pericarditis is upsloping ST segment elevation, whereas in acute MI the ST segment elevation is typically shaped like a dome. Recall in Chapter 10 that we described the ST segment elevation configuration of pericarditis as a "smile" and that of acute MI as a "frown" (**Figure 11-3**). Another helpful clue is that pericarditis usually involves the entire pericardial surface, so you will find ST segment elevation in most, if not all of the leads except aVR and V1 (**Figure 11-4**). By

comparison, acute MI causes ST segment elevation in the contiguous leads that face a region of myocardial necrosis, with ST segment depression often noted in reciprocal leads (see Chapter 10). Pericarditis also involves the atria, resulting in early, transient PR segment elevation in lead aVR, with PR segment depression in other leads. Over a variable period of time, the diffuse ST segment elevation of acute pericarditis resolves, typically followed by T wave inversion that eventually normalizes. Unlike myocardial infarction, diagnostic Q waves do not appear.

 CLINICAL TIP: There are clinical clues to help you differentiate the chest symptoms of acute myocardial infarction from pericarditis. Symptoms of pericarditis are usually more sharp and stabbing than those of acute coronary syndromes, which are typically dull and heavy. Pericardial symptoms are *pleuritic*, meaning they are provoked by inspiration or coughing. The discomfort of acute pericarditis is usually eased by sitting up and made worse by lying supine, whereas ischemic symptoms are unaffected by position. A characteristic auscultative finding is a *friction rub*, a "Velcro-like" sound heard over the precordium. Echocardiography is a vital tool in differentiating acute STEMI from pericarditis. In acute STEMI, a localized wall motion abnormality is typically present that corresponds with the region of the coronary occlusion. In pericarditis, the echocardiogram demonstrates normal wall motion and may also show a pericardial effusion.

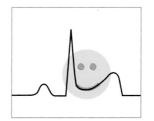 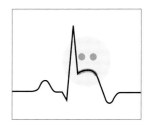

Figure 11-3. Pericarditis (left) typically displays an upsloping "smiling" ST segment whereas acute MI (right) demonstrates an ST segment described as "coved," "domed," or "frowning."

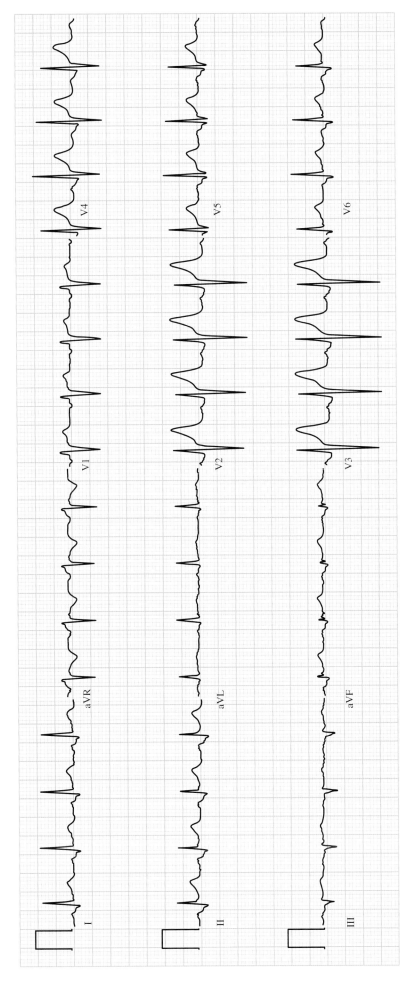

Figure 11-4. ECG of a patient with acute pericarditis. Note the diffuse, upsloping ST segment elevation. Also note the PR segment elevation in lead aVR with PR depression most prominent in leads I, II, aVF, V4-V6.

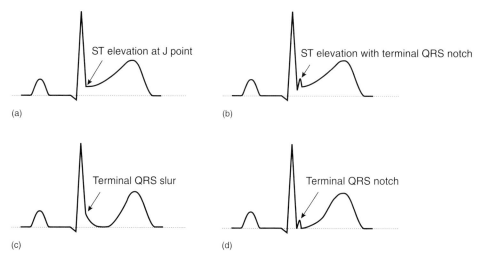

Figure 11-5. Early repolarization is characterized by any findings of J point elevation, an end terminal notch or a slur, which may occur alone or in combination. Examples include (a) ST segment elevation alone, (b) ST segment elevation with a notch, (c) End terminal slur, (d) End terminal notch without ST segment elevation.

Early Repolarization

ST segment elevation may also be present in the absence of clinical symptoms. Considered a variant of normal, asymptomatic early repolarization (ER) has been historically defined by a high J point takeoff that is accompanied by a rapidly upsloping ST segment. Some investigators have recommended that an end-QRS notch or slur is necessary to define the ER pattern, with or without ST segment elevation. The lack of a uniform definition for ER has led to considerable variation in the estimated prevalence of this ECG finding with reports ranging from 1 to 18% of the population. It is most commonly seen in young men (age <40 years), athletes, and individuals of African-American heritage.

The lack of consensus among respected authorities regarding ER doesn't make things easy for the clinical electrocardiographer. But worry not, because I'm going to give you some tips to help you to make an accurate diagnosis. Let's start with some definitions.

- **Early repolarization pattern.** An umbrella term that refers to an asymptomatic patient who has an ECG containing *any* findings of abnormal ST segment elevation, a terminal QRS slur, or notch.
- **Abnormal ST segment elevation.** Defined as ≥1 mm elevation at the J point in two or more contiguous leads. In leads V2 and V3 the criteria for abnormal ST elevation is ≥2 mm in men and ≥1.5 mm in women.

- **Terminal QRS notch.** A low-frequency deflection at the end of the QRS complex. This is distinguished from notching midway or higher on the QRS downslope that may reflect a fragmented QRS complex (see Chapter 10).
- **Terminal QRS slur.** An abrupt change in the slope of the QRS complex as it merges with the ST segment. The slur should appear in the final 50% of the QRS complex.
- **J point.** The position where the QRS complex ends and the ST segment begins. When the J point initiates a notch, some authorities propose separating the J point into the *J onset, J peak,* and *J termination.*
- **J wave.** Refers to any terminal QRS notch or slur. It is best to use a specific description of these findings rather than this catchall term.

You are going to encounter varying forms of the ER pattern (**Figure 11-5**). This will include ST segment elevation with different morphologies, with or without a variety of QRS complex notches and slurs. Most will demonstrate a "smiling" pattern, which resembles that found in acute pericarditis. A helpful clue to differentiate the two entities is to measure the ratio of the amplitude of the ST segment at the J point versus that of the apex of the T wave (**Figure 11-6**). This measurement is preferably made in lead V6 (or V5), using the end of the PR segment as the baseline. Favoring a diagnosis of early repolarization

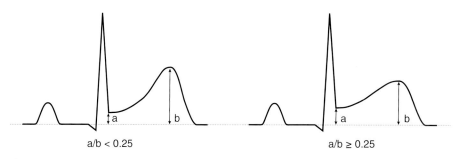

Figure 11-6. Early repolarization versus acute pericarditis. While looking similar, pericarditis is more likely if the J point amplitude is ≥25% of that of the T wave (right), whereas early repolarization is more likely if this ratio is <0.25 (left).

is if the height of the J point is less than 25% of the height of the T wave. With pericarditis, the J point is relatively higher with respect to the T wave, so the ratio is typically ≥0.25.

FOR BOOKWORMS: In the great majority of individuals the ER pattern is a normal variant with no clinical implications. A small subset however, may be at increased risk of lethal cardiac arrhythmias. The *early repolarization syndrome* refers to a patient with the ER pattern who survives idiopathic, ventricular fibrillation with no other explanation for the arrhythmia. Individuals potentially at greater risk are those with an elevated J point in the inferior limb leads, accompanied by a horizontal to downsloping ST segment. In contrast, a rapidly upsloping ST segment after the J point, particularly in the anterior precordial leads, predicts a benign prognosis. This is the most common pattern seen in young athletes.

Differential Diagnosis of the Common ST Elevation Syndromes (**Table 11-1**)

Before moving on, it's worthwhile to review the three most common ECG diagnoses for primary ST segment elevation, namely acute STEMI, pericarditis, and early repolarization. You are going to encounter many patients with symptoms of chest discomfort and ST segment abnormalities, so mastering the findings of each diagnosis is a must. In all cases, make every effort to obtain some clinical information and a previous tracing for comparison.

ST elevation myocardial infarction is characterized by:

- ST segment elevation that is horizontal to downsloping with a pattern described as frowning, domed, or coved.
- ST segment elevation localized to contiguous leads that correspond to the territory supplied by a specific coronary artery (see Chapter 10).
- Reciprocal ST segment depression in contiguous leads that are a mirror image to those with ST elevation.
- Associated T wave abnormalities (early, peaked T waves and later, inverted T waves).

Pericarditis is characterized by:

- ST segment elevation that is horizontal to upsloping with a pattern described as smiling or concave upward.
- ST segment elevation that is diffuse, typically present in all leads except V1 and aVR.

- Early, PR segment elevation may be seen in lead aVR. (PR segment depression in other leads).
- J point/T wave ratio in lead V6 of ≥0.25.

Early repolarization is characterized by:

- ST segment elevation that is typically upsloping, but may be either horizontal or downsloping.
- ST segment elevation that is present in at least two contiguous leads. Common patterns include findings in the anterior precordial leads (V1-V3), the lateral leads (I, aVL, V4-V6) and inferior leads (II, III, aVF), which may appear alone or together.
- A notch or slur in the terminal portion of the QRS complex.
- J point/T wave ratio in lead V6 of <0.25.

The Brugada ECG

The Brugada ECG pattern refers to a QRS complex that resembles a right bundle branch block with an unusual form of ST segment elevation in the right precordial leads (V1 and V2). The *Brugada syndrome* refers to a genetic disorder associated with an increased risk of sudden arrhythmic death in patients who have structurally normal hearts with ECG findings of the Brugada pattern.

Two distinct electrocardiographic Brugada patterns are recognized (**Figure 11-7**). Type 1 is characterized by coved ST segment elevation of ≥2 mm followed by a negative T wave. This is the pattern typically associated with the Brugada syndrome. Type 2 has ST segment elevation of ≥2 mm shaped like a "saddleback" followed by a positive or biphasic T wave. This pattern is not generally associated with sudden cardiac death.

FOR BOOKWORMS: A confounding factor in making this diagnosis is that both types of Brugada patterns can change over time and may be revealed only when the patient is exposed to certain medications, particularly sodium channel blockers (eg, flecainide). The Brugada ECG may be difficult to differentiate from early repolarization and forms of right bundle branch block. There is active research on this topic and I advise the interested reader to review the references at the end of the chapter.

TABLE 11-1	Comparison of ST Elevation Syndromes[a]		
ECG Finding	**Acute MI**	**Pericarditis**	**Early Repolarization**
ST segment shape	Coved (frowning)	Upsloping (smiling)	Upsloping (smiling)
ST elevation location	Corresponds to coronary anatomy	Diffuse (except leads aVR and V1)	Precordial leads
Reciprocal changes	Often present	Absent	Absent
PR segment abnormalities	Absent	PR depression (PR elevation aVR)	Absent
ST/T wave amplitude ratio	Not applicable	≥0.25	<0.25
Evolutionary ST-T wave changes	Yes	Yes	No
Additional findings	Q waves develop	May show PR elevation in lead aVR	QRS may display a terminal notch or slur

[a]*Typical findings listed.*

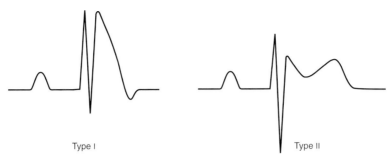

Type I   Type II

Figure 11-7. Brugada ECG pattern, types I and II.

Arrhythmogenic Right Ventricular Cardiomyopathy

Arrhythmogenic right ventricular cardiomyopathy (ARVC) is a genetic disorder characterized by fibrofatty infiltration of the right ventricle that predisposes an individual to ventricular tachyarrhythmias and sudden cardiac death. Like the Brugada pattern, patients with ARVC characteristically have an ECG with an atypical right precordial conduction delay, although the degree of ST segment elevation is comparatively less or may be entirely absent (**Figure 11-8**). T wave inversion in leads V1-V4 may be present. An important diagnostic clue to this condition is the presence of *epsilon waves*, which is an extra notch at the end of the QRS complex or early portion of the ST segment, most commonly seen in leads V1-V3.

Hypothermia

A characteristic ECG feature of profound hypothermia is the *Osborn wave*. Described by Joseph Osborn in 1953, this J wave deflection is seen in approximately 80% of patients with a core temperature of 30°C or less. It is described as a "dome" or "hump" at the end of the QRS complex and may resemble the ST segment elevation of acute MI (**Figure 11-9**). Additional ECG manifestations of hypothermia include shivering artifacts, PR interval prolongation, QT interval prolongation, and marked bradycardia.

Acute Pulmonary Embolus

Even in the presence of a major pulmonary embolus (PE), the ECG is neither a sensitive nor specific indicator of the diagnosis. Rarely, massive PE is associated with transient ST segment elevation, particularly in leads III, aVR, and V1, likely due to acute right heart ischemia. When present, the ECG findings of acute PE are likely to be those other than ST segment elevation (see following discussion).

Hyperkalemia

Moderately elevated potassium may cause ST segment elevation and a pseudoinfarction pattern. This is usually associated with increased T wave amplitude with a peaked, symmetrical "tented" configuration (**Figure 11-10**). Progressive elevations of serum potassium results in QRS prolongation and reduction in P wave amplitude.

Hypercalcemia

Elevated serum calcium reduces the duration of the action potential and characteristically shortens the QT interval. ST segment elevation as well as notching of the terminal portion of the QRS complex may also occur (**Figure 11-11**).

Left Bundle Branch Block

ST segment elevation is a common feature of left bundle branch block. Recall from Chapter 8 that the alteration of depolarization from the conduction delay induces a secondary change in repolarization. The ST segment elevation is prominent in leads with a negative QRS complex, typically V1-V3 (**Figure 11-12**).

Right bundle branch block rarely produces ST segment elevation, but this may occasionally be seen in the inferior leads in the presence of a negative QRS complex.

Ventricular Pacemaker Depolarization and Ectopic Ventricular Complexes

A pacemaker inserted into the right ventricle depolarizes the ventricle with a left bundle branch pattern. This is akin to an "artificial LBBB" as the right ventricle is depolarized first, followed by myocyte-to-myocyte transmission to the remainder of the myocardium. Like LBBB, the alteration of depolarization leads to secondary changes in repolarization with ST segment

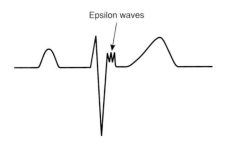

Epsilon waves

Figure 11-8. Arrhythmogenic right ventricular cardiomyopathy. Epsilon waves (arrow) are a specific, but not a sensitive finding.

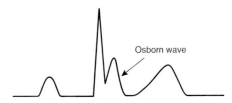

Osborn wave

Figure 11-9. Osborn wave (arrow) of hypothermia.

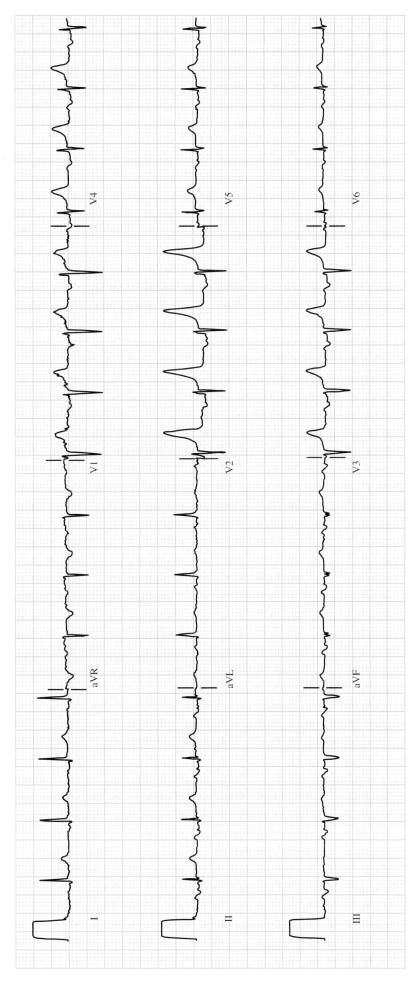

Figure 11-10. Hyperkalemia characteristically causes peaking of the T wave and may also elevate the ST segment, the degree of which depends on the potassium level. Note the tall, "tent shaped" T waves evident in leads V1–V4. ST segment elevation is most prominent in leads V2–V3.

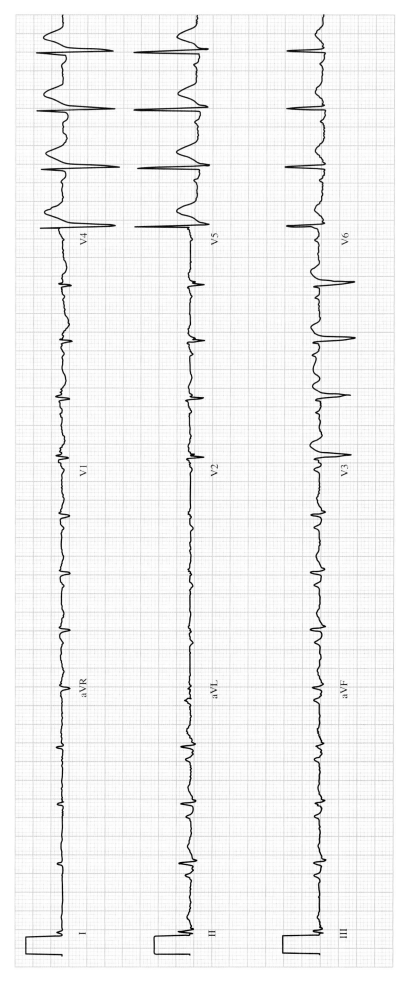

Figure 11-11. Hypercalcemia shortens the QT interval and may cause ST segment elevation (seen here in lead V3).

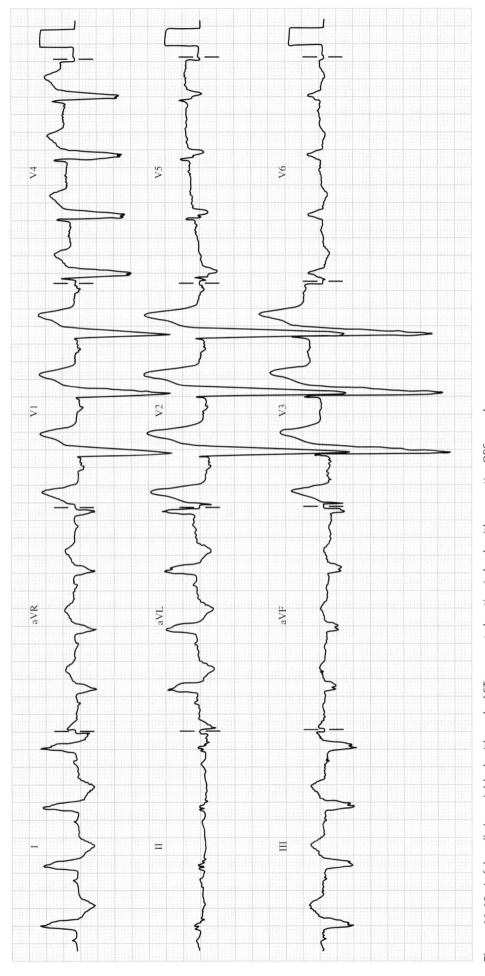

Figure 11-12. Left bundle branch block with marked ST segment elevation in leads with a negative QRS complex.

elevation typically seen in leads with a negative QRS deflection (**Figure 11-13**).

Ectopic ventricular complexes and spontaneous ventricular rhythms will show similar ECG behavior. Leads with a negatively deflected QRS complex may display ST segment elevation.

Preexcitation

Conduction over an atrioventricular bypass connection produces secondary ST segment changes (**Figure 11-14**). Similar to the situation with bundle branch blocks, the alteration of depolarization induces secondary changes in repolarization that may be recorded as ST segment elevation in some leads. Note, however, that ST segment depression and T wave inversion is the more common finding (see following discussion).

Left Ventricular Enlargement/Hypertrophy

Left ventricle enlargement produces predominantly secondary repolarization abnormalities. Recall from Chapter 7 that the increased mass of the left ventricle causes depolarization to be delayed to such a degree that the sequence of repolarization is also altered. ST segment elevation may be present in leads with a deeply negative QRS complex, typically V1 and V2. ST segment depression and T wave inversion may be noted in leads with a tall QRS complex, historically termed the "*left ventricular strain*" pattern (**Figure 11-15**).

▶ NON-ST ELEVATION INFARCTION IMITATORS

There is considerable urgency in correctly identifying an acute STEMI, which is why it is the main focus of this chapter. But we also learned in Chapter 10 that acute STEMI is only one manifestation of coronary artery disease. Unstable angina and other coronary syndromes can produce ST segment depression and T wave inversion, alone or in combination. Similar to the situation with ST segment elevation, there are many conditions unrelated to ischemic heart disease that result in ST segment depression and T wave inversion. Again, these changes may be either primary repolarization alterations or are secondary to depolarization abnormalities. We've already discussed the evaluation of the ST segment, so let's now take the same approach with the T wave.

The Normal and Abnormal T Wave

We learned in Chapter 4 that the T wave represents the continuation of ventricular repolarization (phase 3) (see Figure 11-2). We measure the amplitude of an upright T wave from the upper level of the baseline to the peak of the wave and inverted T waves from the lower level of the baseline to the nadir of the wave. The T wave amplitude should not exceed 6 mm in the limb leads or 10 mm in the precordial leads.

The normal T wave configuration is rounded, smooth, and slightly asymmetric, with the terminal portion exhibiting a steeper downslope. The axis of the T wave parallels that of a normal QRS complex in that lead, usually within 45 degrees of the QRS axis in the frontal plane. Accordingly, leads that

contain a tall R wave will also have an upright T wave. Similarly, leads with a deep S wave will normally have an inverted T wave. In the horizontal plane, the T wave is normally upright in leads V2-V6, and may be either upright or inverted in lead V1.

T wave abnormalities may be characterized by abnormal direction, amplitude, and morphology. The shape of the T wave may be described as peaked, symmetrical, biphasic, flat, or inverted. Ischemic T waves are characteristically deep, symmetrical, and opposite in polarity (>45 degrees) to the main axis of the QRS complex.

OK, now that we've reviewed the T wave, let's go into more detail on imitators of non-STEMI coronary syndromes. ST segment depression and/or T wave inversion may be seen with the following:

- Hypokalemia.
- Digitalis effect.
- RBBB and LBBB.
- Preexcitation.
- Ventricular enlargement/hypertrophy.
- Hypertrophic cardiomyopathy, particularly the apical form.
- Cerebral vascular accidents.
- Juvenile T wave pattern.
- "Memory" T wave inversion.
- Idiopathic global T wave inversion.
- Acute pulmonary embolus.
- Hyperventilation.
- Nonspecific ST segment and T wave abnormalities.

Hypokalemia (**Figure 11-16**) and digitalis (**Figure 11-17**) cause ST segment depression and T wave flattening via primary alterations of repolarization. In contrast, right bundle branch block (**Figure 11-18**), left bundle branch block (see Figure 11-12), preexcitation (see Figure 11-14), and ventricular enlargement (see Figure 11-15) all cause secondary alterations in repolarization that result in ST segment depression and T wave inversion. These findings are discordant to the QRS complex, meaning that the direction of the ST segment depression and T wave inversion is opposite in polarity to the QRS complex.

Marked, diffuse primary T wave inversion may be seen in patients with cerebral vascular accidents, particularly subarachnoid hemorrhage (**Figure 11-19**). Inverted T waves are commonly seen in patients with hypertrophic cardiomyopathy, particularly the apical form. Nonspecific T wave inversion may be present in patients with acute cholecystitis, perforated peptic ulcer, and pancreatitis.

So-called "memory" T wave inversion may be seen after ventricular pacing, transient left bundle branch block, or following a ventricular premature complex.

The persistent juvenile pattern is characterized by T wave inversion in leads V1-V3 in an adult with no other abnormality (**Figure 11-20**). Early in life, T waves are normally inverted across the right and mid-precordial leads. These become upright over time with the exception of lead V1, where T wave inversion may be normally seen.

Rarely, global T wave inversion is present without identifiable case. Interestingly, the amplitude of the T wave inversions can be striking.

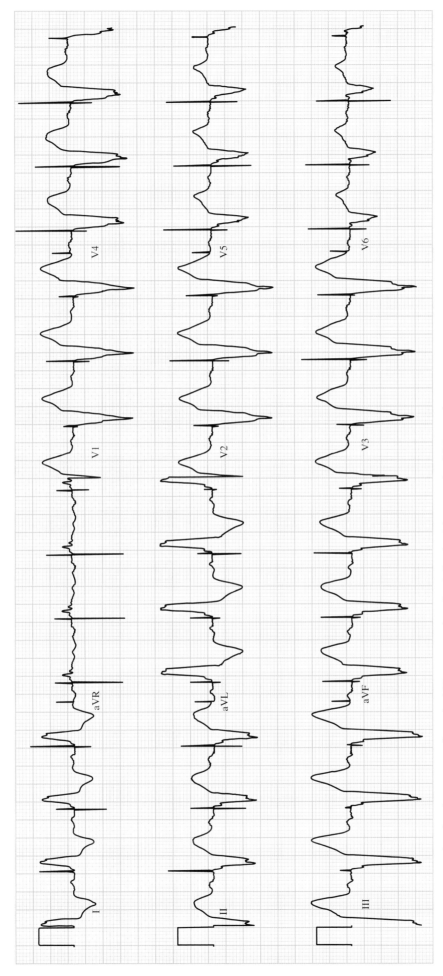

Figure 11-13. Pacemaker depolarization with marked ST segment elevation in leads with a negative QRS complex.

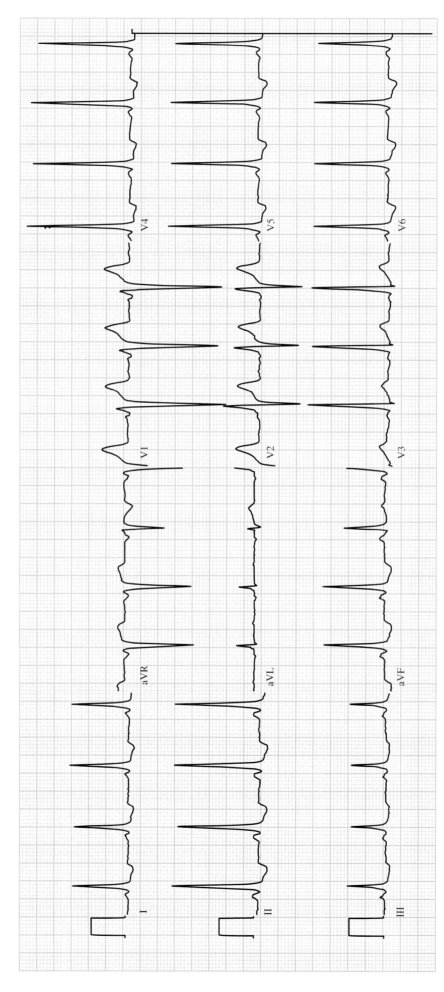

Figure 11-14. Preexcitation via an atrioventricular bypass connection characteristically displays a delta wave with QRS complex prolongation and secondary repolarization findings of ST segment depression and T wave inversion. In some leads, ST segment elevation may be present, seen here in leads V1 and V2.

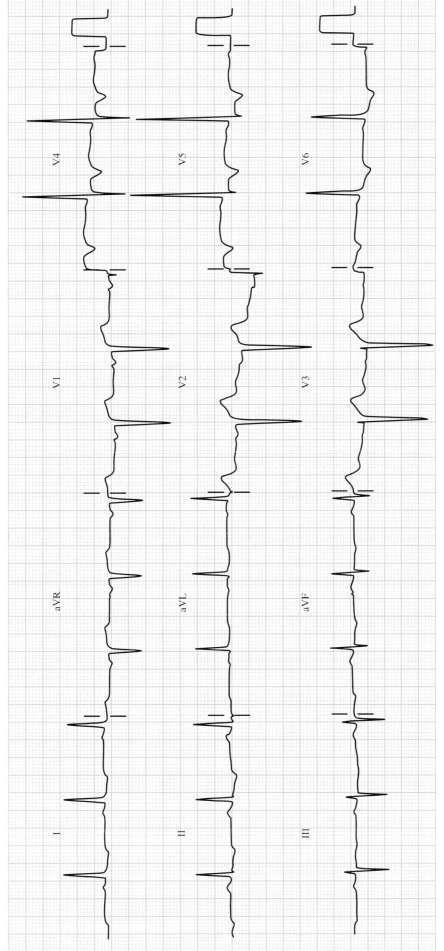

Figure 11-15. Left ventricular enlargement increases QRS voltage with typical findings of ST segment depression and T wave inversion. ST segment elevation may be present in some leads with a negative QRS deflection, seen here in leads V1-V3.

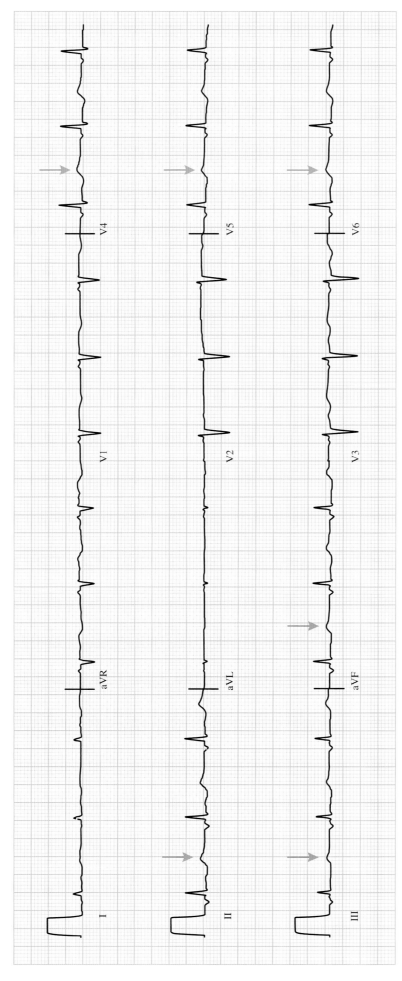

Figure 11-16. Hypokalemia produces ST segment depression, flat or inverted T waves, and prominent U waves (arrows). The ECG findings depend on the degree of potassium reduction. (In this example an AV junctional rhythm is present.)

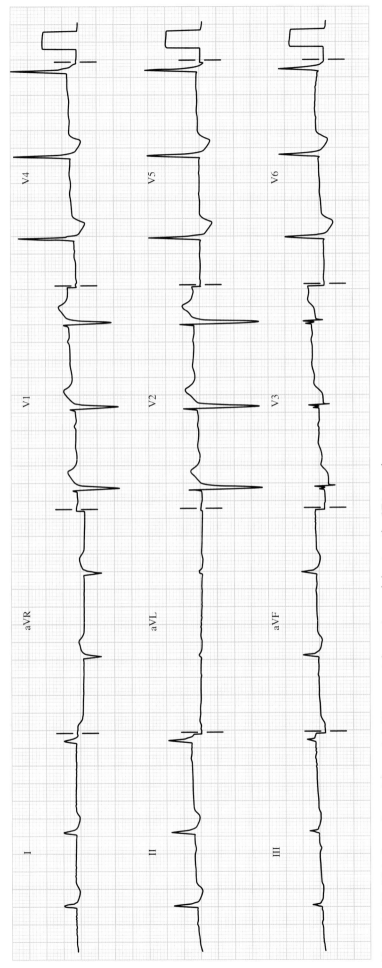

Figure 11-17. Digitalis produces characteristic ST segment depression and shortens the QT interval.

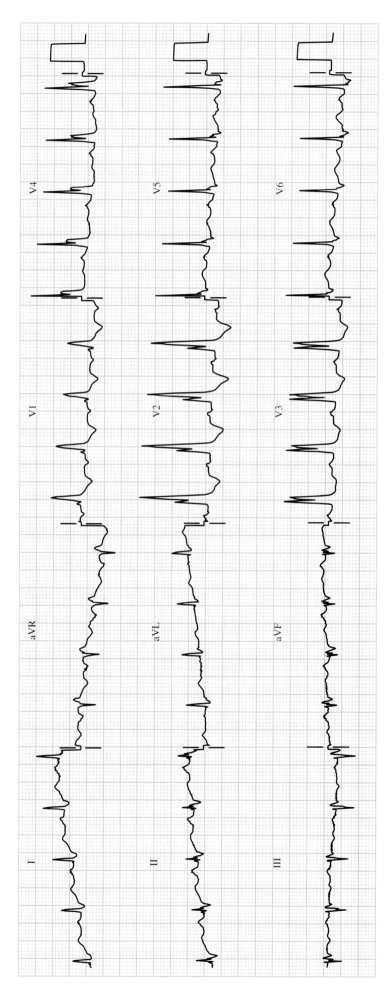

Figure 11-18. Right bundle branch block produces secondary ST segment depression and T wave inversion in the right precordial leads that display the conduction delay, seen here in leads V1-V3.

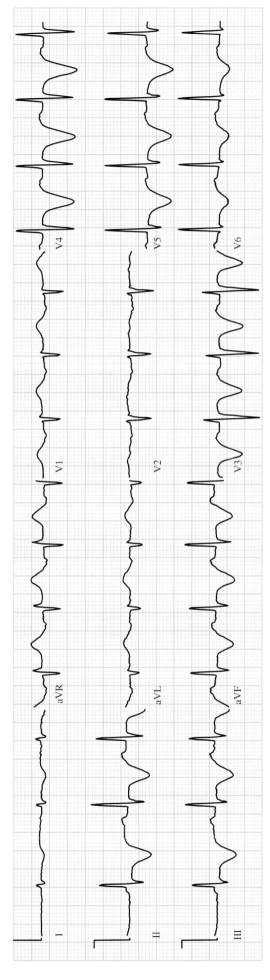

Figure 11-19. Diffuse T wave inversion seen in a patient with acute cerebral hemorrhage.

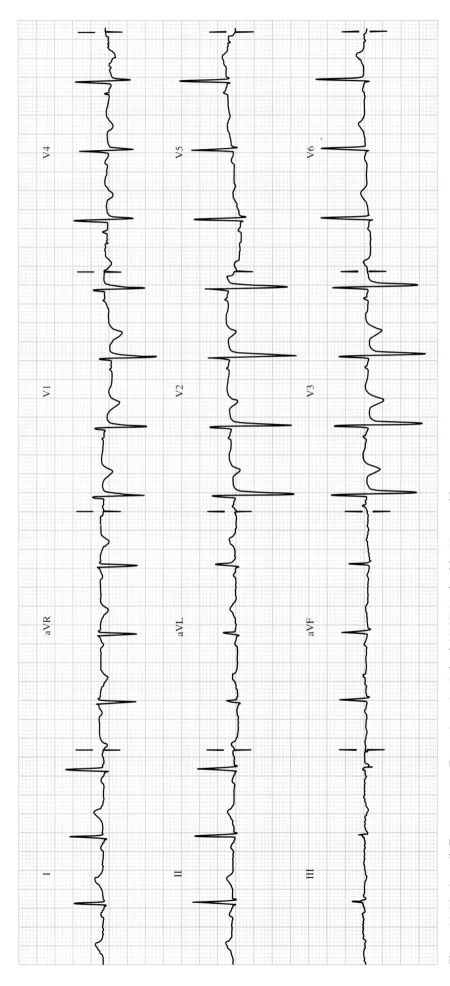

Figure 11-20. Juvenile T wave pattern. T wave inversion in leads V1-V4 in a healthy 29-year-old woman.

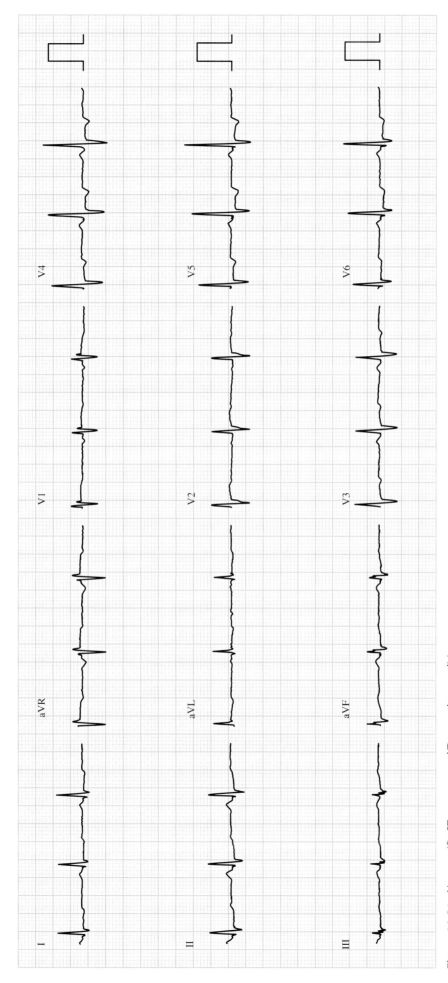

Figure 11-21. Nonspecific ST segment and T wave abnormalities.

Acute pulmonary embolus is more likely to present with ECG findings suggestive of non-STEMI than STEMI. The most common ECG findings include sinus tachycardia and T wave inversion, which may be present in leads III and aVF or the anterior precordial leads (V1-V4). Acute right ventricular pressure overload may induce a rightward axis shift that results in an S wave in lead I and a Q wave in lead III. Other findings that have been associated with pulmonary embolus include either right or left axis deviation as well as a complete or incomplete RBBB. The variety of ECG findings associated with PE makes for difficult decision-making because these patients typically present with chest discomfort and shortness of breath, symptoms also compatible with coronary disease.

T wave inversion may be noted in approximately 10% of healthy adults after 10 to 15 seconds of hyperventilation. After 30 to 60 seconds of hyperventilation the percentage rises to approximately 70%. The mechanism is postulated to involve acid-base and potassium shifts that are induced by the ventilation-induced respiratory alkalosis.

Nonspecific ST segment and T wave abnormalities are frequent findings on the ECG. Simply put, these are minor displacements of the ST segment and alterations of either the amplitude or morphology of the T wave that are not diagnostic of a specific clinical condition (**Figure 11-21**). When present, you should simply comment on the findings and compare them to any previous tracings that are available. Although nonspecific, these seemingly minor ST segment and T wave abnormalities may have prognostic implications, as research indicates a higher incidence of coronary artery disease in patients with these findings.

 BE CAREFUL: If there is no previous tracing for comparison, I recommend you use the term nonspecific ST segment and T wave *abnormalities* to describe the findings. If the findings are *different* from a prior tracing, then it's appropriate to use the term nonspecific ST segment and T wave *changes,* making sure to identify the variances.

▶ SUMMING UP

Making a correct diagnosis of acute STEMI and non-ST elevation coronary syndromes is one of the most important ECG skills you will need to master. This task is made more difficult by the many chameleons that may pose obstacles in your way. You do have the tools at your disposal to help with your decision-making. Always remember to compare the current ECG with any available prior tracing. And even the most skilled electrocardiographer will never fail to take a thorough history, perform a careful physical examination, and review pertinent laboratory data before beginning therapy.

Chapter 11 • SELF-TEST

QUESTIONS

1. Define abnormal ST segment elevation.

2. List at least three causes of ST segment elevation unrelated to acute myocardial infarction due to primary abnormalities of repolarization.

3. List at least three causes of ST segment elevation unrelated to acute myocardial infarction due to secondary abnormalities of repolarization.

4. Describe at least two ECG findings of acute pericarditis.

5. In broad terms, define early repolarization.

6. Describe ECG findings that can be used to differentiate acute pericarditis from acute myocardial infarction.

7. Describe ECG findings that can be used to differentiate acute pericarditis from early repolarization.

8. Describe the characteristic morphology of the "Osborn wave," a finding associated with what condition?

9. Describe the ECG findings of moderate hyperkalemia.

10. ST depression and a prominent U wave are characteristic of what electrolyte abnormality?

11. Hypercalcemia produces what findings on the ECG?

12. Describe the normal T wave.

13. Describe the typical findings of ischemia-induced T wave abnormalities.

14. List at least three ECG diagnoses that characteristically have T wave abnormalities due to secondary alterations of repolarization.

15. What is the persistent juvenile T wave pattern?

16. Define nonspecific ST segment and T wave abnormalities.

ANSWERS

Chapter 11 • SELF-TEST

1. Abnormal ST segment elevation is defined as ≥1 mm elevation at the J point in two or more contiguous leads. In leads V2 and V3 the criteria for abnormal ST segment elevation are ≥2 mm in men and ≥1.5 mm in women.

2. • Pericarditis.
   • Early repolarization.
   • Brugada syndrome.
   • See the chapter for other choices.

3. • Left ventricular enlargement.
   • Bundle branch block.
   • Preexcitation.
   • See the chapter for other choices.

4. • Diffuse, upsloping ST segment elevation.
   • PR segment elevation in aVR (PR depression in other leads).

5. An asymptomatic patient with any ECG findings of abnormal ST segment elevation, a terminal QRS slur, or notch.

6. • Pericarditis: Diffuse, upsloping ST segment elevation without reciprocal ST depression. PR segment elevation in lead aVR with PR depression in other leads.
   • Acute MI: Domed (coved) ST segment elevation in contiguous leads corresponding to the coronary circulation with ST depression in reciprocal leads.

7. • Pericarditis: Relatively higher ST segment elevation amplitude that is ≥25% of the T wave amplitude.
   • Early repolarization: Relatively lower ST elevation amplitude that is <25% of the T wave amplitude.

8. The Osborn wave is a "hump" found at the end of the QRS complex that is associated with hypothermia.

9. Peaked, symmetrical, "tented" T waves, and sometimes, associated ST segment elevation.

10. Hypokalemia.

11. QT interval shortening. ST segment elevation may also occur.

12. The normal T wave configuration is rounded, smooth, and slightly asymmetric, with the terminal portion exhibiting a steeper downslope. The axis of the T wave parallels that of a normal QRS complex in that lead, usually within 45 degrees of the QRS axis in the frontal plane.

13. Ischemic T waves are characteristically deep, symmetrical, and opposite in polarity (>45 degrees) to the main axis of the QRS complex.

14. • Right and left bundle branch block.
    • Preexcitation.
    • Ventricular enlargement.

15. T wave inversion in leads V1-V3 in an adult with no other abnormality.

16. Nonspecific ST segment and T wave abnormalities are minor displacements of the ST segment and alterations of either the amplitude or morphology of the T wave that are not diagnostic of a specific clinical condition.

Further Reading

Antzelevitch C, Brugada P, Borggrefe M, et al. Brugada syndrome: report of the second consensus conference. *Circulation.* 2005;111:659-670.

Antzelevitch C, Yan G-X, Viskin S. Rationale for the use of the terms J-wave syndromes and early repolarization. *J Am Coll Cardiol.* 2011;57:1587-1590.

Bayes de Luna A, Brugada J, Baranchuk A, et al. Current electrocardiographic criteria for diagnosis of Brugada pattern: a consensus report. *J Electrocardiol.* 2012;45:433-442.

Brady WJ. ST segment and T wave abnormalities not caused by acute coronary syndromes. *Emerg Clin N Am.* 2006;24:91-111.

Carrado D, Link MS, Calkins H. Arrhythmogenic right ventricular cardiomyopathy. *N Engl J Med.* 2017;376:61-72.

Digby GC, Kukla P, Zhan ZQ, et al. The value of electrocardiographic abnormalities in the prognosis of pulmonary embolism: a consensus paper. *Ann Noninvasive Electrocardiol.* 2015;20:207-223.

Ginzton LE, Laks MM. The differential diagnosis of acute pericarditis from the normal variant: new electrocardiographic criteria. *Circulation.* 1982;65:1004-1009.

Goldberger AL. ECG simulators of infarction. Part II. Pathophysiology and differential diagnosis of pseudo-infarction ST-T patterns. *PACE.* 1982;5:414-430.

Hanna EB, Glancy DL. ST-segment depression and T-wave inversion: classification, differential diagnosis, and caveats. *Cleve Clin J Med.* 2011;78:404-414.

Hanna EB, Glancy DL. ST-segment elevation: Differential diagnosis, caveats. *Cleve Clin J Med.* 2015;82:373-384.

Huang HD, Birnbaum Y. ST elevation: differentiation between ST elevation myocardial infarction and nonischemic ST elevation. *J Electrocardiol.* 2011;44:494e1-494e12.

Kumar A, Lloyd-Jones DM. Clinical significance of minor nonspecific ST-segment and T-wave abnormalities in asymptomatic subjects: a systematic review. *Cardiol Rev.* 2007;15:133-142.

Macfarlane PW, Antzelevitch C, Haissaguerre M, et al. The early repolarization pattern. *J Am Coll Cardiol.* 2015;66:470-477.

Malhotra A, Dhutia H, Gati S, et al. Anterior T-wave inversion in young white athletes and nonathletes. *J Am Coll Cardiol.* 2017;69:1-9.

Marcus FI, McKenna WJ, Sherrill D, et al. Diagnosis of arrhythmogenic right ventricular cardiomyopathy/dysplasia. *Circulation.* 2010;121:1533-1541.

Obeyesekere MN, Klein GJ, Nattel S, et al. A clinical approach to early repolarization. *Circulation.* 2013;127:1620-1629.

Osborn JJ. Experimental hypothermia: respiratory and blood pH changes in relation to cardiac function. *Am J Physiol.* 1953;175:389-398.

Patton KK, Ellinor PT, Ezekowitz M, et al. Electrocardiographic early repolarization. *Circulation.* 2016;133:1520-1529.

Rautaharju PM, Surawicz B, Gettes LS. AHA/ACCF/HRS recommendations for the standardization and interpretation of the electrocardiogram. Part IV: The ST segment, T and U waves, and the QT interval. *J Am Coll Cardiol.* 2009;53:982-991.

Serra G, Baranchuk A, Bayes de Luna A, et al. New electrocardiographic criteria to differentiate the type-2 Brugada pattern from electrocardiogram of healthy athletes with r′–wave in leads V1/V2. *Europace.* 2014;16:1639-1645.

Shopp JD, Stewart LK, Emmett TW, Kline JA. Findings from 12-lead electrocardiography that predict circulatory shock from pulmonary embolism: systemic review and meta-analysis. *Acad Emerg Med.* 2015;10:1127-1137.

Surawicz B, Macfarlane PW. Inappropriate and confusing electrocardiographic terms. *J Am Coll Cardiol.* 2011;57:1584-1586.

Ullman E, Brady WJ, Perron AD, Chan T, Mattu A. Electrocardiographic manifestations of pulmonary embolism. *Am J Emerg Med.* 2001;19:514-519.

Wang K, Asinger RW, Marriott HJL. ST-segment elevation in conditions other than acute myocardial infarction. *N Engl J Med.* 2003;349:2128-2135.

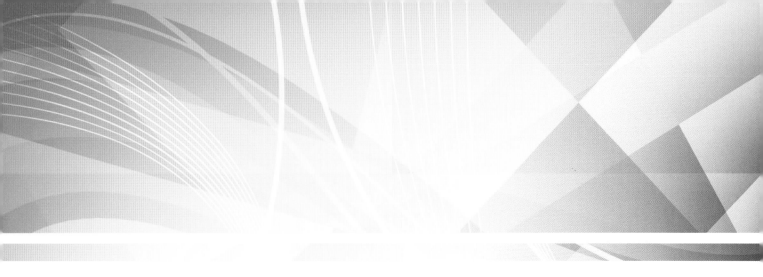

SECTION IV
The Cardiac Rhythms

Laddergrams

We're about to enter the wonderful and sometimes mysterious world of cardiac arrhythmias. This chapter will provide you with a technique to help remove some of the mystery. Ladder diagrams, also known as laddergrams, graphically represent the heart's electrical activity, showing the transmission throughout the cardiac chambers and conduction system. Do you remember when you first studied the rules of grammar, learning the technique of diagramming sentences to match the subject with the verb? Laddergrams are the ECG equivalent, using a diagram to illustrate the transmission of the electrical impulse from one chamber to another.

 FOR HISTORY BUFFS: Ladder diagrams actually predate the discovery of the ECG. Scientists August Chauveau in France, Theodore Engelmann in the Netherlands, Karl Wenckebach in Germany, and Thomas Mackenzie in England all used this technique to depict their clinical observations of cardiac arrhythmias. Thomas Lewis is credited with popularizing ladder diagrams in his classic, *The Mechanism of the Heart Beat*, published in 1911. Accordingly, some references use the term "Lewis diagram," or "Lewis lines" for this form of illustration.

▶ REVIEW OF ELECTROPHYSIOLOGY

Let's take a moment to review some of the material we described in Chapter 4 as it pertains to the construction of laddergrams. The normal cardiac impulse starts in the sinoatrial (SA) node and spreads through the atrial tissue via the interatrial and internodal bundles to the AV node. Transmission follows through the three regions of the AV node (atrionodal, nodal, nodal-His), continuing through the common bundle of His, the bundle branches, and the Purkinje network. These events comprise the PR interval. The electrical impulse now activates the ventricular fibers, which forms the basis of the QRS complex (**Figure 12-1**).

Remember that only some of the steps we just reviewed are visible on the surface ECG. Only the P wave, which represents depolarization of the atria, and the QRS complex, which reflects

the depolarization and early repolarization of the ventricular myocardium, are actually recorded by the ECG. Depolarization of the SA node is too small to be detected and the tracing remains at the baseline. Similarly, the ECG cannot record depolarization of the AV node, the His bundle, the bundle branches, and the Purkinje network, so these events can only be inferred. If that's the case, how do we really know what's going on in these regions of the cardiac conduction system?

Fortunately, we have techniques that allow us to accurately measure these hidden electrical steps. An *electrophysiologic study* (EPS) uses multipolar catheters that are inserted into the heart to record signals from multiple sites and measure electrical events that are not visible on the surface ECG. Recordings can be made of the sinus node discharge and SA conduction time, as well as measurements of the depolarization of the AV node, His bundle, bundle branches, and Purkinje fibers. *His bundle electrocardiography* is a very valuable technique that measures the **atrial-His (AH) interval**, which is an approximation of AV nodal conduction time, the His bundle deflection (**H**), and the **His-ventricular (HV) interval**, which reflects conduction through the His-Purkinje system (**Figure 12-2**). A laddergram can help us understand not only what we observe on the ECG, but also some of the sophisticated measurements made during an EPS.

 CLINICAL TIP: Determining the AH and HV interval can be critical in determining whether a patient with heart block requires a permanent pacemaker. A delay in conduction with prolongation of the HV interval indicates disease in the His-Purkinje system and a risk of life-threatening complete heart block. These patients routinely require a pacemaker. Prolongation of the AH interval is characteristically at the level of the AV node with a more benign prognosis. In normal subjects, the AH interval has a wide range (50-120 msec) and is markedly influenced by the autonomic nervous system. The normal HV interval has a narrow range (35-55 msec) and is not significantly affected by autonomic tone.

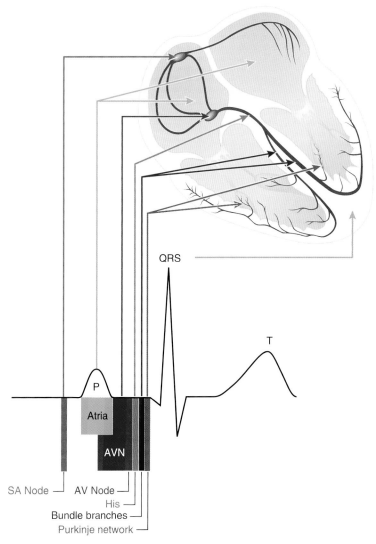

Figure 12-1. The specialized conduction system. Note that the surface ECG records only depolarization of the atria (P wave) and the ventricles (QRS complex). The tracing remains at the baseline during SA node depolarization and transmission through the AV node, bundle of His, bundle branches, and Purkinje network. (The AV node and bundle of His comprise the AV junction.)

Climbing Up and Down the Laddergram

Laddergrams can vary from simple to complex. Each tier of the laddergram represents a level of the cardiac conduction system, drawn as a horizontal line below the ECG (**Figure 12-3**). In its most basic form the laddergram has three levels: one for atrial activation (A), one for AV conduction (AV), and one for ventricular activation (V). We can add additional levels and subdivisions to describe findings of increasing complexity. Vertical or slanted lines are drawn within each level to illustrate transmission of the electrical impulse through the cardiac chambers and conduction system.

Constructing a laddergram is a three-step process. First, diagram what you see at the atrial level. Next, diagram what you see at the ventricular level. Finally, analyze the relationships between the two levels to infer what you cannot see and diagram the connections. Let's now use this method to construct a

basic laddergram and discuss some of the conventions we use for illustration.

Figure 12-3 shows a tracing with normal sinus rhythm. Notice that every P wave is followed by a QRS complex. Below we have drawn three tiers representing levels for the atria, AV conduction, and the ventricles. Steps one and two are to diagram what we see at the atrial and ventricular levels, so we draw a vertical line within the atrial tier below the onset of each P wave and another vertical line within the ventricular tier at the beginning of each QRS complex. Step three is to determine if there is a relationship between the P waves and QRS complexes, and if so, connect the two vertical lines. Here it looks like every P wave relates to a QRS complex, so we connect each atrial line to its corresponding ventricular line. We've now taken what we see on the ECG and graphically illustrated atrial depolarization (P wave), AV conduction

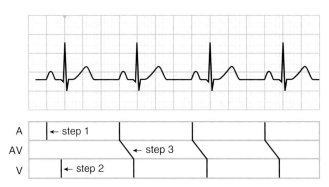

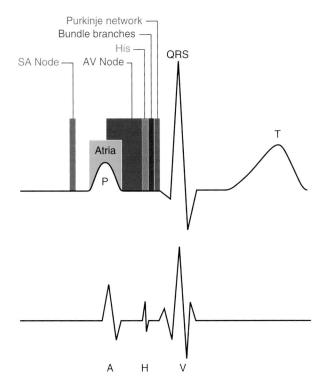

Figure 12-2. His bundle recording. The atrial-His (AH) interval is an approximation of the AV nodal conduction time. Conduction through the His-Purkinje system is estimated by the His-ventricular (HV) interval.

Figure 12-3. The basic laddergram contains three elements representing depolarization of the atria (A), AV conduction (AV), and ventricles (V). The three-step process involves (1) identifying the P waves, (2) identifying the QRS complexes, and (3) diagramming the relationship between the two elements.

(PR interval), and ventricular depolarization (QRS complex). That was easy!

We have a few different options to illustrate the same electrocardiographic process (**Figure 12-4**). The first complex of Figure 12-4 illustrates normal sinus rhythm using solid lines to represent depolarization of the atria, ventricles, and AV conduction. Depending on your style and illustration needs, other features can be added. You can add a dot to represent the site of origin (complex b). It's reasonable to place the dot at the top line, or even slightly above, to indicate that the depolarization actually started in a "higher" position in the conduction system than the atrial level we've depicted, namely the SA node.

If desired, place an arrow to show the direction of transmission (complex c). Depolarization of the cardiac chambers is not instantaneous, so it's technically most accurate to slightly slope the vertical lines below the P waves and QRS complexes to reflect the passage of time (complex d). Most people find it easier to draw the lines vertically and omit the slope (me too!). It's often helpful to indicate the timing intervals of the laddergram components in milliseconds (complexes e and f). You will see some authors indicate the intervals in hundredths of a second rather than milliseconds. All of these choices are acceptable and you can "mix and match" these options depending on what you are trying to illustrate.

We know that cardiac electrophysiology is far more complicated than what we just diagrammed with three levels, so how do we show additional detail? The answer is to add additional tiers to the laddergram to suit our needs. **Figure 12-5** illustrates normal sinus rhythm with an expanded laddergram that includes levels for the SA node depolarization, SA conduction time, the atria, AV conduction (divided further into AH, H, and HV tiers), and the ventricles. The expanded laddergram uses the same system as before, first drawing in what we can see, namely the P waves and QRS complexes. But this time we add more inferred items, namely the sinus node depolarization, SA conduction time, and the AH, H, and HV intervals. Remember

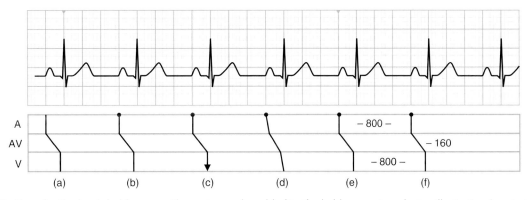

Figure 12-4. Options for the basic laddergram. Elements may be added to the laddergram to enhance illustration (see text for details).

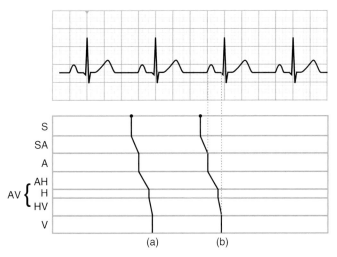

Figure 12-5. The expanded laddergram adds levels for the sinus node depolarization (S) and sinoatrial conduction time (SA), also dividing the AV conduction tier (AV) into the atrial-His (AH), His bundle, and His-ventricular (HV) intervals. The dotted lines in complex (b) refer to elements that comprise the PR interval.

that none of these inferred items are evident on the surface ECG and can be measured only in the electrophysiologic laboratory. In most cases, a simple laddergram with three tiers will suffice to illustrate the rhythm in question. But in some cases, the expanded laddergram will prove invaluable for helping you to understand the mechanism of the findings.

We now have the skills to diagram the path of a normal cardiac impulse as the depolarization travels from the sinus node to the ventricles. Oh, if life (and electrocardiography) were this easy. Cardiac arrhythmias, like the rules of grammar, have nuances and complexities, so we need some other tools to illustrate the mechanisms. Let's add some other items to our laddergram toolbox.

Illustrating the Site of Origin

Thus far we have shown examples of normal sinus rhythm, where the depolarization begins in the SA node and conducts normally to activate the ventricles. But as we know from previous chapters, the electrical impulse can originate from any other cell of the myocardium. Let's look at **Figure 12-6** to see how to illustrate those situations.

Laddergram (a) of Figure 12-6 illustrates a normal sinus complex. Panel (b) of this figure depicts a non-sinus depolarization

that originates within the atrial tissue. We indicate the atrial origin of the impulse with a dot placed within the atrial tier, rather than on the top line. Some authors use an asterisk (*) to highlight that this is an ectopic focus, but I prefer a simple dot. Laddergram (c) shows a complex that originates in the AV junction. The next panel (d) illustrates a complex of ventricular origin with transmission backward through the AV junction to the atrium. Some authors use a rectangle to illustrate the wide complexes originating from the ventricles, but again, I prefer the simplicity of a solid dot.

Illustrating Intracardiac Conduction

Both our simple and expanded laddergrams (see Figures 12-4 and 12-5) show the normal passage of the cardiac impulse from a "higher" chamber (eg, the sinus node or atria) to a "lower" chamber (eg, the ventricles). The lines illustrating this top-to-bottom process represent **antegrade conduction**. The transmission of cardiac impulses in health and disease is more complex than this, so we will need a variety of graphical options. At every step of the way, the electrical impulse can be modified, interrupted, or even reversed. Think of the depolarization as a traveler, determined to find his way from his departure point in the sinus node to his eventual destination in the ventricles. On the way he may find delays and obstacles; so let's take a look at the many potential fates of our intrepid voyager and how we should illustrate the journey (**Figure 12-7**).

Laddergram (a) of Figure 12-7 shows normal AV conduction. In panel (b) the slope in the AV junction is more gradual, indicating an **AV conduction delay**. In (c) AV transmission is **blocked**. Panel (d) illustrates options for depicting **aberrant conduction** where the QRS morphology is widened, a topic we will be exploring in later chapters. In each of these examples (a-d) conduction is antegrade.

The next two laddergrams (e and f) show examples of **retrograde conduction**, where a depolarization originating in the ventricle is transmitted *backwards* through the conduction system. In (e) the impulse originates in the ventricle and travels retrograde through the AV tier until depolarizing the atrial tissue. In (f) there is **retrograde block**, as the impulse fails to propagate through the AV junction. Accordingly, the atria fail to depolarize and a P wave is absent.

Both antegrade and retrograde conduction may occur simultaneously from the same focus, often at different speeds.

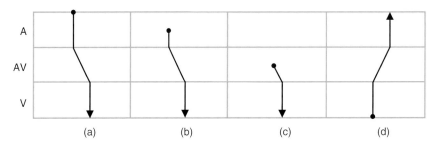

Figure 12-6. Site of impulse origin. A laddergram illustrating origin of the impulse: Sinus (a), atrial (b), AV junctional (c), and ventricular (d).

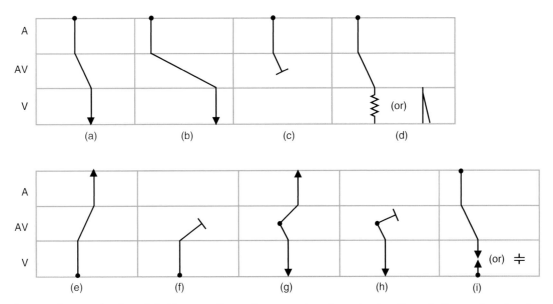

Figure 12-7. Intracardiac conduction. A laddergram illustrating examples of conduction through the cardiac chambers: Normal (a), delayed (b), blocked (c), aberrant (d), retrograde (e), blocked retrograde (f), combined antegrade and retrograde (g), normal antegrade with blocked retrograde (h), fusion of supraventricular and ventricular complexes (i).

Laddergram (g) shows an impulse originating in the AV junction with rapid antegrade conduction to the ventricle and relatively slower retrograde conduction to the atrium. The next panel shows an AV junctional complex with normal antegrade transmission, but blocked retrograde conduction. In this example, no P wave would be evident. Finally, laddergram (i) shows the concept of fusion, where depolarizations from two sites fire concurrently and the electrical impulses merge. I like to illustrate fusion as the meeting of two arrowheads, but you may also see this depicted as two horizontal lines.

 CLINICAL TIP: Fusion complexes most frequently occur in the ventricles, where a supraventricular focus competes with one of ventricular origin. In patients with

wide complex tachycardia of unclear origin, a fusion complex strongly suggests the arrhythmia is ventricular tachycardia.

***

More Nuts and Bolts

Sometimes it's helpful to use other tools to illustrate "virtual" electrical processes that are not visible on the surface ECG. **Figure 12-8** shows just such a situation where the normal sinus impulse is obscured by a ventricular premature complex. Remember back in Chapter 5 where we calculated the atrial rate by counting a P wave that we couldn't see (see Figure 5-7)? We can illustrate this on the laddergram with an open circle to represent the P wave buried within the QRS complex. Here, AV

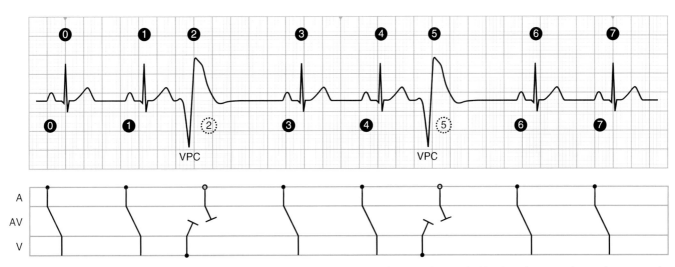

Figure 12-8. Virtual or hidden findings. An open dot can be used to illustrate findings that are hidden by other complexes. The ventricular premature complex hides the underlying sinus depolarization.

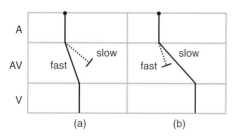

Figure 12-9. Dual AV nodal pathways. Illustration of two AV nodal pathways with different conduction properties.

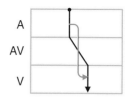

Figure 12-10. Preexcitation. The blue bracket represents transmission over an accessory pathway that directly connects the atrial and ventricular myocardium, bypassing the AV node. At the same time, the sinus impulse proceeds normally through the AV node and His-Purkinje system, which results in a hybrid QRS complex.

transmission from the atrial impulse is blocked because the AV junction and ventricles are rendered refractory by the premature ventricular depolarization.

Another tool is to use a dotted line to indicate the presence of a hidden conduction pathway. Such a situation may exist when there are *dual AV nodal pathways*. We're going to learn more about this when we discuss supraventricular tachycardia (SVT), but the laddergram illustration concept is introduced here. **Figure 12-9** shows a solid line through the AV tier to illustrate one pathway and a dotted line to indicate the presence of a second, hidden pathway. Note that the slope of the line is different for each pathway, reflecting differing conduction velocities. AV transmission may alternate between one pathway and another with the solid and dotted lines used accordingly to illustrate either the active or virtual pathway.

 CLINICAL TIP: Dual AV nodal pathways with different conduction velocities and refractory periods play an important role in the genesis of SVT. In many patients with SVT, an EPS with radiofrequency ablation is used to interrupt transmission in the slow pathway and eliminate the substrate for the arrhythmia.

In Chapter 9 we learned about *bypass connections* that allow transmission from the atria to the ventricles without passing through the AV node and the normal His-Purkinje system. In the WPW pattern, the impulse travels over *both* the accessory tract and through the AV node, eventually fusing within the ventricles to form a hybrid QRS complex (**Figure 12-10**).

Factoring in Refractory Periods

In Chapter 3 we spent considerable time discussing refractory periods of the conduction system. We don't usually depict

refractory periods on the laddergram, but doing so can prove useful to illustrate concepts of intracardiac conduction. Recall that after each depolarization the myocyte becomes temporarily refractory to further stimulation. Each component of the cardiac conduction system has different refractory properties. At each step, if the next impulse arrives during that cell's *effective refractory period* no further depolarization is possible and the impulse will be "blocked." If the impulse arrives during the *relative refractory period* the transmission through that fiber is altered and the impulse will be delayed. Let's go back to our traveling analogy and think of the refractory periods as parts of a stoplight. An impulse reaching an intersection within the conduction system must stop at a red light (effective refractory period), slow at a yellow light (relative refractory period), and is free to travel during a green light (no longer refractory and fully recovered).

 BE CAREFUL: Remember that many references interchange the terms *absolute refractory period* and *effective refractory period*. If a stimulus arrives during the absolute refractory period of the action potential *absolutely* nothing happens. The effective refractory period encompasses some additional time beyond the absolute refractory period when a new stimulus results in a weak, ineffective depolarization such that *effectively* nothing happens. In either case, the impulse will not propagate further through the conduction system, so for the purpose of this discussion the terms are equivalent.

Figure 12-11 illustrates the concept of refractory periods using pairs of supraventricular complexes. After each complex, the ability of a second supraventricular depolarization to conduct through the AV junction depends on whether it arrives during the effective refractory period (red), relative refractory

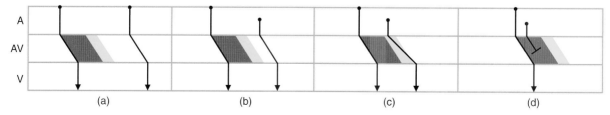

Figure 12-11. Refractory periods. Transmission of a premature depolarization depends on whether it arrives during the effective refractory period (red), relative refractory period (yellow), or after full recovery (see text for details).

TABLE 12-1	Key of Laddergram Symbols	
Symbol	**Representation**	**Comment**
●	Site of origin	For sinus origin, place at top of highest depicted level.
● (or) ✱	Ectopic site	For ventricular origin, place at bottom of ventricular level. For other non-sinus origin, place within appropriate tier.
○	Virtual (hidden) complex	
|	Atrial or ventricular conduction	May add arrows for clarification.
＼ (or) ↘	Antegrade conduction	Degree of slope indicates speed of conduction.
⅄	Blocked antegrade conduction	
／ (or) ↗	Retrograde conduction	Degree of slope indicates speed of conduction.
⅄	Blocked retrograde conduction	
⇕ (or) ⊢	Fusion	
⦚ (or) ∧	Aberrancy	
⁄ ˙ ˙ ⁀	Virtual (hidden) antegrade and retrograde conduction	
⦚	Atrioventricular bypass connection	Represents conduction via both the normal and accessory route.

period (yellow), or afterwards, when the cells are fully recovered. Panel (a) shows two normal sinus complexes with the refractory periods of the AV junction indicated with our stoplight colors. In panel (b) a premature complex originating in the atria arrives at the AV junction well beyond both refractory periods and the impulse conducts normally. Panel (c) shows an atrial premature complex arriving during the relative refractory period, causing AV conduction to be delayed. In panel (d) the premature supraventricular impulse is blocked because it

arrives during the effective refractory period when no further transmission is possible.

Remember that a laddergram is simply a tool to help you illustrate and better understand what you see on the surface ECG. You can mix and match different laddergram styles to suit your needs. You might even come up with a system that works better for you than what I've presented here. **Table 12-1** is a key of the laddergram symbols that you will see used throughout this book.

QUESTIONS

Chapter 12 • SELF-TEST

1. List the components of the specialized cardiac conduction system.
2. Depolarization of which structures are visible on the surface ECG?
3. Depolarization of which structures are hidden on the surface ECG?
4. Name the three-step process to construct a laddergram.
5. Depolarization that travels from a "higher" to a "lower" cardiac chamber is called _____.
6. Depolarization that travels from a "lower" to a "higher" cardiac chamber is called _____.
7. The cardiac impulse will be blocked if it reaches cells that are in what period of the action potential?
8. The cardiac impulse will be delayed if it reaches cells that are in what period of the action potential?

ANSWERS

Chapter 12 • SELF-TEST

1. The SA node, the interatrial and internodal bundles, the AV node, the bundle of His, the bundle branches (right and left), and the Purkinje fibers. (The AV node and bundle of His comprise the AV junction).
2. The atria and the ventricles.
3. The SA node, the AV node, the bundle of His, the bundle branches, the Purkinje fibers.
4. • Step one: Denote atrial depolarizations.
   • Step two: Denote ventricular depolarizations.
   • Step three: Analyze the relationship between the atrial and ventricular depolarizations and make the connections.
5. Antegrade conduction.
6. Retrograde conduction.
7. Effective refractory period.
8. Relative refractory period.

Further Reading

Friedman HH. *Diagnostic electrocardiography and vectorcardiography.* 3rd ed. New York, NY: McGraw-Hill; 1985:419-420.

Jacobson C. Tools for teaching arrhythmias: wide QRS beats and rhythms-part I; P waves, fusion, and capture beats. *AACN Adv Crit Care.* 2006;17:462-465.

Johnson JB, Chun SK. Arrhythmia conference. *JAMA.* 1969;61:362-364.

Johnson NP, Denes P. The ladder diagram (A 100+ year history). *Am J Cardiol.* 2008;101:1801-1804.

Mariott HJL, Conover MHB. *Advanced Concepts in Arrhythmias.* St. Louis, MO: Mosby; 1983: 167-189.

Shapiro, E. Engelmann and his laddergram. *Am J Cardiol.* 1977;39: 464-465.

Suazo NL. Laddergrams: A useful approach for analyzing complex rhythm disturbances. *Crit Care Update.* 1983;10:36-37.

Wagner GS. *Marriott's Practical Electrocardiography.* 11th ed. Philadelphia, PA: Wolters Kluwer/Lippincott Williams & Wilkins; 2008: 256-257.

Mechanisms of Arrhythmias

It's now time to begin our discussion of arrhythmias, one of the most important aspects of clinical electrocardiography. In the last chapter, we reviewed the fate of the normal sinus depolarization, using either a simple or expanded laddergram to illustrate passage of the impulse through the AV node and the remainder of the specialized conduction system until activating the ventricles (**Figure 13-1**). A cardiac arrhythmia may be defined as any disruption or aberration of this normal electrical sequence from start to finish.

 FOR HISTORY BUFFS: There has been some debate regarding the proper term to describe abnormalities of the cardiac rhythm—*arrhythmia* or *dysrhythmia*. The ancient Greek meaning of *rhythmos* is "proportion, order, or symmetry." Applying the prefix "*a*" indicates the *absence* of these characteristics. Therefore in the purest sense, the term arrhythmia means "no rhythm." Using the prefix *dys* suggests *ill, bad, or defective*. One may then conclude that dysrhythmia should be the preferred choice to describe an abnormality of the cardiac rhythm. However, arrhythmia has the benefit of widespread usage and tradition. I consider the terms interchangeable, so you have my permission to use whichever term you prefer.

▶ ACTION POTENTIAL REVIEW

In Chapter 3 we reviewed in detail the components of the action potential and the two different types of cardiac cells, pacemaker and nonpacemaker. Let's take another look to help us understand the mechanisms of arrhythmias.

In nonpacemaker cells the action potential is divided into five phases (0, 1, 2, 3, 4) (**Figure 13-2a**). Phase 0 represents rapid depolarization, which begins when an adjacent cell provides a stimulus that raises the membrane potential from a resting potential of –90 mV to the threshold potential of –60 mV to –70 mV. Phases 1, 2, and 3 represent repolarization and phase 4 is the resting phase between depolarizations. Nonpacemaker cells constitute the atrial and ventricular myocardium and

cannot normally initiate spontaneous depolarization without an outside stimulus.

In pacemaker cells the action potential has only three phases (0, 3, 4) (see **Figure 13-2b**). Pacemaker cells possess the property of **automaticity**, characterized by a phase 4 that slopes gradually upward from a maximum diastolic potential in the range of –60 mV until reaching the threshold potential of –30 mV to –40 mV, thereby *spontaneously* initiating depolarization. Pacemaker cells are present in the SA node, the primary pacemaker of the heart. Latent, subsidiary pacemakers are present in portions of the right atrium, the proximal and distal portions of the AV junction, and the remainder of the His-Purkinje system. These secondary pacemakers are normally inhibited due to *overdrive suppression* by the more rapid primary pacemaker activity of the SA node.

Figure 13-3 depicts the normal sequence of sinus rhythm, illustrating the representative action potentials as each area of

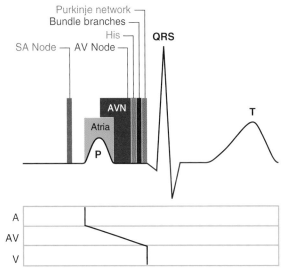

Figure 13-1. Laddergram depicting the normal sequence of conduction during sinus rhythm.

(a)

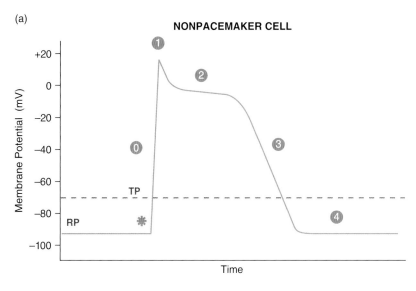

(b)

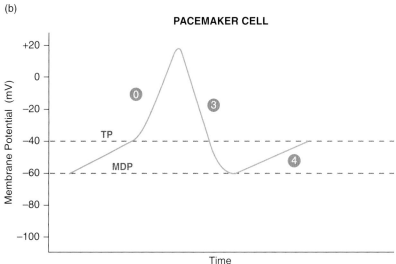

Figure 13-2. Action potential of a nonpacemaker cell (a) and pacemaker cell (b). A nonpacemaker cell requires an outside stimulus (*) to raise the membrane potential from the resting potential (RP) to the threshold potential (TP), thereby initiating depolarization (phase 0). Pacemaker cells have the property of automaticity, which intrinsically increases the voltage from the maximum diastolic potential (MDP) until reaching the threshold potential.

the heart is depolarized in turn. Temporary physiologic abnormalities (eg, electrolyte disturbance, myocardial ischemia, drug effect) or permanent injury (eg, myocardial infarction) may induce membrane changes and alterations in the action potential that result in cardiac arrhythmias.

▶ CLASSIFICATION OF ARRHYTHMIAS

There are a number of ways to classify cardiac arrhythmias. One way is according to their underlying mechanism, which may be broadly grouped into (1) disorders of impulse formation (automaticity and triggered activity), (2) disorders of impulse conduction (conduction delay and reentry), or (3) combinations of both (**Table 13-1**). We can also describe an arrhythmia based on the site of origin (supraventricular or ventricular), heart rate (tachycardia-fast or bradycardia-slow), discharge

type (premature, late, paroxysmal, fibrillation, and others), and AV relationship (heart block) (**Table 13-2**). These different descriptions have clinical utility and can be used either alone or in combination.

Disorders of Impulse Formation

Arrhythmias related to disorders of impulse formation are caused by two major factors (1) disordered automaticity and (2) triggered activity. Disordered automaticity is further subdivided into alterations of normal automatic mechanisms and those involving abnormal automaticity. Triggered activity refers to abnormal membrane oscillations called *afterdepolarizations* that are defined as either early or late according to where they fall within the action potential.

Disordered (altered) normal automaticity The normal rate of discharge of both dominant and latent pacemaker cells

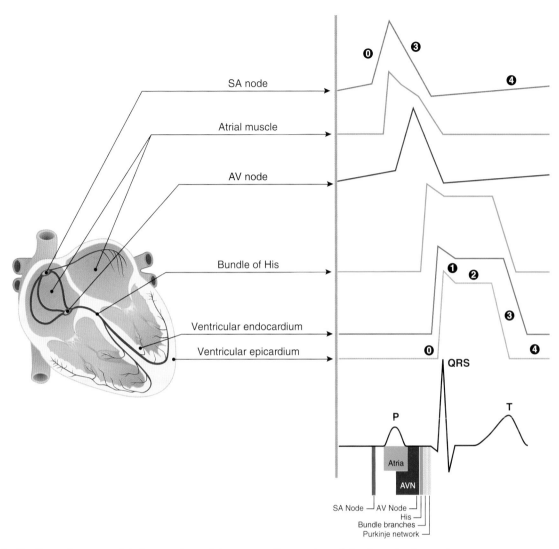

Figure 13-3. Cardiac action potentials from regions of the myocardium and specialized conduction system.

depends on three primary variables. These are (1) the slope of phase 4 diastolic depolarization, (2) the level of the maximum diastolic potential, and (3) the level of the threshold potential (**Figure 13-4**). Disordered "normal" automaticity typically reflects a change in the slope of phase 4, without other ionic disturbance of the action potential. This results in either a "hyper-automatic" (accelerated) or "hypo-automatic" (decelerated) alteration of the depolarization rate. For example, inappropriate sinus tachycardia or bradycardia reflects an alteration of the normal discharge of the SA node with a rate that is respectively either too fast or too slow relative to the physiologic requirement. Another example of disordered normal automaticity is an accelerated discharge of a latent pacemaker in the AV junction that overcomes the usual inhibition of overdrive suppression. Let's look at how this might occur.

Recall from Chapter 3 that both native and latent pacemaker cells are under the influence of the autonomic nervous system. Parasympathetic (vagal) effects decrease the slope of phase 4 of the SA node, which prolongs the time to reach the threshold potential, thereby slowing the heart rate (see **Figure 13-4a**). Contributing to a slower heart rate is that parasympathetic effects lower the maximum diastolic potential (more negative) and raise the threshold potential (more positive), both of which increase the time it takes to depolarize the cell (see **Figure 13-4b** and **c**). If the dominant pacemaker in the SA node is sufficiently suppressed, a subsidiary pacemaker lower in the conduction system hierarchy may emerge as an *escape complex*. Continued suppression of the dominant pacemaker may allow the subsidiary pacemaker to persist as an *escape rhythm*. These are examples of arrhythmias caused by depressed (hypo-automatic), but otherwise normal automaticity. In simple terms, phase 4 has been prolonged, but the remainder of the action potential remains unaffected.

Sympathetic catecholamines (epinephrine and norepinephrine) increase the slope of SA nodal phase 4 depolarization (**Figure 13-5a**). This reduces the time it takes to reach the threshold potential and raises the normal sinus rate, an effect opposite to that of parasympathetic influence (see **Figure 13-5b**). Contributing to a faster heart rate is that sympathetic stimulation lowers the threshold potential (more negative) toward the maximum diastolic potential, reducing the time it takes to depolarize the cell. High levels of catecholamines may also enhance the automaticity of a latent pacemaker

TABLE 13-1	Cardiac Arrhythmias Categorized by Mechanism		
	Mechanism	Type	Clinical Example
DISORDERS OF IMPULSE FORMATION	Disordered normal automaticity	Hypo-automatic (Decelerated)	Sinus bradycardia, pauses, atrial and junctional escape complexes and rhythms
		Hyper-automatic (Accelerated)	Sinus tachycardia, accelerated ectopic atrial and junctional rhythms Automatic and multifocal atrial tachycardias
	Abnormal automaticity		Accelerated idioventricular rhythm early in MI[a]
	Triggered activity	Early afterdepolarizations	Torsades de pointes
		Late afterdepolarizations	Digitalis-induced atrial, junctional, and ventricular arrhythmias
DISORDERS OF IMPULSE CONDUCTION	Nonreentry unidirectional or bidirectional conduction block	Pathological (transient or fixed)	SA block
			AV block
			Bundle branch block
		Functional	Nonconducted supraventricular premature complexes
			Aberrantly conducted supraventricular premature complexes
	Unidirectional block and reentry		Sinus node reentrant tachycardia
			Reentrant atrial tachycardias
			AV nodal reentrant tachycardia
			Atrioventricular reentrant tachycardia (involving an accessory pathway)
			Atrial flutter
			Atrial fibrillation[b]
			Ventricular tachycardia[b]
			Ventricular fibrillation[b]
COMBINED DISORDERS	Disordered automaticity with unidirectional entrance block		Parasystole
	Phase 4 depolarization and conduction		Bradycardia-induced aberrancy

[a]Mechanism not confirmed.
[b]Multiple mechanisms involved.

such that the rate of depolarization becomes greater than that of the sinus node, allowing an *accelerated, ectopic* rhythm to assume control. These are examples of arrhythmias caused by increased (hyper-automatic), but otherwise normal automaticity. Here, phase 4 has been shortened with the remainder of the action potential again left undisturbed.

Here's an analogy to help you understand this potentially confusing topic. Disordered normal automaticity is like an automobile driver who is incorrectly using the gas pedal and the brake. There's nothing really wrong with the engine, but the driver is either pressing too hard on the accelerator, or pushing too hard on the break, causing the car to travel either above or below the normal speed limit.

 BE CAREFUL: You will encounter the term, *enhanced automaticity* for *all* disorders of ionically normal automatic arrhythmias. I find this misleading. To me the word "enhanced" implies "improved, strengthened,

or better," which is clearly not the case when it results in an arrhythmia. And as we reviewed in the preceding discussion, altered normal automaticity may result in both tachyarrhythmias from *hyper-automaticity* that accelerates and bradyarrhythmias from *hypo-automaticity* that decelerates the rate of impulse generation. That is the reason I prefer to utilize the term *disordered normal automaticity,* that is, either hyper-automatic (accelerated) or hypo-automatic (decelerated) to indicate that the ion currents of the action potential are intrinsically normal, but the rhythm is not.

Abnormal automaticity Abnormal automaticity affects impulse formation via *ionically abnormal* pacemaker mechanisms. The changes in the action potential typically reflect alterations in the membrane potential that markedly affect the natural depolarization properties of the cell. One example is when diseased, nonpacemaker cells outside the specialized

TABLE 13-2	Cardiac Arrhythmias Categorized by Site of Origin					
Sinus Node Arrhythmias	Supraventricular Arrhythmias and Complexes	AV Junctional Arrhythmias and Complexes	Ventricular Arrhythmias and Complexes	Pacemaker Rhythms and Complexes	AV Conduction Abnormalities	Miscellaneous AV Relationships
Sinus bradycardia	Atrial premature complexes (conducted normally, aberrantly, or nonconducted)	Wandering atrial pacemaker to the AV junction	Ventricular premature complexes	Single-chamber atrial pacemaker rhythm or complexes	AV block, first-degree	Ventriculophasic sinus arrhythmia
Sinus arrhythmia	Ectopic atrial rhythm	AV junctional premature complexes	Ventricular escape complexes	Single-chamber ventricular pacemaker rhythm or complexes	AV block, second-degree, Mobitz type I (Wenckebach)	AV dissociation
Sinus tachycardia	Wandering atrial pacemaker	AV junctional escape complexes	Ventricular tachycardia	Dual-chamber pacemaker rhythm or complexes	AV block, second-degree, Mobitz type II	Reciprocal (echo) complexes
Sinus arrest or pause	Multifocal atrial rhythm	AV junctional escape rhythm	Accelerated idioventricular rhythm	Pacemaker-mediated tachycardia	AV block, second-degree, 2:1	Retrograde atrial activation from a ventricular focus
Sinoatrial exit block	Multifocal atrial tachycardia	AV junctional rhythm	Ventricular fibrillation		AV block, high-grade	Fusion complexes
Sinus node reentrant tachycardia	Atrial tachycardia	AV junctional rhythm, accelerated	Torsades de pointes		AV block, third-degree or complete	Ventricular capture complexes
Wandering atrial pacemaker within the sinus node	AV nodal reentrant tachycardia Atrioventricular reentrant tachycardia Supraventricular tachycardia (unspecified)	Junctional tachycardia	Ventricular parasystole		Enhanced AV conduction (short PR interval pattern with normal QRS complex in sinus rhythm)	Interpolation of ventricular premature complexes
	Atrial flutter				Ventricular preexcitation (WPW pattern)	Concealed conduction
	Atrial fibrillation					

conduction system develop automaticity, a property they do not normally possess when healthy. The precise mechanism and clinical relevance of abnormal automaticity is controversial, but might occur in the setting of myocardial ischemia or infarction. One theory is that the membrane of the injured nonpacemaker cell becomes "leaky," which allows ions to pass more freely and less able to maintain a concentration gradient. If the resting potential rises to a level above −60 mV (ie, less negative), the action potential of the nonpacemaker cell begins to resemble that of a pacemaker cell and may acquire a degree of spontaneous depolarization. This is the proposed mechanism behind some atrial and ventricular arrhythmias.

Let's again use our automobile driver analogy to explain this mechanism. Abnormal automaticity is as if the gas pedal were moved to the back seat, giving control of the automobile to a passenger where it was never intended.

Triggered activity Unlike automatic rhythms, which arise *de novo* in the absence of prior electrical activity, arrhythmias related to triggered activity occur in response to a preceding impulse (the trigger). Triggered activity results from *afterdepolarizations*, which are oscillations of membrane voltage consequent to a preceding action potential (**Figure 13-6**). These occur either during repolarization (early afterdepolarizations) or shortly after full repolarization (late afterdepolarizations). The afterdepolarizations may then trigger further impulses that may be either isolated or sustained.

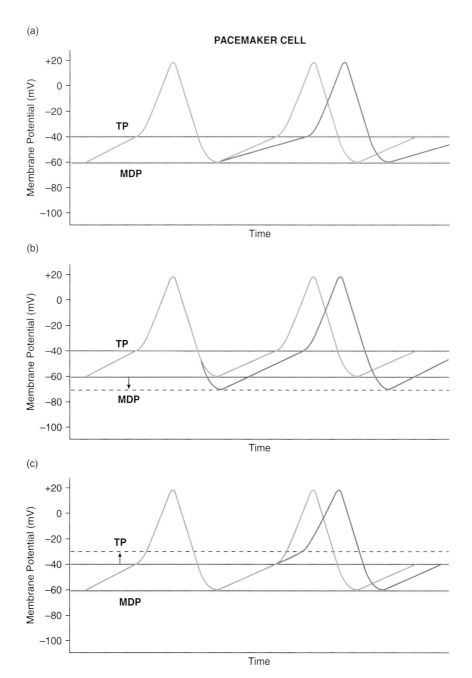

Figure 13-4. Normal sinus node depolarization (blue) and examples of variables that will lower the heart rate (red). Decrease in phase 4 slope (a). Reduction in maximum diastolic potential (MDP) (b). Increase in threshold potential (TP) (c). All increase the time between depolarizations.

CLINICAL TIP: Early afterdepolarizations are more likely to occur in conditions that prolong repolarization (and hence the QT interval). Examples include hypokalemia, hypomagnesemia, class IA and class III antiarrhythmic drugs, and hereditary long QT syndromes. This may lead to a polymorphic ventricular tachycardia called *torsades de pointes* (see Chapter 19). Late afterdepolarizations are associated with conditions that increase intracellular calcium, including digitalis toxicity, hypercalcemia, and catecholamine excess. This may lead to digitalis-related and catecholamine-associated atrial and ventricular arrhythmias.

Disorders of Impulse Conduction

Conduction block Conduction block or delay represents either a failure (block) or slowing (delay) of an impulse to propagate further through the conduction system (**Figure 13-7**). Conduction block may be *unidirectional* (conduction inhibited in one direction, but able to conduct a different impulse at another time in reverse), or *bidirectional* (conduction impeded in both directions). Pathological impairment of conduction may be transient due to a temporary physiologic abnormality or fixed due to permanent fibrosis. Alternatively, altered conduction may be *functional*, resulting from the normal refractory properties of the cell.

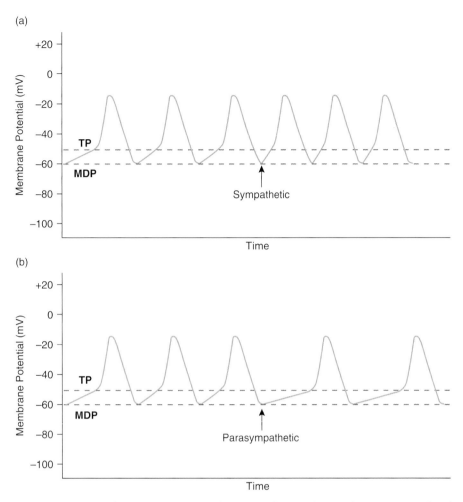

Figure 13-5. Autonomic nervous system influences. With sympathetic stimulation, phase 4 slope increases, thereby raising the heart rate (a). Under parasympathetic influence, the slope of phase 4 depolarization decreases, which lowers the heart rate (b).

Two critical factors determine the ability of the impulse to conduct from one cardiac cell to another. These are (1) the effectiveness of the stimulus and (2) the excitability of the receiving fibers.

The effectiveness of the stimulus to propagate from one cardiac cell to another is directly related to the amplitude and rate of rise of depolarization. Cells depressed by disease may have an action potential with a lower amplitude and velocity of phase 0 such that conduction is either slowed or stopped entirely.

More commonly, conduction is functionally impaired because the fibers receiving the stimulus are normally refractory and no longer excitable. We learned in Chapter 3 that after each depolarization there is a period of time where the cell is rendered either completely or partially refractory to any further stimulus (**Figure 13-8**). The *effective refractory period* (ERP) begins at phase 0 and extends partially into phase 3. If the cell receives a stimulus during this period, it **cannot** generate a new action potential and conduction fails. At the very end of phase 3 is the *relative refractory period* (RRP) when the cell has been repolarized to a range approaching the threshold potential. A stimulus received during this period can depolarize the cell, but the resulting action potential is weaker than usual, with a lower amplitude and rate of rise of phase 0, resulting in a conduction delay.

Let's describe how refractory periods impact impulse transmission as if the process were a relay race. Consider the action potential in each cell as a runner, transferring the stimulus like a baton to the next competitor. Under normal circumstances, the first sprinter transfers the baton to the next in line with optimal timing. But if the competitor lunges and tries to pass the baton prematurely before the next athlete is fully prepared (ie, during the RRP), the exchange is bobbled and the following runner starts slowly. Now if one of the racers attempts an even earlier baton transfer when the next competitor is completely unprepared (ie, during the ERP), the exchange fails and the race is over.

 CLINICAL TIP: An example of functional, physiologic conduction failure is a blocked (nonconducted) atrial premature complex. In contrast, most forms of atrioventricular (AV) block are pathological abnormalities of impulse conduction due to transient or permanent impairment of the specialized conduction system.

Reentry Reentry is a special type of impulse conduction disorder that is responsible for the majority of cardiac arrhythmias. Normally, the cardiac impulse sequentially activates the entire heart, depolarizing each cell in turn until the stimulus is

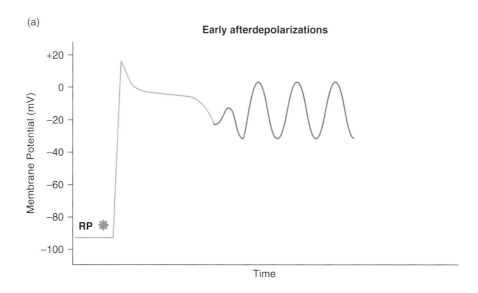

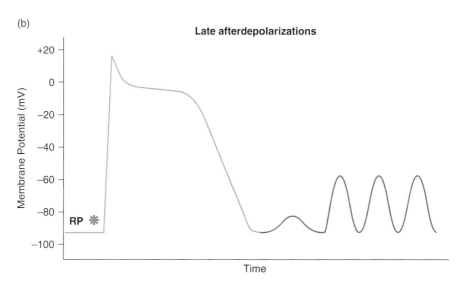

Figure 13-6. Afterdepolarizations (shown in red) may occur either early during repolarization (a) or during a late phase of the cardiac action potential (b). Abbreviations: RP = resting potential, (*) = stimulus.

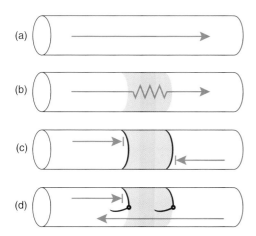

Figure 13-7. Conduction delay and block. (a) Normal conduction. (b) Slowed conduction. (c) Bidirectional block. (d) Unidirectional block.

extinguished and surrounded by refractory tissue. In time the cells repolarize and may be activated by a new impulse. Under the circumstances reviewed in the following discussion, the initial propagating impulse may fail to extinguish and persist, allowing it to return and reexcite tissue that has just been activated. This process is called **reentry**.

For reentry to occur, an *initiating trigger* must encounter *all* of the following factors.

1. The presence of at least two functionally or anatomically distinct pathways that are connected to form a circuit.

2. Unidirectional block in one of the pathways.

3. Slow conduction.

Let me walk you through the steps of the necessary conditions for reentry anywhere in the heart (**Figure 13-9**). Panel (a) shows a cardiac fiber that divides into **two limbs**, labeled

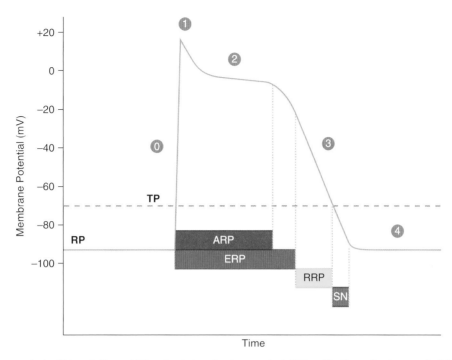

Figure 13-8. Refractory periods. Abbreviations: ARP = absolute refractory period. ERP = effective refractory period. RRP = relative refractory period. SN = supernormal period.

(α) and (β), which **connect distally**. If both pathways have identical properties, any impulse reaching the branch point (x) will travel down both limbs to conduct both distally and toward each other, meeting simultaneously at the connection (panel b). Each stimulus extinguishes at the connection, unable to proceed as it meets refractory tissue depolarized from the other direction. So the mere presence of two pathways is not enough to produce reentry. Panel (c) illustrates limb β with **unidirectional block**, showing the impulse impeded when traveling in a forward (antegrade) direction, but allowing backward (retrograde) transmission. Is this enough for reentry? Nope, reentry will not occur because the retrograde impulse conducts rapidly and will find the tissue beyond the block *refractory* to further stimulation. Functionally, it's as if limb β had bidirectional block (panel d), because the impulse meets tissue that is unexcitable. Panel (e) illustrates the effect of isolated **slow conduction** in limb α, which again is insufficient alone to allow reentry. But when slow conduction is *combined* with unidirectional block, the setting is ripe for reentry (panel f). A fortuitously timed impulse may find the β pathway refractory, allowing conduction only through the α limb. The added time for the original impulse to cross the area of slow conduction provides a sufficient delay such that the returning impulse meets a zone that is **no longer refractory**. The tissue is now **reexcitable** and the **original impulse reenters** the α pathway to begin a new cycle. The returning impulse also has the opportunity to pass retrograde in the direction of the original stimulus.

Anatomical reentry involves distinct anatomical circuits, such as might occur in the presence of an accessory bypass connection or dual AV nodal pathways. In these circumstances, the anatomically different pathways have unique electrophysiological differences in conduction and refractoriness that are the substrates for reentry. *Functional reentry* does not involve distinct anatomic structures, but results from electrical heterogeneity of small regions of myocardium. And as we will learn in later chapters, a premature impulse that encounters a temporarily refractory fiber will typically be the stimulus for the reentrant arrhythmia.

 CLINICAL TIP: Arrhythmias associated with reentry include most supraventricular tachycardias, accessory pathway-related tachycardias (WPW), and reciprocal rhythms (atrial and ventricular echo complexes). A reentry mechanism is also implicated in the generation of atrial fibrillation, atrial flutter, and ventricular tachycardia.

 FOR HISTORY BUFFS: The basic physiologic concepts of reentry were introduced in 1914 by English physiologist George Mines, who coined the term *reciprocating rhythm.* He suggested that a "circulating excitation" (subsequently known as a *circus movement*) might be responsible for some cases of paroxysmal tachycardia.

Combined Disorders of Impulse Generation and Conduction

Arrhythmias may involve abnormalities of both impulse generation and impulse conduction. One example is *parasystole*, which is characterized by a persistent ectopic impulse

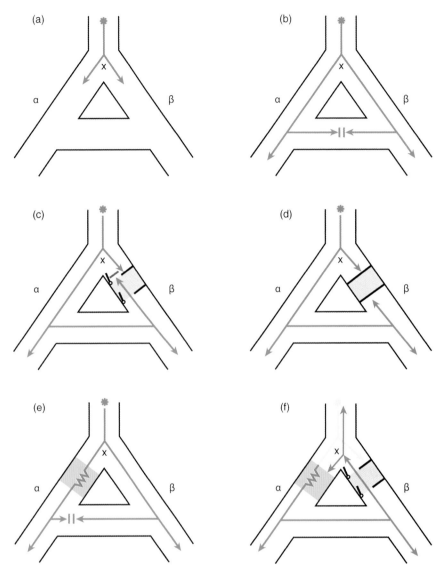

Figure 13-9. Mechanism of reentry (see text for details). (a) A depolarizing stimulus (*) splits at point (x). (b) The split impulse meets at the branch point. (c) Unidirectional block allows conduction to pass antegrade in only one limb. The retrograde impulse cannot proceed because it meets tissue that remains refractory from the initial antegrade depolarization (red bar). (d) Bidirectional block prevents conduction both antegrade and retrograde. (e) A zone of slow conduction (yellow) delays conduction in the (α) limb. (f) The combination of slow conduction and unidirectional block provides the substrate for reentry. The original stimulus (blue) returns to find tissue that is no longer refractory, which allows it to be depolarized again (green arrow).

(disordered automaticity) that is surrounded by a protective zone of depressed tissue (unidirectional entrance block). This allows the ectopic impulse to fire independently of the normal sinus depolarization. Parasystole is most commonly described in the ventricles, but may be present in the atria, AV junction, or the SA node. We will review this topic in more detail in a later chapter. An unusual combined disorder is bradycardia-induced (phase 4) conduction delay, again a topic we will cover later when we discuss aberrant conduction.

▶ SUMMARY

You now understand the underlying mechanisms of cardiac arrhythmias and how they can be categorized. In the next chapters we will use these concepts to analyze all the principal classes of rhythm disorders. Our learning adventure will culminate in a comprehensive, step-by-step method of interpretation.

Chapter 13 • SELF-TEST

1. Identify the five phases of the action potential of a nonpacemaker cell action potential and what they represent.
2. Identify the three phases of the action potential of a pacemaker action potential and what they represent.
3. Define automaticity.
4. Arrhythmias may be classified into which three broad categories?
5. What is the effect of catecholamines on the pacemaker action potential?
6. What is the effect of vagal influence on the pacemaker action potential?
7. Define triggered activity.
8. Name two primary factors that determine conduction.
9. What is the consequence of a stimulus that arrives during the following phases of the action potential?
   • The effective refractory period.
   • The relative refractory period.
10. What are the three electrophysiological requirements for reentry?

Chapter 13 • SELF-TEST

1. • Phase 0 (rapid depolarization).
   • Phase 1 (early rapid repolarization).
   • Phase 2 (plateau).
   • Phase 3 (terminal rapid repolarization).
   • Phase 4 (resting).
2. • Phase 0 (depolarization).
   • Phase 3 (repolarization).
   • Phase 4 (diastolic depolarization).
3. Automaticity is the property of a cell to initiate spontaneous depolarization.
4. Arrhythmias may be classified broadly into disorders of impulse formation, impulse conduction, and combinations of the two.
5. Catecholamines (epinephrine and norepinephrine) raise the slope of phase 4 depolarization and thereby raise the heart rate.
6. Vagal influences decrease the slope of phase 4 depolarization and thereby lower the heart rate.
7. Triggered activity is the presence of afterdepolarizations that are a consequence of a preceding impulse.
8. Conduction is affected by the effectiveness of the stimulus and the excitability of the receiving fibers.
9. • An impulse arriving during the effective refractory period will fail to propagate.
   • An impulse arriving during the relative refractory period will conduct with a weaker, delayed response.
10. Along with an initiating trigger, reentry requires:
    • The presence of at least two functionally or anatomically distinct pathways that connect to form a circuit.
    • Unidirectional block in one of the pathways.
    • Slow conduction.

Further Reading

Antzelevitch C, Burashnikov A. Overview of basic mechanisms of cardiac arrhythmia. *Card Electrophysiol Clin.* 2011;3:23-45.

Gaztanaga L, Marchlinski FE, Betensky BP. Mechanism of cardiac arrhythmias. *Spanish J Cardiol* (Engl ed). 2012;65:174-185.

Hoffman BF, Rosen MR. Cellular mechanism for cardiac arrhythmias. *Circ Res.* 1981;49:1-15.

Issa ZF, Miller JM, Zipes DP. Electrophysiological mechanisms of cardiac arrhythmias. In: *Clinical Arrhythmology and Electrophysiology.* 2nd ed. Philadelphia, PA: Elsevier; 2012:36-61.

Marriott HJL, Conover M. Arrhythmogenic mechanisms and their modulation. In: *Advanced Concepts in Arrhythmias.* 3rd ed. St. Louis, MO: Mosby; 1998:47-68.

Vetulli HM, Elizari MV, Naccarelli GV, Gonzalez MD. Cardiac automaticity: basic concepts and clinical observations. *J Interv Electrophysiol.* 2018;52:263-270.

Wit AL. Cellular electrophysiologic mechanisms of cardiac arrhythmias. *Cardiol Clin.* 1990;8:393-409.

Wit AL, Rosen MR. Cellular electrophysiology of cardiac arrhythmias I. Arrhythmias caused by abnormal impulse generation. *Mod Concepts Cardiovasc Dis.* 1981;50:1-8.

Wit AL, Rosen MR. Cellular electrophysiology of cardiac arrhythmias II. Arrhythmias caused by abnormal impulse conduction. *Mod Concepts Cardiovasc Dis.* 1981;50:7-12.

Zipes DP. Mechanisms of clinical arrhythmias. *J Cardiovasc Electrophysiol.* 2003;14:909-912.

Sinus Rhythms

▶ NORMAL SINUS RHYTHM

Let's start our discussion of the cardiac rhythms at the very beginning by learning about normal sinus rhythm and its abnormalities. Sinus rhythms originate in the sinoatrial (SA) node, located within the wall of the high right atrium near the inlet of the superior vena cava (**Figure 14-1**). From this anatomical location, the SA node first depolarizes the right atrium in a leftward, inferior, and anterior direction, followed by the left atrium in a leftward, inferior, and posterior direction (**Figure 14-2**). The mean axis of the normal P wave in the frontal plane is between 0 and +75 degrees. Accordingly, we see normal sinus P waves that are positive in leads I, II, and aVF with a negative P wave in lead aVR. Remember that the SA nodal depolarization is too small to be seen on the surface ECG so our first evidence of this discharge is the appearance of a normal P wave, indicating successful depolarization of the atria. By convention, the normal sinus rate is defined as 60 to 100 bpm. The term *normal sinus rhythm* implies depolarization by the SA node at a standard rate with normal atrial depolarization, followed by transmission through the AV node and His-Purkinje system to the ventricles (**Figure 14-3**). This results in a normal P wave that is accompanied by a normal PR interval (0.12-0.20 sec). The P-P interval between complexes is regular, with any variation between the longest and shortest cycle lengths no more than 0.12 seconds or 10% (**Figure 14-4**).

SA nodal discharge is sensitive to modulation by the autonomic nervous system. Sympathetic influences increase and parasympathetic (vagal) effects decrease the heart rate (HR). Temperature and metabolic status also influence HR. The rate of SA nodal discharge increases with elevated environmental and body temperature as well as with hyperthyroidism. Cold ambient and body temperature and hypothyroidism slow the HR.

Sinus bradycardia describes an otherwise normal sinus rhythm with a HR <60 bpm (see **Figure 14-5**). Note that some authors define sinus bradycardia as <50 bpm. Sinus bradycardia may be due to physiologically enhanced vagal tone, such as might occur in a trained athlete or during sleep. Conversely, a pathological increase in vagal tone with profound bradycardia

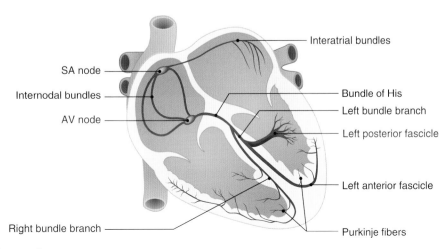

Figure 14-1. The cardiac conduction system.

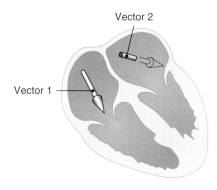

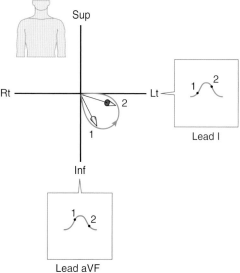

Frontal Plane

Figure 14-2. In the frontal plane, the normal P wave is upright leads I, II, and aVF. Vector 1 represents right atrial depolarization and vector 2 left atrial depolarization.

may be seen in acute nausea with inhibition of sinus node output. Sinus bradycardia may be present in inferior wall myocardial infarction due to ischemia of the SA node. Medications such as beta blockers and verapamil commonly result in sinus bradycardia.

Sinus tachycardia is an otherwise normal sinus rhythm with a HR >100 bpm (Figure 14-5). This occurs during exercise and as a physiological response to shock or hypoxia as the body tries to maintain cardiac output and oxygen delivery. Medications such as epinephrine and isoproterenol produce sinus tachycardia by sympathetic stimulation. Other stimulants such as caffeine and nicotine also increase the sinus rate, as do abused drugs such as cocaine and amphetamines. Atropine produces sinus tachycardia by inhibiting parasympathetic action.

 CLINICAL TIP: The most common cause of sinus tachycardia is *physiological sinus tachycardia*, with the elevated HR responding secondary to the hemodynamic or environmental stressors mentioned in the preceding discussion. *Inappropriate sinus tachycardia* (IST) is defined as a persistent, nonphysiological resting HR without an obvious pathological stress. In this condition, the HR typically

normalizes during sleep. *Postural orthostatic tachycardia syndrome* (POTS) is an abnormal sinus tachycardia that is triggered by upright posture and relieved by recumbency. Importantly, orthostatic hypotension is not present. Emerging data suggests that both IST and POTS may result post COVID-19 infection. *Sinus node reentrant tachycardia* is a sudden paroxysm of sinus tachycardia that is commonly both triggered by and terminated with an atrial premature depolarization.

Criteria for Normal Sinus Rhythm
- P wave of sinus origin.
  - Normal P wave configuration (upright in leads I, II, and aVF, and inverted in aVR).
  - Normal mean axis (between 0 and +75 degrees).
- Normal PR interval (0.12-0.20 seconds).
- Consistent P wave configuration and PR interval in each lead.
- Constant P-P cycles with only minor variation.
  - Variation between the longest and shortest cycles of ≤0.12 seconds or ≤10%.
- HR of 60 to 100 bpm.

Criteria for Sinus Bradycardia
- Normal sinus rhythm except for HR.
- HR <60 bpm (some authors define it as <50 bpm).

Criteria for Sinus Tachycardia
- Normal sinus rhythm except for HR.
- HR >100 bpm.

▶ SINUS ARRHYTHMIA

In *sinus arrhythmia*, the sinus rate periodically slows and speeds, with a P-P interval that varies between the maximum and minimum cycle length either by >0.12 seconds or by >10%. *Respiratory sinus arrhythmia* is a phasic change in the P-P interval that is associated with the respiratory cycle, decreasing with inspiration and increasing with expiration (**Figure 14-6**). Vagal tone normally decreases with inspiration and increases with expiration causing the HR to increase as one inhales and decrease as one exhales. You can remember this by thinking, "I'm inspired to increase my heart rate." This normal physiological response is common in the young and can be extinguished by breath-holding. *Nonrespiratory sinus arrhythmia* is a phasic variation in the P-P interval that does not fluctuate with breathing. This form of sinus arrhythmia is more common in individuals with heart disease and as a consequence of digitalis toxicity. *Ventriculophasic sinus arrhythmia* is a form of nonphasic sinus arrhythmia characteristically associated with complete heart block (**Figure 14-7**). The P-P intervals that contain a QRS complex are shorter than those without. The mechanism is uncertain and this may be observed whether the origin of the ventricular depolarization is from the native myocardium or via an electronic pacemaker. *Sinus bradyarrhythmia* is the term used to describe sinus arrhythmia when the HR is <60 bpm.

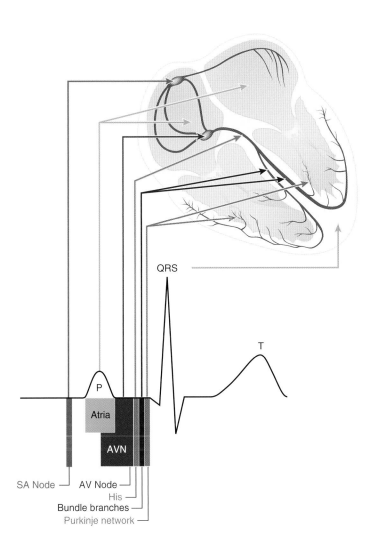

Figure 14-3. The surface ECG records only depolarization of the atria (P wave) and the ventricles (QRS). The tracing remains at the baseline during SA node depolarization and transmission through the AV node, bundle of His, bundle branches, and Purkinje network.

Criteria for Sinus Arrhythmia

- P wave of sinus origin with normal P wave morphology and axis.
- Normal HR.
- Phasic variability of P-P intervals.
- P-P intervals vary from the shortest to longest cycle by either:
  - >0.12 seconds.
  - >10%.
    - Determine this percentage by dividing the difference between the two numbers by the average of the two numbers, then multiplying by 100 to convert to percent.
    - Difference between the two numbers: (Maximum P-P interval − Minimum P-P interval).
    - Average of the two numbers: (Maximum P-P interval + Minimum P-P interval) ÷ 2.
    - Comment: The cycles used in the above calculation do not need to be consecutive.
- Sinus arrhythmia may be further characterized as respiratory, nonrespiratory, ventriculophasic, and combined with bradycardia (sinus bradyarrhythmia).

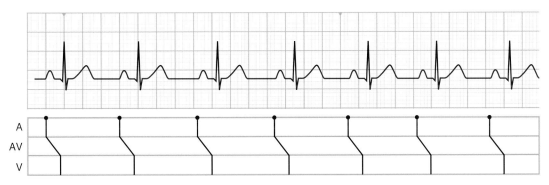

Figure 14-4. Normal sinus rhythm. The laddergram depicts the normal depolarization of the sinus impulse through the atria, AV junction, and ventricles.

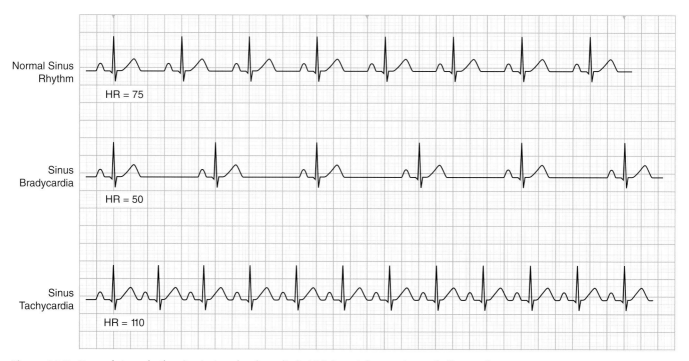

Figure 14-5. Normal sinus rhythm (top), sinus bradycardia (middle), and sinus tachycardia (bottom).

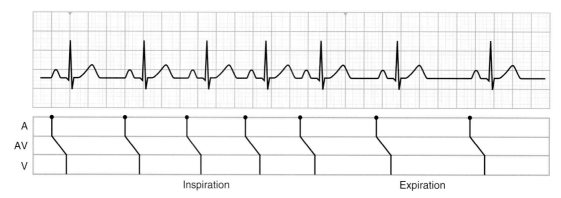

Figure 14-6. Respiratory sinus arrhythmia is characterized by P-P cycles that shorten with inspiration and lengthen with expiration. The nonrespiratory form of sinus arrhythmia does not vary with the respiratory cycle.

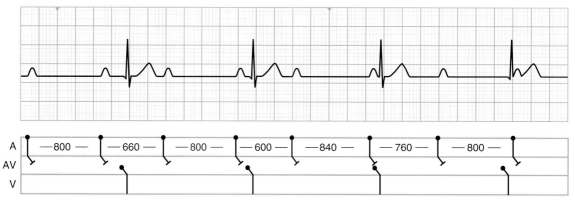

Figure 14-7. Ventriculophasic sinus arrhythmia. This tracing demonstrates sinus rhythm with complete AV block. The P waves are independent of a subsidiary AV junctional escape rhythm that depolarizes the ventricles. Note that the P-P intervals that contain a QRS complex are considerably shorter than those without (time intervals are in msec).

▶ SINUS NODE DYSFUNCTION

Abnormalities of sinus node function may be due to either abnormal impulse formation within the sinus node or failure of a normal sinus impulse to conduct through the perinodal tissues. Causes include degenerative or inflammatory processes that result in fibrosis of the sinus node or surrounding tissues. Myocardial ischemia or infarction may temporarily or permanently damage the sinus node. Commonly used medications such as beta blockers, nondihydropyridine calcium channel blockers (verapamil, diltiazem), and clonidine also may interfere with sinus node function.

Sinus Arrest or Pause

The terms sinus arrest and sinus pause are used interchangeably to describe a temporary failure of impulse formation within the sinus node. P waves do not appear as expected and end either with the return of the normal P wave or with an escape complex from a subsidiary pacemaker of a different origin. **Figure 14-8** illustrates this concept using an expanded laddergram to show the "behind the scenes" process you can't see on the ECG. The pause is sudden without the phasic change in cycle length seen with sinus arrhythmia. A characteristic feature is that the pause is **not** an exact multiple of the normal cycle length, which differentiates this entity from the various forms of SA block (see following discussion).

 CLINICAL TIP: Short sinus pauses are common during sleep, in trained athletes, and very common in patients with obstructive sleep apnea. Whereas there is no universal definition of what constitutes an abnormal sinus pause, a delay of >2 seconds raises the suspicion of abnormal sinus node function. Pauses >3 seconds are rare; however, even this finding may not represent pathology that requires intervention. For the interested reader, please review the reference material provided at the end of this chapter.

 FOR BOOKWORMS: Sinus node function can be evaluated in the electrophysiology lab with analysis of the sinus node recovery time (SNRT). In this procedure, the atrium is temporarily paced in the region of the sinus node at a rate greater than the intrinsic rhythm. The stimulus is stopped and a measurement is then made of the time it takes the sinus node to resume function. The normal SNRT is typically <1500 msec. Because the SNRT depends on the native cycle length prior to the pacing stimulus, a correction value is used (cSNRT = SNRT − native cycle length), with a normal value typically <550 msec.

Criteria for Sinus Arrest or Pause
- Sinus rhythm with sudden absence of P waves at the expected time/cycle.
- P waves and QRS complexes are absent during the pause (except for the emergence of a subsidiary pacemaker).
- The resulting pause is not an exact multiple of the normal cycle length.

 CLINICAL TIP: The sick sinus syndrome represents a constellation of symptoms associated with rhythm abnormalities of the sinus node. Concomitant AV nodal disease is also commonly present. Symptoms of fatigue, dyspnea, lightheadedness, or syncope may result from profound sinus bradycardia, sinus arrest or pause, or SA block. If so, pacemaker therapy is typically required. Often there are accompanying tachyarrhythmias such as paroxysmal supraventricular tachycardia, atrial fibrillation or flutter, coining the term "tachy-brady syndrome." These rapid arrhythmias often terminate with a prolonged pause (>3 seconds), which may be symptomatic. This "conversion pause" is yet another manifestation of abnormal sinus node function. Accordingly, the tachyarrhythmia cannot be suppressed pharmacologically without implantation of a permanent pacemaker to protect against medication-exacerbated bradyarrhythmia.

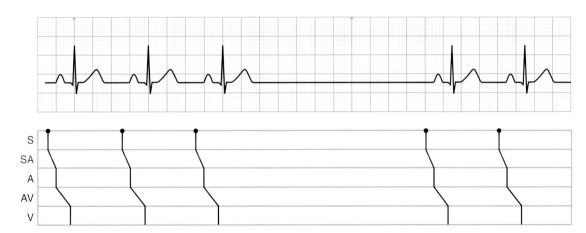

Figure 14-8. Sinus arrest represents a sudden failure of SA nodal depolarization. The pause is not a multiple of the native sinus rate.

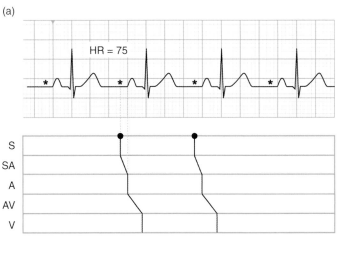

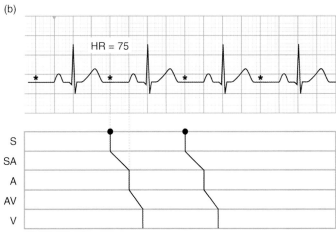

Figure 14-9. First-degree SA block. Normal sinus depolarization (a) and first-degree SA block (b) appear identical on the surface ECG. In first-degree SA block, sinus depolarization occurs normally (*) followed by a prolonged SA conduction time that can be detected only in the electrophysiology laboratory. (The time between the dotted lines highlights the prolongation).

Sinoatrial Exit Block

In sinoatrial (SA) exit block, the sinus node discharges at the normal rate, but some impulses are blocked within the sinus node or perinodal tissue and unable to depolarize the atria. Accordingly, the sinus depolarization does not produce a P wave. SA block is termed *exit block* since the sinus impulse does not "exit" from its site of depolarization. Because the sinus depolarization is not evident on the surface ECG, the various forms of SA block are inferred from their effect on the visible P waves. SA block is divided into first, second, and third degrees.

First-degree SA block This represents a fixed prolongation of the SA conduction time (**Figure 14-9**). This form of SA block cannot be recognized on the surface ECG and can be differentiated from normal sinus rhythm only in the electrophysiologic laboratory.

Second-degree SA block This is an intermittent failure of the sinus impulse to exit the sinus node and depolarize the atria. Unlike a sinus pause, there is a recognizable pattern to the absent P waves. Two types of second-degree SA block are

described, type I and type II. It's a little easier to understand type II second-degree SA block than type I, so let's discuss this in reverse order.

In type II, there is a sudden failure of the sinus impulse to exit the node and depolarize the atrium, with the resulting pause *an exact multiple* (two or more) of the preceding normal P-P interval. In **Figure 14-10** you see sinus rhythm followed by a series of pauses. The first pause is exactly three times and the second pause is twice that of the normal sinus interval.

In type I, there is a *progressive delay* of SA conduction until it fails. In **Figure 14-11a** the first two and last two complexes show normal conduction from the SA node. But beginning with the third complex, SA conduction begins to delay until it eventually blocks. The clue that this is type I, second-degree SA block is by recognizing that the P-P intervals progressively shorten until a pause becomes evident. Also note that the P-P interval of the pause is *less than* the sum of any two consecutive short cycles. This characteristic pattern is termed the *Wenckebach* phenomenon, a topic we will visit again in more detail when we discuss AV block

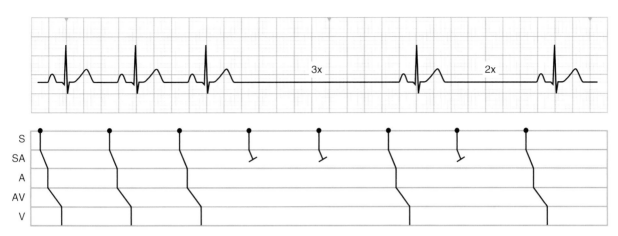

Figure 14-10. Second-degree SA block, type II. The SA node fires normally, followed by a sudden failure of SA conduction. The resulting pause is an exact multiple of the native cycle.

(see Chapter 17). Another very helpful clue to the diagnosis is that the cycles often repeat in a pattern of *group beating* (**Figure 14-11b**).

Third-degree SA block In this instance, the total absence of P waves is due to the failure of conduction of the sinus impulse out of the sinus node (**Figure 14-12a**). Note that in the presence of a junctional escape rhythm third-degree SA block cannot be distinguished on the surface ECG from sinus arrest caused by failure of impulse formation (see **Figure 14-12b**).

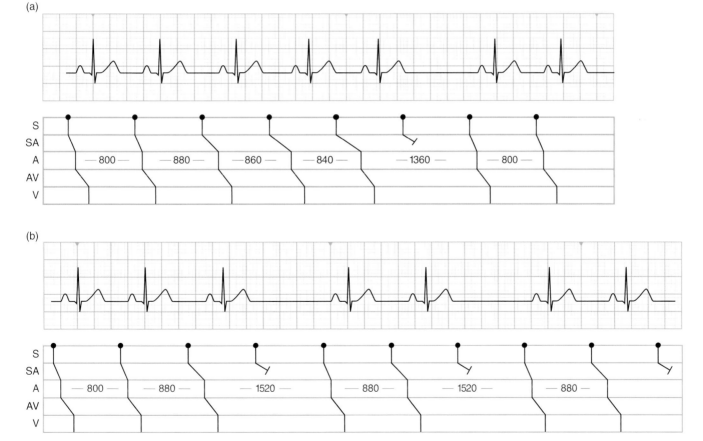

Figure 14-11. Second-degree SA block, type I (Wenckebach). (a) The SA node fires normally with progressive prolongation of SA conduction beginning with the third complex until failure (see text for details). The P-P interval gradually shortens until a pause appears. Normal conduction is present in the first two and last two complexes. (b) Normal SA depolarization with prolonged SA conduction that begins with the third complex, the pattern repeating for several cycles. Note the "group beating" representing three sinus depolarizations per two P wave-QRS complexes characteristic of a 3:2 SA Wenckebach pattern.

(a)

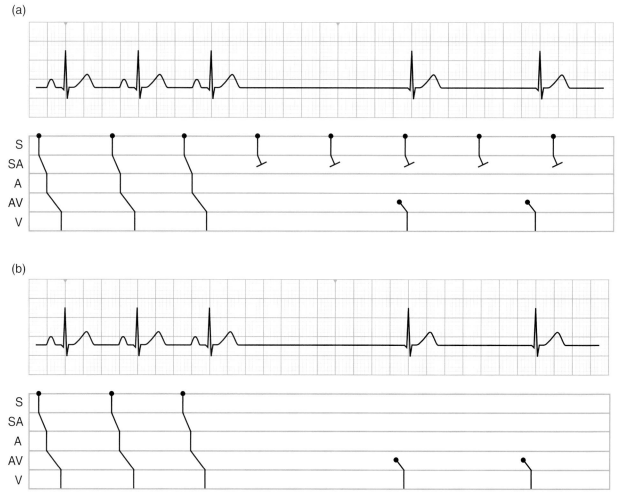

(b)

Figure 14-12. Third-degree SA block (a). There is complete failure of SA conduction with the emergence of a subsidiary junctional escape rhythm. In this circumstance, third-degree SA block cannot be differentiated on the surface ECG from sinus arrest (b).

 BE CAREFUL: Remember that in all forms of SA block the PR interval does not change. The diagnosis is made by analyzing the P-P intervals. Don't confuse this with AV block, where the conduction abnormality affects the PR intervals.

Criteria for Second-Degree SA Block, Type I (Wenckebach)

- Sinus rhythm with normal P wave morphology and axis.
- Normal PR interval.
- Progressive shortening of the P-P interval that is followed by a pause.
- The pause is less than the sum of any two consecutive short cycles.
- Supporting criteria:
  - Group beating is common.

Criteria for Second-Degree SA Block, Type II

- Sinus rhythm with normal P wave morphology and axis.
- Normal PR interval.
- Constant P-P interval with sudden absence of the P wave.
- The pause is an exact multiple (two or more) of the normal cycle length.

Wandering Pacemaker Within the Sinus Node

The sinus mechanism can originate from different sites within the sinus node. Wandering pacemaker within the sinus node is characterized by the presence of gradual variation in the P wave morphology and PR interval during sinus rhythm (**Figure 14-13**). Although slightly different in configuration, all of the complexes have a P wave axis and PR interval in the normal range, indicating that the origin of the impulse remains within the sinus node. At times, the pacemaker impulse may shift more distally into either the atrium or AV junction, as evidenced by an inverted P wave and relative shortening of the PR interval. If this occurs the rhythm is reported as a *wandering atrial pacemaker* or a *wandering pacemaker to the AV junction* (see Chapter 18).

 FOR BOOKWORMS: The sinus node is a tadpole-shaped, subepicardially located structure with a complex anatomy. The exit site of the pacemaker depolarization depends on autonomic tone, shifting the focus superiorly with adrenergic stimulation and inferiorly under vagal influence.

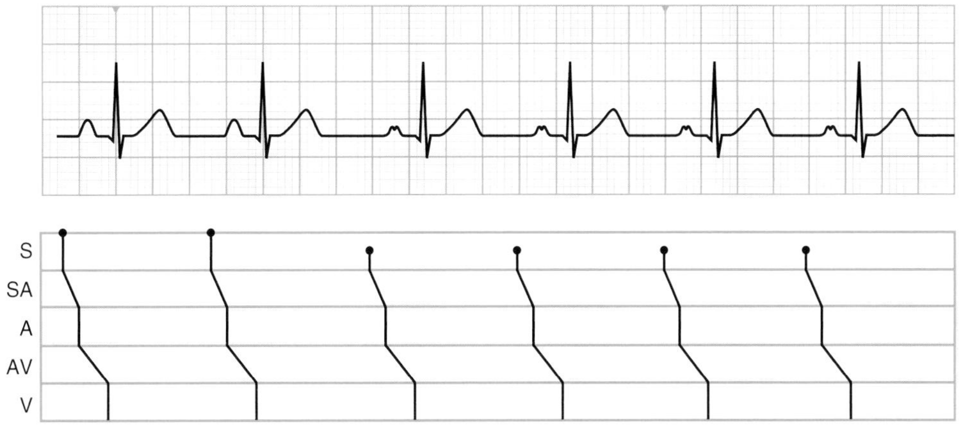

Figure 14-13. Wandering pacemaker within the sinus node. After a slight pause, a new pacemaker emerges with the third complex from a different focus within the sinus node. Note the slightly different P wave configuration and amplitude that results from changes in the P wave vector. The P wave axis and PR interval remain within the normal range.

Criteria for Wandering Atrial Pacemaker
Within the Sinus Node

- P wave of sinus origin with normal P wave axis.
- Varying P wave configuration, but remaining upright in leads I, II, and aVF and inverted in lead aVR.
- Constant P-P intervals with minor, normal variation.
- PR interval may have slight variation, but remains within the normal range (0.12-0.20 seconds).

 BE CAREFUL: Slight variations in P wave configuration with a normal PR interval may be seen with changes in posture and with respiration. But in these circumstances, the patterns of the QRS complexes and T waves usually vary with the P waves in tandem.

Chapter 14 • SELF-TEST

1. List the criteria for normal sinus rhythm.
2. The P wave represents depolarization of which cardiac chambers?
3. The QRS complex represents depolarization of which cardiac chambers?
4. True or false? SA nodal discharge can be detected on the electrocardiogram.
5. Define sinus arrhythmia.
6. In ventriculophasic sinus arrhythmia, the P-P cycles that contain a QRS are longer or shorter?
7. In respiratory sinus arrhythmia, the heart rate increases or decreases with inspiration?
8. Define second-degree SA block, type I.
9. Define second-degree SA block, type II.
10. Define wandering pacemaker within the sinus node.

QUESTIONS

ANSWERS

Chapter 14 • SELF-TEST

1. P wave of sinus origin with normal axis in the frontal plane (between 0 and +75 degrees) accompanied by a normal PR interval (0.12-0.20 seconds).

2. The atria.

3. The ventricles.

4. False.

5. Sinus rhythm with variation between the longest and shortest P-P cycle by >0.12 seconds or by >10%.

6. Shorter.

7. Increases (P-P interval decreases).

8. Sinus rhythm with a normal PR interval with progressive shortening in the P-P interval until a pause. The pause is less than the sum of any two consecutive short cycles.

9. Sinus rhythm with a normal PR interval until a pause. The pause is an exact multiple of the normal P-P cycle.

10. Sinus rhythm with a slight variation of the P wave morphology that maintains a normal axis. The PR interval must remain within the normal range.

Further Reading

Ahmed A, Pothineni NVK, Charate R, et al. Inappropriate sinus tachycardia: etiology, pathophysiology, and management. *J Am Coll Cardiol* 2022;79:2450-2462.

Alboni P, Malcarne C, Pedroni P, Masoni A, Narula OS. Electrophysiology of normal sinus node with and without autonomic blockade. *Circulation*. 1982;65:1236-1242.

De Marneffe M, Gregoire JM, Waterschoot P, Kestemont MP. The sinus node function: normal and pathological. *Eur Heart J*. 1993;5:649-654.

Hilgard J, Ezri MD, Denes P. Significance of ventricular pauses of three seconds or more detected on twenty-four-hour Holter recordings. *Am J Cardiol*. 1985;55:1005-1008.

Hingorani P, Karnard DR, Rohekar P, Kerkar V, Lokhandwala YY, Kothari S. Arrhythmias seen in baseline 24-hour Holter ECG recordings in healthy normal volunteers during phase 1 clinical trials. *J Clin Pharmacol*. 2016;56:885-893.

Ilson BE. Cardiovascular monitoring in normal healthy adults: a literature review and recommendations for the reporting of disturbances of cardiac rhythm. *Am J Ther*. 1995;2:983-899.

John RM, Kumar S. Sinus node and atrial arrhythmias. *Circulation*. 2016:133:1892-1900.

Murphy C, Lazzara R. Current concepts of anatomy and electrophysiology of the sinus node. *J Interv Card Electrophysiol*. 2016;46:9-18.

Oshansky B, Sullivan RM. Inappropriate sinus tachycardia. *J Am Coll Cardiol*. 2013;61:793-801.

Schuessler RB. Abnormal sinus node function in clinical arrhythmias. *J Cardiovasc Electrophysiol*. 2003;14:215-217.

Schuessler RB, Boineau JP, Bromberg BI. Origin of the sinus impulse. *J Cardiovasc Electrophysiol*. 1996;7:263-274.

Senturk T, Xu H, Puppala K, et al. Cardiac pauses in competitive athletes: a systematic review examining the basis of current practice recommendations. *Europace*. 2016;18:1873-1879.

Wajngarten M, Grupi C, Bellotti GM, Lemos da Luz P, Gastao do Serro Azul L, Pileggi F. Frequency and significance of cardiac rhythm disturbances in healthy elderly individuals. *J Electrocardiol*. 1990;23:171-176.

Yusuf S, Camm AJ. Deciphering the sinus tachycardias. *Clin Cardiol*. 2005;28:267-276.

Zehender M, Meinrtz T, Keul J, Just H. ECG variants and cardiac arrhythmias in athletes: clinical relevance and prognostic importance. *Am Heart J*. 1990;119:1378-1391.

Complex Cornucopia

▶ INTRODUCTION

In normal sinus rhythm the heart is depolarized in a sequential, predictable fashion. From the sinoatrial (SA) node, the impulse first depolarizes the atria on its way to the AV node and then travels through the specialized conduction system to ultimately activate the ventricles. Each cell of the heart is depolarized on time, recorded on the ECG as the P wave, PR interval, and QRS complex, something that we can display graphically with a ladder diagram (**Figure 15-1**). But to liberally paraphrase Scottish poet Robert Burns, *"The best laid plans of mice and men and the sinus node go oft awry."* With that introduction, let's now discuss the subject of ectopic complexes.

Terminology of Ectopy

Any electrocardiographic complex that originates from a focus *outside* of the SA node may be termed **ectopic**. This is a large subject that is made more difficult by a lack of uniformity in nomenclature. But fear not, because I'm going to help you simplify the process. I recommend you follow a convention that describes the complexes by (1) the site of origin, (2) the timing relative to the native rhythm, and (3) with additional descriptors as needed. Depending on the situation, the modifiers may be placed either before or after you name the complex by origin and timing. The three-step method is summarized as follows:

- Step one: Identify the site of origin.
  - Atrial.
  - AV junctional.
  - Ventricular.
- Step two: Analyze the timing.
  - Premature (early).
  - Escape (late).
- Step three: Add descriptors as required.
  - Normally conducted.
  - Nonconducted (blocked).
  - Aberrantly conducted.
  - Retrograde conduction.
  - Interpolated.
  - Late (end) diastolic.
  - Fusion.
  - Concealed.
  - Reciprocal (echo).
  - Uniform/Multiform.
  - Repetitive or in a pattern.

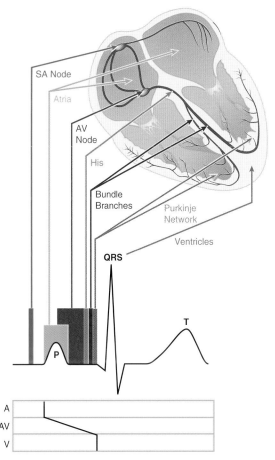

Figure 15-1. Laddergram depicting a normal sinus complex and the relationship to the cardiac conduction system.

For example, we can use the convention above to describe an ectopic complex that originates in the ventricles and occurs earlier than the next expected sinus complex as a *ventricular premature complex* (VPC). We first name the site of origin (the ventricles) and then the timing (premature). That was easy! In many texts, you will find the same complex described as a premature ventricular complex (PVC) instead of a VPC. It's perfectly reasonable to identify the timing first and the origin second because both VPC and PVC are equivalent. But the "origin first-timing second" naming convention is something we can use consistently for both early and late complexes and the one I think is best.

Ectopy Schmectopy, What's in a Name?

Even when using the recommended order, you are going to encounter many other ways to describe the same VPC. These include ventricular premature beat (VPB), ventricular premature contraction (VPC), ventricular premature systole (VPS), and ventricular premature depolarization (VPD). All of these terms are flawed. The ECG records electrical complexes, not a heartbeat, heart contraction, or cardiac systole. Extrasystole is yet another term sometimes used that is also a misnomer, because not every ectopic complex is "extra." Depolarization comes closest to being acceptable and it is a depolarization that initiates the favored term of complex. However, I prefer to reserve depolarization when describing electrophysiology, and use complex for what we see recorded on the ECG. OK, I think I've made my case for using the proper terminology, so now let's get to work.

▶ PART I. PREMATURE COMPLEXES

Premature complexes are those that occur *early* in relation to the native rhythm. They can arise from the atrium, AV junction, or ventricle. Using our convention in the preceding discussion, we refer to these as an **atrial premature complex** (APC), **junctional premature complex** (JPC), and **ventricular premature complex** (VPC). The electrophysiologic basis for most premature complexes is either disordered automaticity or reentry. Let's review each type of premature complex in turn beginning with the ventricles.

Ventricular Premature Complex

Origin and morphology A VPC originates in the ventricular Purkinje fibers or ventricular muscle. The depolarization spreads throughout the ventricle via myocyte-to-myocyte transmission, outside of the specialized conduction system. As we learned in the chapter on bundle branch block, this type of transmission produces a wide (≥0.12 seconds) QRS complex with secondary ST segment and T wave abnormalities directed opposite to that of the dominant R wave (**Figure 15-2**). VPCs with the same QRS morphology are termed *uniform* and typically arise from one ventricular site (unifocal). Those with different morphologies are termed *multiform* typically arising from multiple sites (multifocal). The shape of the VPC provides some clues as to its origin. VPCs arising from the left ventricle resemble a RBBB configuration and those from the right ventricle or interventricular septum resemble a LBBB pattern.

Timing VPCs occur early relative to the cycle length of the normal sinus rhythm (or R-R interval in the setting of atrial fibrillation). VPCs arise independently of the sinus mechanism; therefore, they are electrically unrelated to any preceding P wave. This is one of the defining characteristics of ventricular ectopy. The term *coupling interval* refers to the time between the onset of the VPC and the QRS of the preceding complex. Ectopic complexes from one focus tend to have the same coupling interval, whereas those from multiple locations have different coupling intervals (see Figure 15-2).

In most circumstances, the VPC does not conduct retrograde to depolarize and reset the SA node, so the sinus rhythm continues on its merry way as if nothing happened. The SA node keeps depolarizing the atria, but you usually can't see the P wave because it is hidden in the ventricular complex (**Figure 15-3**). Furthermore, the normal sinus impulse cannot travel through the specialized conduction system to produce a QRS complex because the ventricles (and likely the AV junction) are rendered refractory after ventricular depolarization. Accordingly, the next P wave and related QRS complex appear when they are expected. In Figure 15-3, note on the laddergram that the missing P wave is presented as a "virtual" or "hidden" depolarization. Now, look at the gap after the VPC until the return of the next sinus complex, which arrives right on time. This *fully compensatory pause* between the VPC and the normal sinus complex that follows is another of the characteristic features of a VPC. An easy way to check for this phenomenon is to take your calipers and confirm that the R-R (or P-P) interval containing the VPC is exactly twice

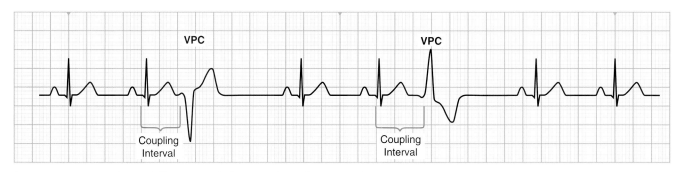

Figure 15-2. VPCs with two different morphologies and coupling intervals.

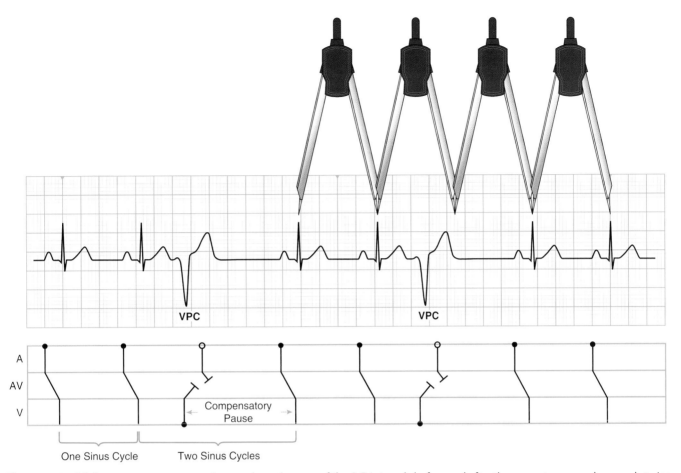

Figure 15-3. A fully compensatory pause is one where the sum of the R-R intervals before and after the premature complex equals twice that of the native sinus cycle (see text for details).

that of the normal cycle length. If so, the post-ectopic pause is fully compensatory.

 CLINICAL TIP: VPCs may either be totally asymptomatic or cause a sensation of palpitation. The ectopic impulse may not generate a palpable pulse or blood pressure. The patient may feel as if the "heart stopped," following which they experience a strong heartbeat in the chest or throat after the pause.

VPCs may be present in healthy individuals or occur in the setting of significant clinical illness. Some causes of VPCs include heart failure, coronary ischemia, hypoxia, acidosis, medications, electrolyte disturbances, alcohol, and stimulants such as catecholamines or caffeine.

VPC Conduction Modifiers and Variants

VPCs are not all the same and interact with the rest of the cardiac conduction system. We can describe these relationships with a variety of modifiers.

Retrograde ventriculoatrial activation At times the ventricular depolarization can "reverse course" through the entire specialized conduction system to depolarize the atria (**Figure 15-4**). If so, a retrograde inverted P (P′) wave may be seen in leads II,

III, and aVF. Alternatively, the P′ wave may be hidden within the ST segment or T wave of the VPC. Note that this retrograde P′ wave is distinguished from a normal sinus P wave because it is inverted and occurs earlier than expected. If the retrograde impulse travels through the atria to depolarize the SA node, the normal sinus rhythm will be reset. Accordingly, in this situation the post-VPC pause is not fully compensatory (noncompensatory). Depending on the recovery time of the sinus node, the noncompensatory post-ectopic pause may be either shorter or longer than the native sinus cycle.

Interpolated VPC An *interpolated* VPC is one that appears interposed between two normal sinus impulses (**Figure 15-5**). A typical finding of an interpolated VPC is prolongation of the PR interval of the following sinus complex. This is due to *concealed retrograde conduction* of the ventricular depolarization into the AV junction, causing partial refractoriness and a delay in antegrade conduction of the following sinus impulse. The retrograde conduction is considered "concealed" because it is not visible on the surface ECG, but may be inferred because of the effect on the following complex. Interpolated VPCs are more frequently seen when the native sinus rhythm is relatively slow.

VPC with reciprocal (echo) complex On occasion, retrograde transmission of the ventricular impulse may return

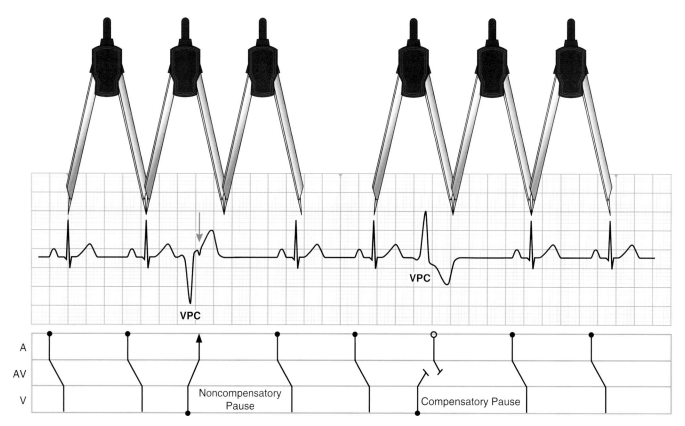

Figure 15-4. The VPC on the left demonstrates retrograde activation of the atria (arrow). The SA node resets, resulting in a noncompensatory pause. Depending on the time it takes for SA nodal recovery, the post-ectopic pause may be either shorter or longer than the native sinus cycle. The VPC on the right does not reset the sinus node and the post-ectopic pause is fully compensatory.

to depolarize the ventricle as a *reciprocal* or *echo* complex (**Figure 15-6**). This is a form of reentry, which as we discussed in Chapter 13 requires a second AV pathway with different conduction characteristics. The mechanism involves entry of the retrograde impulse through a second, slowly conducting pathway in the AV node. With sufficient delay, the impulse can return antegrade through the now recovered fast pathway to depolarize the ventricles. This results in an early, narrow complex appearing after the VPC.

Late (end) diastolic VPC Sometimes the VPC has a coupling interval late in the cardiac cycle such that it occurs just after the P wave (**Figure 15-7**). This is called a *late or end-diastolic* VPC. Remember in this situation that even though you see a P wave, it did not *initiate* the following QRS complex, which is that of the VPC. A *fusion complex* may be seen if there is just enough time for the sinus impulse to travel through the specialized conduction system to merge with the VPC. This complex is wider than the normal QRS, but narrower than that of the

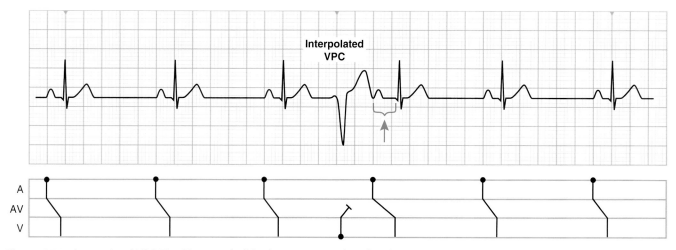

Figure 15-5. Interpolated VPC. The PR interval of the first sinus complex after the VPC is prolonged (arrow) due to concealed retrograde conduction into the AV junction, which renders the region partially refractory.

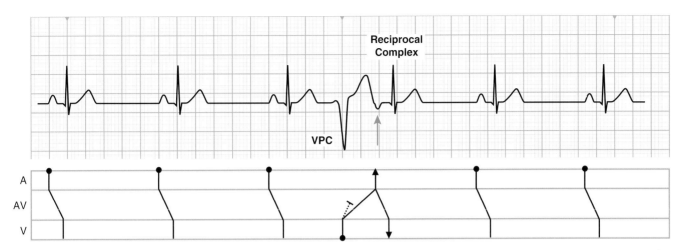

Figure 15-6. VPC with reciprocal (echo) complex. Retrograde AV conduction via a slowly conducting pathway produces an inverted P′ wave on the ECG (arrow). The impulse returns antegrade via another faster-conducting pathway to depolarize the ventricles a second time.

VPC, reflecting the blending of the two waves of depolarization, one supraventricular and the other ventricular.

Post-VPC T wave change On occasion, the sinus complex that follows a VPC will demonstrate a change in the T wave configuration compared with normal (**Figure 15-8**). This is a nonspecific response of unclear etiology that does not appear to have clinical implications.

R on T phenomenon A VPC with a short coupling interval may fall on or near the T wave of the preceding complex. This is during the repolarization phase of the action potential, historically considered a *vulnerable period* that might precipitate ventricular tachycardia. Clinical experience suggests this risk is small (see Figure 15-8).

Repetitive VPCs, or occurring in a pattern VPCs may occur alone (*isolated*), grouped repetitively, or present in a pattern related to the native sinus complex. Two VPCs in a row are termed a ventricular *couplet* or *pair*. The morphology of the two complexes may either be uniform or multiform. A group of three rapid VPCs in a row defines *ventricular tachycardia*, a topic we will review in Chapter 19. *Ventricular bigeminy* describes VPCs that alternate with each sinus complex. VPCs appearing every third complex are said to have a pattern of *ventricular trigeminy*.

Parasystole Ventricular parasystole is a unique form of ventricular ectopy (**Figure 15-9**). In classic parasystole, an automatic ventricular focus fires completely independent of the sinus mechanism. A zone of unidirectional *entrance block* "protects" the abnormal site from outside depolarization while allowing the impulse to exit and capture the ventricles when they are not refractory. The best analogy is to think of the parasystolic focus as akin to an electronic fixed-rate pacemaker, unable to sense the native rhythm and firing at set intervals.

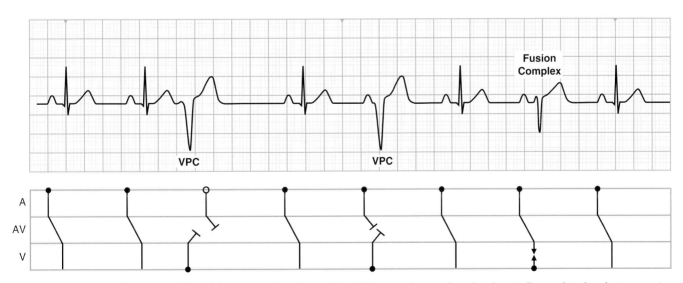

Figure 15-7. Late (end) diastolic VPC and fusion complex. The middle VPC occurs late in diastole, electrically unrelated to, but appearing just after inscription of the P wave. The VPC on the right occurs slightly later, producing a fusion complex that represents merging of the ventricular and normal sinus depolarizations. The three VPCs alternate with normal sinus complexes in a pattern of bigeminy.

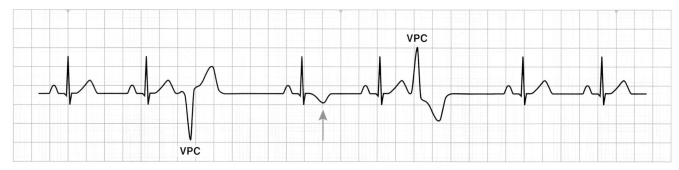

Figure 15-8. Post-VPC T wave change and R on T phenomenon. The first complex after the VPC on the left demonstrates T wave inversion (arrow). The VPC on the right has a short coupling interval such that the R wave of the premature complex falls on the downslope of the T wave of the preceding sinus complex.

The clues to ventricular parasystole are premature complexes that vary in relationship to the sinus mechanism (variable coupling intervals), longer interectopic intervals that are multiples of the shortest interectopic interval, and the presence of interpolated and fusion complexes. There are many complex variants of parasystole, which may originate in areas other than the ventricles. For more information, please review the suggestions for further reading at the end of this chapter.

Criteria for Ventricular Premature Complex

- The complex occurs early relative to the native rhythm and is not preceded by a P wave.
- QRS duration ≥0.12 seconds.
- Secondary ST segment and T wave abnormalities directed opposite to that of the dominant R wave.
- Supporting criteria:
  - A fully compensatory pause is present.
- Exceptions and modifications (see text for details).
  - Interpolated VPC.
  - Late (end) diastolic. VPC.

Atrial Premature Complex

Origin and morphology   An APC can originate anywhere in the atrial myocardium outside of the sinus node. The morphology of the P′ wave is either unchanged or different from the normal P wave, reflecting its ectopic location (**Figure 15-10**). If the depolarization arises near the sinus node, the configuration will be nearly normal. If originating near the AV node, it will be inverted reflecting retrograde depolarization of the atria. The morphology of the P′ wave in different leads may be notched, biphasic or isoelectric, depending on its source located in either atrium. The impulse is transmitted through the AV node and His-Purkinje system as usual, producing a P′R interval that is either normal, or slightly shorter depending on its proximity to the AV node. At times, the premature impulse may find the AV node partially refractory whereupon the associated P′R interval will be prolonged over baseline. In the absence of aberrant ventricular conduction, the QRS complex that follows will be identical to the native rhythm.

Timing   APCs appear early in relation to the cycle length of the native sinus rhythm. The ectopic atrial depolarization

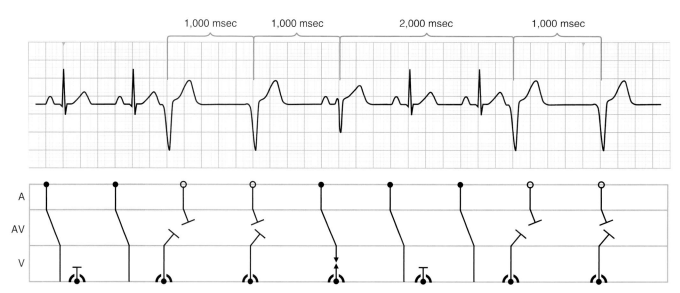

Figure 15-9. Ventricular parasystole. A parasystolic focus, protected by entrance block, depolarizes the ventricles when not refractory. The fifth complex from the left represents fusion of the sinus and parasystolic impulses. The longest interectopic interval (2000 msec) is a multiple of the shortest interectopic interval (1000 msec).

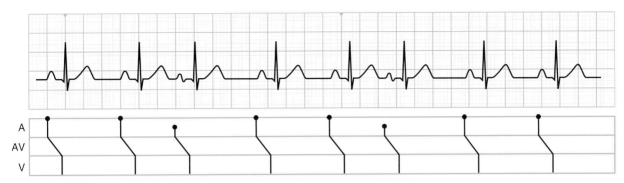

Figure 15-10. Atrial premature complexes.

typically depolarizes the SA node, resetting the native rhythm. This produces a post-ectopic pause that is *not fully compensatory* (*noncompensatory*) (**Figure 15-11**). Compare this with the *compensatory pause* we see with a VPC where the SA node is usually unaffected by the premature impulse.

 CLINICAL TIP: APCs may be found in normal individuals, but are particularly common in patients with chronic obstructive pulmonary disease (COPD) and the elderly. Like VPCs, atrial ectopy is often due to electrolyte

disturbance, caffeine and other stimulants, alcohol, heart failure, valve disease, and medications. They may be asymptomatic or produce a sensation of palpitation.

APC Conduction Modifiers and Variants

The fate of the APC depends on the state of the conduction system distal to the premature depolarization. To reach the ventricular myocardium, the impulse must conduct through the AV junction, the bundle branches, and the Purkinje fibers. However, recall from Chapter 3 that after every depolarization,

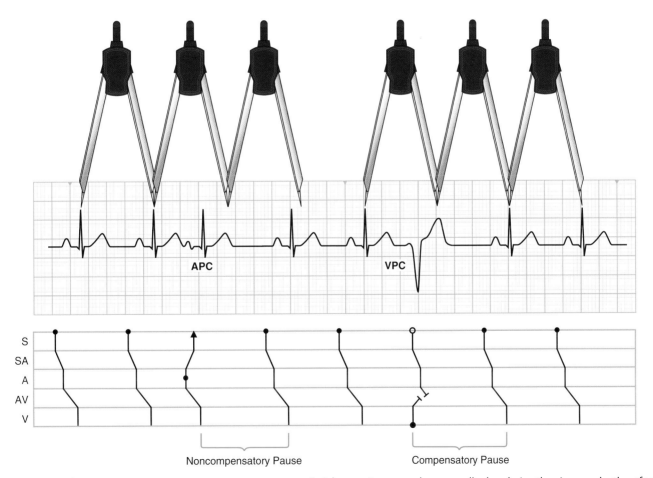

Figure 15-11. Compensatory versus noncompensatory pauses. Atrial premature complexes usually depolarize the sinus node, therefore the post-ectopic pause is noncompensatory. Ventricular premature complexes typically do not reset the sinus node, resulting in a post-ectopic pause that is fully compensatory.

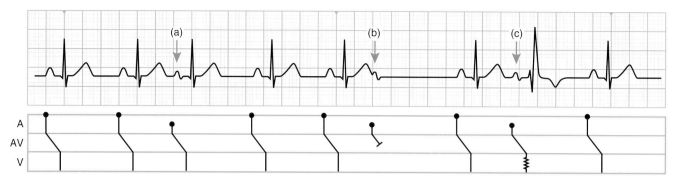

Figure 15-12. Depending on the timing relationship with the normal cardiac cycle, an atrial premature depolarization may be conducted normally (a), blocked (b), or show aberrant morphology (c). (See text for details.)

there is a period of time when each myocyte becomes either partially or completely refractory to further stimulation. Accordingly, a premature impulse may find these cells either partially or completely inhibited to further conduction. **Figure 15-12** reviews the potential options. With normal conduction we see a P′ wave with a nearly normal P′R interval and a QRS identical to the native complex. Variations occur as follows:

Nonconducted (blocked) APC If the premature depolarization occurs early such that it arrives at the AV node during the effective refractory period, the impulse will be *nonconducted* or "*blocked*." An early P′ wave is present but without a following QRS complex.

 BE CAREFUL: It's important to remember that a premature impulse that fails to conduct distally because it encounters tissue that is physiologically refractory represents **normal** behavior.

APC with prolonged PR interval Sometimes a premature impulse arrives at the AV node during the relative refractory period, resulting in a delay of conduction and PR prolongation. A prolonged PR interval may also result if the APC originates in the left atrium with an intra-atrial conduction delay.

APC with aberrant ventricular conduction In this situation, the APC conducts normally through the AV node and bundle of His, but finds one of the bundle branches refractory from the previous impulse, resulting in a wide complex. In most circumstances, this *aberrant conduction* has the morphology of a right bundle branch block, because the refractory period of the right bundle branch is intrinsically longer than the left bundle branch. Accordingly, a premature impulse is more likely to find the left bundle branch fully recovered and the right bundle branch refractory, producing a QRS with RBBB morphology.

 BE CAREFUL: There may be times when the P′ wave appears to be absent, but is actually hidden in the T wave of the previous complex. A careful inspection of the T waves in every lead will often reveal the "missing" P′ wave.

  An APC with aberrant conduction is often mistaken for a VPC. Look for clues that can help you differentiate the two including searching for a P′ wave, a noncompensatory

pause, and RBBB morphology, all of which favor a supraventricular premature complex with aberrancy (see Chapter 16).

APC with reciprocal (echo) atrial complex Reciprocal complexes are more common with APCs than VPCs. As with a ventricular echo complex, this is a form of reentry typically involving dual AV nodal pathways with different conduction properties. The premature atrial depolarization blocks in the fast pathway and conducts with an antegrade delay through the slow pathway **(Figure 15-13)**. Retrograde transmission of the impulse via the now recovered fast pathway returns to re-excite the atrium. The ECG demonstrates an initial premature atrial complex followed by a second inverted P′ wave. As we will review in Chapter 18, this is frequently the trigger for supraventricular tachycardia.

Repetitive APCs or occurring in a pattern Like VPCs, atrial ectopy may occur alone (*isolated*), grouped repetitively, or present in a pattern related to the native sinus complex. Two APCs in a row is an atrial *couplet* or *pair*. A group of three rapid APCs in a row is a form of *supraventricular tachycardia*. *Atrial bigeminy* describes APCs alternating with each sinus complex. APCs appearing every third complex are said to have a pattern of *atrial trigeminy*.

Criteria for Atrial Premature Complex
- The complex appears early relative to the native rhythm.
- A nearly normal P′ wave is present, but may be biphasic or inverted.
- The P′R interval is typically within the normal range (0.12-0.20 seconds), but may be shorter or longer than that of the baseline sinus complex.
- The P′ wave is followed by a QRS complex identical to the native rhythm.
- Supporting criteria:
  - The complex is followed by a noncompensatory pause.
- Exceptions and modifiers (see text for details).
  - Nonconducted (blocked) APC.
  - APC with aberrant conduction.

AV Junctional Premature Complex

Origin and morphology JPCs originate in the AV node or bundle of His. Retrograde conduction to the atrium results in an inverted P (P′) wave, seen best in leads II, III, and aVF

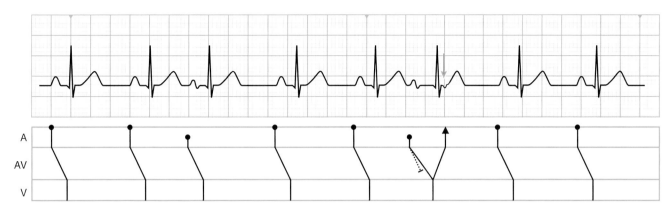

Figure 15-13. APC with reciprocal (echo) complex. The premature depolarization finds one pathway blocked, conducting more slowly antegrade via a second pathway. The impulse now finds the first pathway recovered allowing retrograde conduction to reexcite the atrium. A retrograde P´ wave is faintly seen after the QRS (arrow).

(**Figure 15-14**). The retrograde P´ wave may appear before, after, or hidden within the QRS complex depending on two factors (1) the relative speed of both antegrade and retrograde conduction and (2) the location within the AV junction (**Figure 15-15**). When the P´ wave appears prior to the QRS, the P´R interval is short (<0.12 seconds), which differentiates a JPC from an APC. In the absence of aberrant ventricular conduction, the associated QRS complex will be identical to the native rhythm.

Timing JPCs appear early relative to the normal sinus rhythm. The post-ectopic pause is highly variable. Retrograde depolarization of the SA node may occur, resetting the native rhythm and resulting in a post-ectopic pause that is not fully compensatory (noncompensatory). If the JPC and the normal sinus depolarization occur nearly simultaneously, the complexes may fuse and a fully compensatory pause will be evident. Alternatively, retrograde block may prohibit reset of the sinus node by the junctional depolarization.

JPC Conduction Modifiers and Variants

The fate of the JPC depends on both antegrade and retrograde conduction (**Figure 15-16**).

JPC with blocked antegrade conduction An inverted P´ wave is present but without a following QRS complex. Because there is no P´R interval, it is not possible to distinguish this from a nonconducted APC that is low in the atrium and near the AV junction.

JPC with blocked retrograde conduction A normal QRS complex is present without a retrograde P´ wave. Because a P´ wave is absent, this is indistinguishable on the ECG from a P´ wave that is hidden within the QRS complex.

JPC with both blocked antegrade and retrograde conduction (concealed JPC) In this unusual situation, the depolarization is not evident on the ECG (concealed) and is inferred by the effect on another complex such as delay or failure of expected conduction.

JPC with aberrant ventricular conduction A P´ wave is present, followed by a QRS complex that is wide compared with the native complex (see discussion in APC section).

JPCs may also appear in groups, patterns, and with reciprocal complexes as discussed earlier with APCs.

Criteria for AV Junctional Premature Complex
- The complex appears early relative to the native rhythm.
- An inverted, retrograde P´ wave is present that may appear before, within, or after the QRS complex.
- When present before the QRS complex, the P´R interval is short (<0.12 seconds).
- The P´ wave is followed by a QRS complex identical to the native rhythm (unless aberrant conduction).
- Exceptions and modifiers.
  - Abnormalities of both antegrade and retrograde conduction may be present (see text for details).

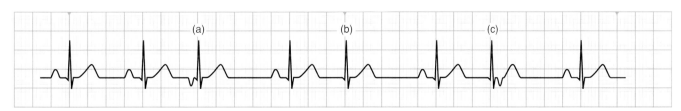

Figure 15-14. Junctional premature complexes. The inverted, retrograde P´ wave may be present: before (a), hidden within (b), or after the QRS complex (c). In this example, the retrograde impulse conducts to the atrium but fails to depolarize the SA node; therefore, the post-ectopic pause is fully compensatory.

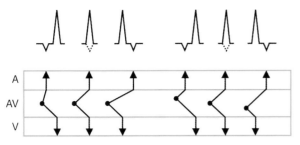

Figure 15-15. P´–QRS relationship of junctional premature complexes. The position of the inverted retrograde P´ wave vis-à-vis the QRS complex depends on both the relative rates of antegrade and retrograde conduction (left) and the location of the impulse within the AV junction (right).

A Brief Pause About Pauses

Before we move on, let's take a moment to review the terminology of the pauses associated with premature complexes. If you struggle to grasp the difference between a pause that is fully compensatory versus one not fully compensatory (noncompensatory), you're not alone. Here's the bottom line: If the sinus node cycle remains intact, the post-ectopic pause should be fully compensatory. The pause after a VPC is typically fully compensatory because the sinus mechanism is unaffected (**Figure 15-17**). But, if the VPC *does* conduct retrograde to depolarize the SA node, or is interpolated, the pause will be noncompensatory. Similarly, a noncompensatory pause is typically seen after an APC, because the SA node is reset (**Figure 15-18**). But if the APC *fails* to reset the sinus node, the pause is fully compensatory.

Here's a nautically inspired memory tool that may help you. Think of the SA node as the "commander of conduction." If the commander sails the ship safely through the conduction system, then payment for the voyage is made in full (fully compensated). But if another "impulsive underling" prematurely grabs the helm, the commander is docked some salary (not fully compensated). An APC is nearby the SA node commander and has more opportunity to temporarily take control. A VPC is below decks and unlikely to do so.

FOR BOOKWORMS: There are some exceptions to the concepts reviewed in the preceding discussion. A compensatory pause may not be equal to two sinus cycles in the presence of underlying sinus arrhythmia where the sinus cycle varies. In this setting, the compensatory pause will potentially be either longer or shorter than expected. The post-ectopic interval of a noncompensatory pause is typically equal to that of the native sinus cycle, reflecting reset of the SA node. An exception is when the premature depolarization temporarily depresses automaticity of the SA node, prolonging the return to sinus rhythm.

▶ PART II. LATE (ESCAPE) COMPLEXES

Escape complexes are those that arise from a subsidiary pacemaker following a pause in the native rhythm *longer* than the normal cycle length. They have all the same morphologic characteristics as premature complexes, but emerge only when a faster, more dominant pacemaker has failed. Using our convention of origin-first, timing-second we name these as **atrial escape complexes**, **AV junctional escape complexes**, and **ventricular escape complexes**, adding additional modifiers as necessary.

Cells within portions of the atria, AV junction, and the remainder of the His-Purkinje system have the property of *automaticity*, which give them the capacity for spontaneous depolarization. Normally, they are inactive because the intrinsic depolarization rate of the SA node is greater, inhibiting the discharge of these secondary pacemakers by *overdrive suppression*. The natural automatic rate of the SA node is 60 to 100 bpm, the AV junction 40 to 60 bpm, and the Purkinje system 20 to 40 bpm.

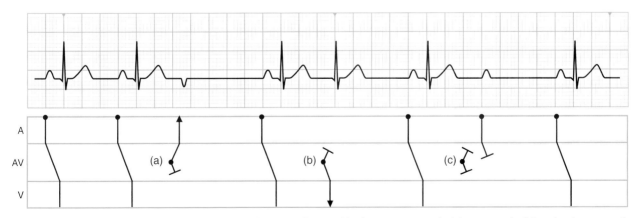

Figure 15-16. Junctional premature complexes may exhibit conduction block in an antegrade (a), retrograde (b), or both antegrade and retrograde direction (c). See text for details.

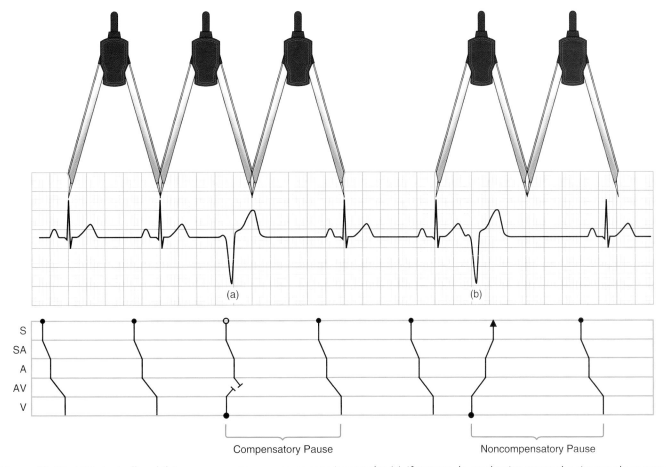

Figure 15-17. VPCs typically exhibit a compensatory pause, as seen in complex (a). If retrograde conduction resets the sinus node as seen in complex (b), a noncompensatory pause will result.

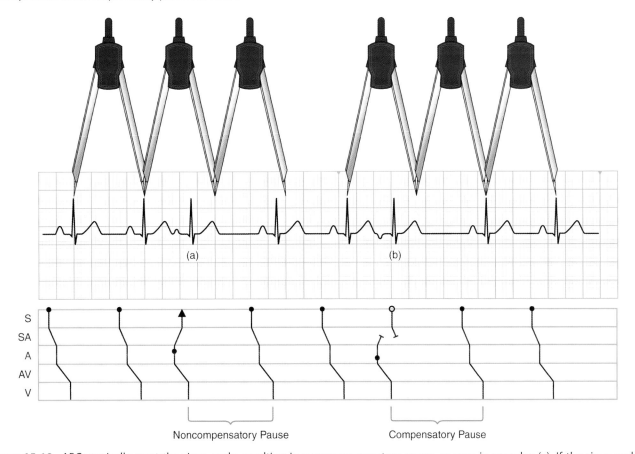

Figure 15-18. APCs typically reset the sinus node, resulting in a noncompensatory pause, as seen in complex (a). If the sinus node is undisturbed as seen in complex (b), a fully compensatory pause will result.

Escape complexes result from either primary depression or failure of the sinus depolarization (eg, sinus bradycardia, sinus arrest) or conduction failure of the sinus impulse distal in the conduction system (eg, SA block, AV block). They may also be present after prolonged pauses that occur after the termination of rapid atrial arrhythmias. Escape complexes are most often of AV junctional origin. Ventricular escape complexes are less frequent and those originating in the atria are uncommon.

Like premature complexes, a number of modifiers can apply to escape complexes, but with some important differences. A pattern of two or more consecutive escape complexes is called an *escape rhythm* (eg, AV junctional or ventricular escape rhythm). Escape complexes may exhibit aberrant ventricular conduction, but the mechanism of aberrancy of these late complexes is different from those that are premature, something we will review in detail in Chapter 16.

AV Junctional Escape Complex

Origin and morphology AV junctional escape complexes arise from either the upper or lower AV junction (not the actual AV node). A retrograde P′ wave is usually absent because the cycle rate of the AV junctional escape complex is nearly synchronous with the normal sinus cycle, which interferes with retrograde conduction (**Figure 15-19**). If retrograde depolarization does occur, an inverted P′ wave may be present before, after, or within the QRS complex, depending on the relative characteristics of antegrade and retrograde conduction (see Figure 15-15). In the absence of aberrant ventricular conduction, the QRS complex will be identical to the native morphology.

Timing AV junctional escape complexes appear late relative to the normal rhythm. The spontaneous rate of depolarization of the AV junction is 40 to 60 bpm. If the sinus mechanism falls below this rate, AV junctional escape complexes may emerge. AV junctional escape complexes are often seen

in the setting of sinus pause or arrest, marked sinus bradycardia with sinus arrhythmia, prolonged pauses after a premature complex, and AV block. Note that the native rhythm may not be sinus as AV junctional escape complexes and rhythm can be present in patients with atrial fibrillation and concomitant AV block.

Criteria for AV Junctional Escape Complex

- The complex appears late relative to the cycle of the normal rhythm, emerging due to a failure of a normally faster physiologic pacemaker.
- P′ waves are commonly absent.
- If present, an inverted, retrograde P′ wave may appear before, within, or after the QRS complex.
- When present before the QRS complex, the P′R interval of the junctional complex is short (<0.12 seconds).
- The QRS complex is identical to the native rhythm.

Ventricular Escape Complex

Origin and morphology Ventricular escape complexes originate below the bundle of His, typically in the Purkinje fibers that intertwine with the cells of the ventricular myocardium. Less frequently, ventricular escape complexes may derive from the bundle branches. The actual ventricular myocardial cells do not normally possess the property of automaticity. Like VPCs, the QRS morphology is wide (≥0.12 seconds) with secondary ST segment and T wave abnormalities (**Figure 15-20**).

Timing Ventricular escape complexes appear late relative to the native rhythm. The intrinsic rate of depolarization of Purkinje cells is 20 to 40 bpm. If the rate of the native rhythm falls below this level, ventricular escape complexes may emerge. The appearance of ventricular escape complexes implies dysfunction not only of the sinus mechanism but also that of the AV junction because normally that site would serve as the next subsidiary pacemaker.

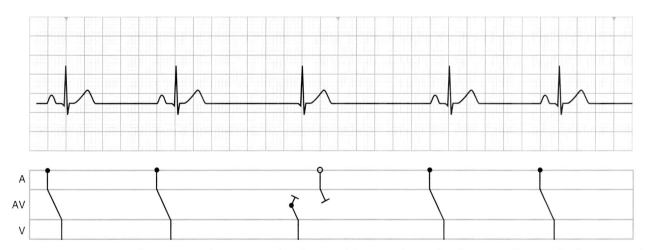

Figure 15-19. Sinus pause with AV junctional escape complex. Slowing of the normal sinus depolarization allows a subsidiary pacemaker to emerge from the AV junction.

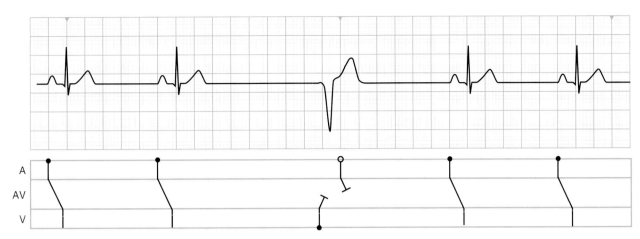

Figure 15-20. Sinus pause with ventricular escape complex. One would expect the AV junction would emerge as the next subsidiary pacemaker; therefore, the presence of a ventricular escape complex implies significant disease in the AV junction.

Criteria for Ventricular Escape Complex

- The complex appears late relative to the cycle of the normal rhythm, emerging due to a failure of a normally faster physiologic pacemaker.
- The complex is wide (≥0.12 seconds) with secondary ST segment and T wave abnormalities.
- There is no relationship to a P wave.

Atrial Escape Complex

Origin and morphology Atrial escape complex may rarely arise from localized areas of the atria, particularly in the region of the crista terminalis. Depending on its proximity to the AV node, the ectopic P′ wave may appear nearly normal, or inverted. The P′R interval remains within the normal range (0.12-0.20 seconds). The depolarization typically conducts normally so the QRS complex morphology will be identical to the native rhythm (**Figure 15-21**).

Timing Atrial escape complexes appear late relative to the native rhythm. The intrinsic rate of depolarization of the atrial focus is approximately 50 bpm. This rate is usually very similar to the native rhythm, with the escape complex emerging in the setting of sinus bradycardia or after a brief pause. In most circumstances, the AV junction is the next subsidiary pacemaker to emerge; therefore, isolated atrial escape complexes are unusual.

Criteria for Atrial Escape Complex

- The complex appears late relative to the cycle of the normal rhythm, emerging due to a failure of a normally faster physiologic pacemaker.
- The P′ wave is nearly normal relative to the native P wave, but may be inverted.
- The P′R interval remains within the normal range (0.12-0.20 seconds).
- The QRS complex is identical to the native rhythm.

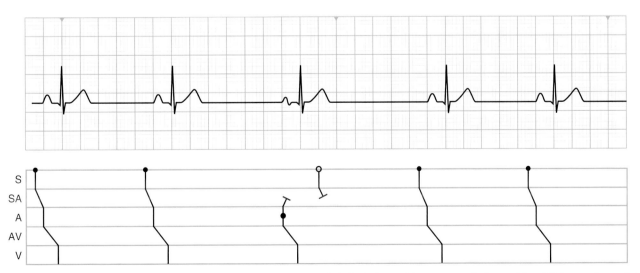

Figure 15-21. Sinus pause with an atrial escape complex. Note the slightly different P′ wave morphology with a P′R interval remaining within the normal range.

Q U E S T I O N S

Chapter 15 • SELF-TEST

1. Ectopic complexes are named according to what recommended convention?

2. What is the term given to an ectopic complex that originates in the ventricles and occurs early compared with the normal sinus cycle?

3. What is the term given to an ectopic complex that originates in the AV junction and occurs late compared with the normal sinus cycle?

4. What is the term used to describe the interval between the last normal complex and the premature ectopic complex?

5. What is the difference between a fully compensatory pause and a noncompensatory pause?

6. Any premature complex that does not reset the sinus node would be expected to exhibit which type of post-ectopic pause?

7. Any premature complex that resets the sinus node would be expected to exhibit which type of post-ectopic pause?

8. What is the term used to describe a VPC that appears sandwiched in between two normal sinus complexes?

9. What is the term used to describe a VPC that appears electrically unrelated to, but just after the appearance of the P wave?

10. An atrial premature complex with aberrant conduction is most likely to have a morphology that resembles what type of bundle branch block?

11. AV junctional complexes characteristically demonstrate what type of P′ wave morphology?

12. What two factors determine the location of the retrograde P′ wave with regards to its relationship to the QRS complex?

13. What is a fusion complex?

14. The SA node is the primary pacemaker of the heart. What other areas have the property of automaticity and may emerge as subsidiary pacemakers?

15. What is the normal automatic rate of the sinus node, AV junction, and the Purkinje system?

Chapter 15 • SELF-TEST

ANSWERS

1. • The site of origin.
   • The timing relative to the native rhythm.
   • With additional descriptors as needed.

2. Ventricular premature complex.

3. AV junctional escape complex.

4. Coupling interval.

5. A compensatory pause "compensates" for the prematurity of the ectopic complex. The sum of the coupling interval and the pause equals two normal sinus cycles. A noncompensatory pause does not compensate for the prematurity of the ectopic complex, such that the sum of the coupling interval and the pause is either longer or shorter than two normal sinus cycles.

6. Compensatory.

7. Noncompensatory.

8. Interpolated.

9. Late (end) diastolic VPC.

10. Right bundle branch block.

11. Inverted.

12. The relative speed of antegrade and retrograde conduction and the location of the focus within the AV junction.

13. A complex that represents the merging of depolarization from two separate foci.

14. Regions within the atria, the upper and lower portions of the AV junction, and the remainder of the His-Purkinje system.

15. • Sinus node: 60 to 100 bpm.
    • AV junction: 40 to 60 bpm.
    • Purkinje system: 20 to 40 bpm.

Further Reading

Bagliani G, DellaRocca DG, DePonti R, Capucci A, Padeletti M, Natale A. Ectopic beats. *Card Electrophysiol Clin.* 2018;10:257-275.

Chung EKY. Parasystole. *Prog Cardiovasc Dis.* 1968;11:64-81.

Engel TR, Meister SG, Frankl WS. The "R-on-T" phenomenon: an update and critical review. *Ann Intern Med.* 1978;88:221-225.

Fisch C, Zipes DP, McHenry PL. Electrocardiographic manifestations of concealed junctional ectopic impulses. *Circulation.* 1976;53:217-223.

Janse MJ. The premature beat. *Cardiovasc Res.* 1992;26:89-100.

Kennedy HL, Whitlock JA, Sprague MK, Kennedy LJ, Buckingham TA, Goldberg RJ. Long-term follow-up of asymptomatic healthy subjects with frequent and complex ventricular ectopy. *N Engl J Med.* 1985;312:193-197.

Leonelli FM, DePonti R, Bagliani G. Electrocardiographic approach to complex arrhythmias: P, QRS, and their relationships. *Card Electrophysiol Clin.* 2019;11:239-260.

Mond HG, Haqqani HM. The electrocardiographic footprints of atrial ectopy. *Heart Lung Circ.* 2019;28:1463-1471.

Mond HG, Haqqani HM. The electrocardiographic footprints of ventricular ectopy. *Heart Lung Circ.* 2020;29:988-999.

Pick A, Langedorf R. Parasystole and its variants. *Med Clin North Am.* 1976;60:125-146.

Wang K, Hodges M. The premature complex as a diagnostic aid. *Ann Intern Med.* 1992;117:766-770.

Aberrant Conduction

► INTRODUCTION

A supraventricular impulse results in a narrow QRS complex by virtue of rapid synchronous conduction through the His-Purkinje system, finally reaching the ventricular myocardium. As we have learned previously, a fixed conduction delay or interruption in the bundle branches or their divisions produces abnormalities of QRS complex morphology that we know as bundle branch block or fascicular block. The ECG findings include alterations in QRS complex duration, amplitude, configuration, and axis. The term **aberration** (or aberrant ventricular conduction) is used to describe *transient* bundle branch block and fascicular block that are unrelated to preexisting bundle branch block, preexcitation, or the effects of drug or electrolyte abnormalities. This temporary alteration of conduction, also called *phasic aberrant ventricular conduction*, is due to differential refractoriness of the bundle branches combined with variances in cycle length, concepts that we will now review.

Refractory Period Review

In Chapter 3 we learned that the action potential of a nonpacemaker myocyte is divided into five phases (0,1,2,3,4) (**Figure 16-1**). Phase 0 (rapid depolarization) is the rapid upstroke from the negative resting membrane potential (RP) that begins depolarization. A stimulus from an adjacent cell opens sodium channels to reach the threshold potential (TP), further inducing the rapid influx of positively charged sodium ions. Phase 1 (early rapid repolarization) is the initial reversal of the transient positive overshoot of depolarization from phase 0. Phase 2 (plateau) is the delay in repolarization resulting from a balance of inward-flowing calcium ions and outward-flowing potassium ions. Phase 3 (terminal rapid repolarization) continues repolarization toward the baseline membrane potential. Phase 4 (resting) is the time between action potentials, during which the stable negative resting potential is established, preparing the cell for the next stimulus.

During each action potential, there is a period of time when the cell is either partially or completely unable to respond to a new stimulus. These *refractory periods* are dependent on the number of sodium channels available for opening, which are depleted with depolarization and restored with repolarization. The **absolute refractory period** (ARP) comprises phases 1 and 2 of the action potential, during which time the cell cannot generate a new action potential, no matter how great the stimulus. The **effective refractory period** (ERP) includes the ARP and the early portion of phase 3. Any arriving stimulus produces a weak, ineffective response that will not produce a new depolarization (**Figure 16-2**). Recall that I like to think of this portion of the action potential as the "ineffective" refractory period because any impulse arriving during this time will not propagate further. The fundamental reason is that not enough sodium channels have regenerated to permit for a new

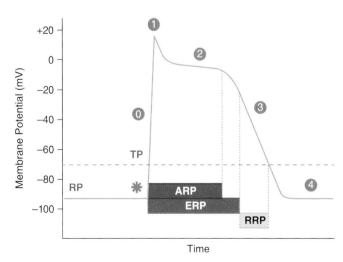

Figure 16-1. Action potential of a nonpacemaker cell showing the phases and refractory periods (see text for details). ARP = absolute refractory period, ERP = effective refractory period, RP = resting potential, RRP = relative refractory period, TP = threshold potential, (*) = stimulus.

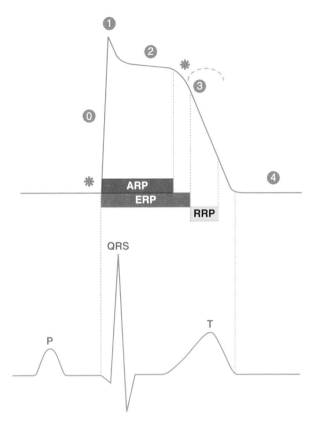

Figure 16-2. A stimulus (˚) arriving during either the ARP or ERP will not propagate. The ERP extends into phase 3 of the action potential, which correlates on the ECG with the first portion of the T wave.

action potential. On the ECG, we see this as a failure of conduction (block), which is the origin of the term **phase 3 block**. The **relative refractory period** (RRP) encompasses the latter portions of phase 3, during which a stimulus can depolarize the cell, but with a weaker and slower than normal response. Of course we can't see refractory periods on the ECG, but in practical terms, phase 3 begins with the first portion of the T wave (see Figure 16-2).

> **BE CAREFUL:** Remember that a premature impulse that fails to conduct distally because it encounters tissue that is physiologically refractory represents normal behavior.

I find it helpful to think of the phases of the action potential as the lights of a traffic signal. During phase 4 the light is green, where a depolarization may proceed at greatest speed. The light is yellow during the RRP, where a new impulse may advance, but more slowly. A red light represents the ERP that includes phases 1, 2, and the first portion of phase 3, where any arriving impulse is compelled to stop.

Figure 16-3 illustrates the concept of refractory periods using pairs of supraventricular complexes. After each complex, the ability of a second supraventricular impulse to conduct through the AV node depends on whether it arrives during the ERP (red), RRP (yellow), or afterwards when the cells are fully recovered. Panel (a) shows two normal sinus complexes with the refractory periods of the AV node indicated with our stoplight colors. In panel (b) a premature complex originating in the atria arrives at the AV node well beyond both refractory periods and the impulse conducts normally. Panel (c) shows an atrial premature complex arriving during the RRP, resulting in a delay in AV conduction. In panel (d) the premature impulse fails to conduct because it arrives during the ERP when no further transmission is possible.

Different segments of the cardiac conduction system have refractory period properties that differ from one another. As seen in Figure 16-3, conduction through the AV node is typically graded, exhibiting either unimpeded transmission, conduction delay, or block, the outcome dependent on the timing between the supraventricular impulses. In contrast, the His-Purkinje system usually exhibits an "all or nothing" response (**Figure 16-4**).

> **FOR BOOKWORMS:** At slower heart rates, the ERP of the AV node is shorter than that of the bundle branches. Therefore, a premature impulse may conduct normally through the AV node and then be blocked more distally (see Figure 16-4). At faster heart rates, both refractory periods shorten, but that of the His-Purkinje system does so to a much greater degree than the AV node. This means that during supraventricular tachyarrhythmias, the AV node typically becomes the limiting factor whether the supraventricular impulse conducts through to the ventricles.

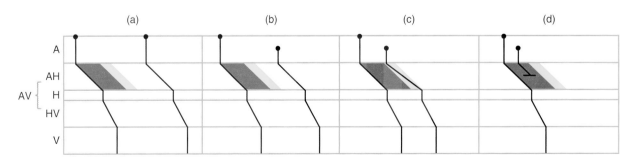

Figure 16-3. Laddergrams showing transmission of impulses through the AV node. Panel (a) shows normal conduction. In panel (b) a premature impulse falls outside the refractory periods of the first complex and conducts normally. In panel (c), the premature impulse falls within the RRP (yellow) and conducts with a delay. In panel (d) the impulse arrives during the ERP (red) and is blocked. Laddergram abbreviations: A = atrium, AH = atrial-His, H = His, HV= His-Purkinje, V = ventricle, AV = AV conduction.

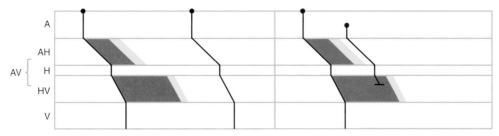

Figure 16-4. Refractory periods are different throughout the conduction system. The premature impulse may pass through the AV node only to be blocked more distally.

Mechanism of Aberrant Intraventricular Conduction

Aberrant ventricular conduction of a supraventricular impulse results from three primary mechanisms: (1) depolarization arriving during phase 3 of the action potential (phase 3 aberration), (2) stimulation during phase 4 of the action potential (phase 4 aberration), and (3) concealed retrograde trans-septal conduction. Aberrancy may accompany any supraventricular complex or rhythm including sinus, atrial, AV junctional, supraventricular tachycardias, atrial flutter, and atrial fibrillation.

▶ PHASE 3 ABERRANCY

Unequal Bundle Branch Refractoriness and Critically Timed Impulses

The key underlying mechanism of phasic aberrant ventricular conduction is unequal refractoriness of the bundle branches. Up to now, we have depicted the bundle branch system as having one refractory period. In actuality, the ERP of the bundle branches and their divisions are not the same. The ERP of the right bundle branch is typically longer than that of the left bundle branch, and that of the anterior fascicle of the left bundle branch longer than the posterior fascicle. Aberrant conduction results when a supraventricular impulse encounters one (but not all) of the bundle branches or fascicles during its ERP. The impulse blocks in the refractory structure (usually the right

bundle branch) and conducts through the unblocked fascicle(s). **Figure 16-5** illustrates the process. Notice that the right bundle branch ERP is longer than that of the left bundle branch. If an impulse arrives beyond the ERP of *both* bundle branches, the impulse will conduct normally with a narrow QRS complex (panel a). Conversely, if a premature impulse arrives when *both* bundle branches are refractory, the supraventricular impulse will be blocked (panel b), resulting in a P′ wave that is not followed by a QRS complex. But if a premature impulse arrives when *only* the right bundle branch is refractory, conduction will proceed normally through the left bundle branch, the QRS complex appearing with a RBBB morphology (panel c).

So now you can see that aberrant conduction depends on two factors (1) differential refractoriness of the bundle branches and (2) a critically timed impulse. This represents normal, physiologic behavior of the cardiac conduction system.

Dependence on Cycle Length

The ERP of the His-Purkinje system is not fixed, but is proportional to the duration of the **preceding** cycle length (R-R interval) (**Figure 16-6**). With faster heart rates (shorter cycle length), the ERP of the bundle branches shorten. Conversely, with slower heart rates (longer cycle length), the ERP lengthens. Of note is that at slower heart rates the ERP of the right bundle branch exceeds that of the left bundle, but at higher heart rates the reverse is true. This explains why in the same patient, a premature impulse may conduct aberrantly

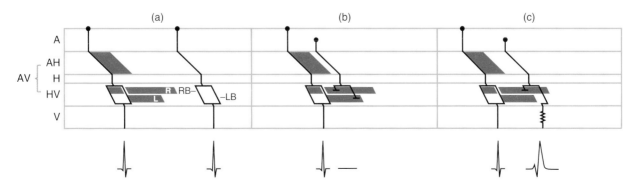

Figure 16-5. At normal heart rates, the ERP of the right bundle branch (RB) is longer than that of the left bundle branch (LB). Another impulse arriving beyond the refractory periods of both bundle branches will conduct normally with a narrow QRS complex morphology (panel a). A premature impulse will fail to conduct if it arrives when both bundle branches are refractory (panel b). Aberrant conduction will result when the premature impulse arrives during the ERP of one, but not both of the bundle branches (panel c). In this example, the second impulse finds the right bundle branch refractory and transmits normally through the left bundle branch. The ECG shows aberrant conduction with a right bundle branch block morphology.

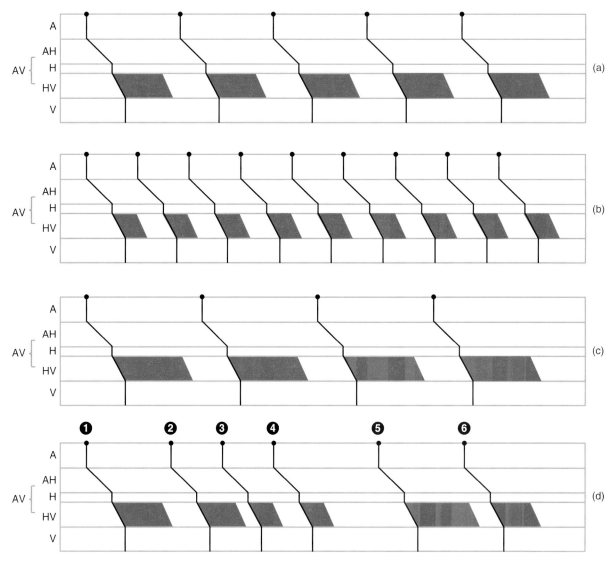

Figure 16-6. The refractory period varies with the cycle length, shortening as the heart rate rises (shorter cycle length) and lengthening as the heart rate slows (longer cycle length). Laddergrams depict refractory periods of the His-Purkinje system for cycle lengths at baseline (a), shorter (b), longer (c), and with variable cycle lengths (d). The refractory period of each complex is proportional to the preceding cycle length. In panel (d) notice how the refractory periods following each complex vary according to the cycle length between that complex and the one before. The refractory periods of complex 2 and complex 6 are identical because the preceding cycle lengths are the same. The same is true for complexes 3 and 4.

with the morphology of a RBBB at one heart rate and a LBBB at another.

The relationship between the refractory period and preceding cycle length is particularly important when the heart rhythm is irregular (**Figure 16-7**). A long R-R interval followed by a short R-R interval (long-short cycle) facilitates aberrancy (or block) as the short cycle complex that follows the long interval encounters cells with a longer refractory period. Does this situation sound familiar? It should because we described this phenomenon in Chapter 15 when we considered the potential fates of atrial premature complexes (**Figure 16-8**). Now you understand why different premature complexes that have the same coupling intervals may have different fates depending on the refractoriness of the tissue they encounter.

FOR HISTORY BUFFS: In a 1947 publication of the American Heart Journal, James Gouaux and Richard Ashman described aberrant conduction in the setting of atrial fibrillation, where variable R-R intervals are the norm. The *Ashman phenomenon* is the eponym used to describe an aberrantly conducted complex precipitated by a long-short cycle.

Acceleration-Dependent Aberrancy

Acceleration-dependent aberration is a form of rate-related bundle branch block that develops as heart rate increases (**Figure 16-9a**). Also called tachycardia-dependent aberrancy, it reflects a failure of the ERP of one of the bundle branches to shorten sufficiently to allow normal conduction in response to an increasing heart rate. As opposed to the physiologic phase

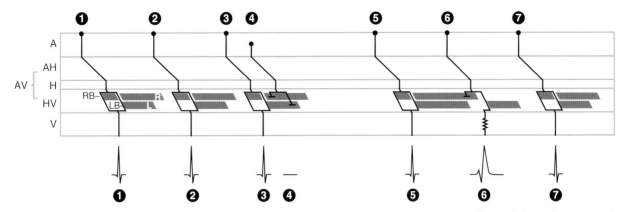

Figure 16-7. A premature impulse (complex 4) arrives when both the right bundle branch (RB) and left bundle branch (LB) are refractory and is blocked. The resulting pause lengthens the ERP of the following complex (complex 5), setting the stage for aberrant conduction in the following impulse (complex 6). The normal timing of complex 6 returns the ERP to baseline, which permits a narrow complex 7 to follow.

3 aberration that we discussed earlier, acceleration-dependent phase 3 BBB often reflects a diseased His-Purkinje system. This is particularly true when the BBB occurs at relatively slow heart rates (<70 bpm), displays LBBB morphology, and appears with a gradual, rather than abrupt change in cycle length. The *critical rate or cycle* is the term given to the heart rate or cycle length at which the bundle branch appears during acceleration and disappears during slowing. The critical rate that the bundle branch block develops is typically faster than the one where it resolves (see **Figure 16-9b**).

▶ PHASE 4 DECELERATION-DEPENDENT ABERRANCY

Another form of rate-related ventricular aberration is deceleration-dependent bundle branch block. Also called phase 4 or bradycardia-dependent aberrancy, this form of aberrant conduction becomes manifest as the heart rate slows (**Figure 16-10**). Hmmm, that seems odd. Why would conduction be impaired when the stimulus arrives beyond the refractory period, a time when the cell should be fully responsive? The postulated mechanism is that cells of the conduction system exhibit slow, phase 4 depolarization, which reduces responsiveness (**Figure 16-11**). Normally, a supraventricular impulse arriving during this time

progresses through the conduction system without delay, with any subsidiary pacemakers staying inactive by virtue of overdrive suppression. But injured cells may develop abnormal automaticity, depolarizing at a faster rate than would normally be expected. So after a long cycle, abnormally automatic cells of the His-Purkinje system begin to depolarize, the next sinus impulse reaching the region at a less negative membrane potential. Just like with phase 3 block, if there are insufficient sodium channels available for depolarization, conduction will fail. Deceleration-dependent aberrancy is uncommon and usually shows a LBBB pattern, reflecting structural heart disease that affects the left bundle branch.

▶ CONCEALED TRANS-SEPTAL CONDUCTION ABERRANCY

We have just learned that the ERP of the His-Purkinje system is proportional to the preceding cycle length. A long-short cycle favors aberrant conduction in the complex ending the short cycle because the supraventricular depolarization encounters fibers with a longer refractory period. This aberrantly conducted complex has a preceding short cycle with a shorter ERP, so we expect that the complex that follows will conduct

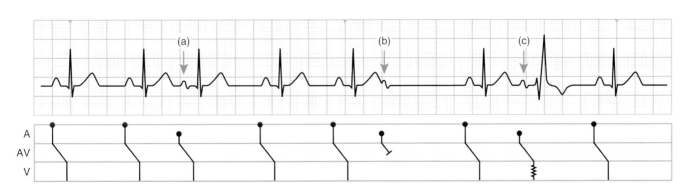

Figure 16-8. Depending on the timing relationship with the preceding cardiac cycle, an atrial premature complex may be conducted normally (a), blocked (b), or conducts with aberrant morphology (c). Complexes (a) and (c) have the same degree of prematurity, but complex (c) conducts aberrantly because it encounters cells with a longer refractory period.

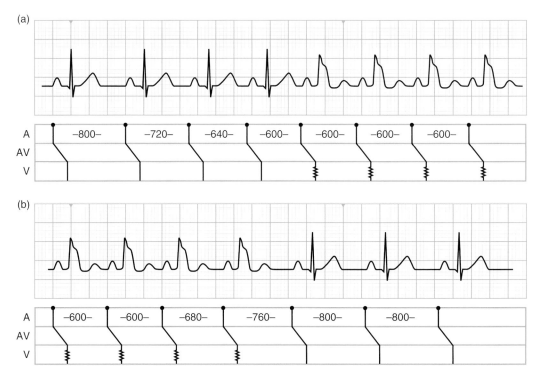

Figure 16-9. Acceleration-dependent aberrant conduction with characteristic left bundle branch morphology. The aberrancy typically appears at a shorter cycle length (600 msec) during acceleration (a) than when it resolves (760 msec) as the heart rate slows (b).

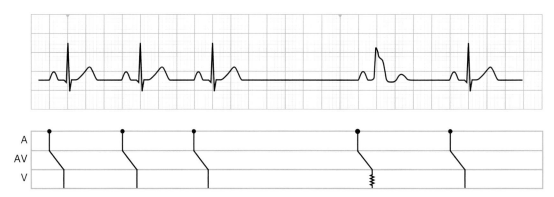

Figure 16-10. Deceleration-dependent aberrancy with typical left bundle branch morphology.

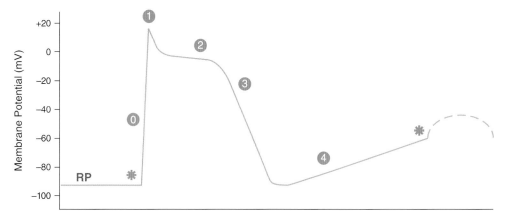

Figure 16-11. Deceleration-dependent aberrancy is believed due to abnormal, spontaneous phase 4 depolarization, which renders the cell incapable of propagating an impulse (see text for details).

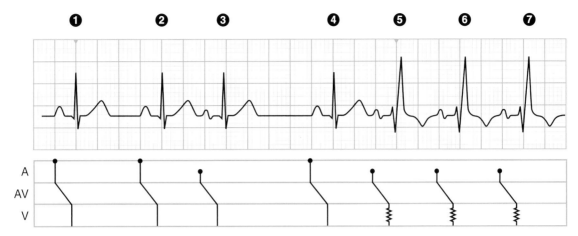

Figure 16-12. Persistent aberrant conduction. The first atrial premature complex (complex 3) conducts normally. After a pause, three premature atrial complexes appear in sequence, all with aberrant conduction (complexes 5, 6, and 7).

normally (see Figures 16-7 and 16-8). If that's the case, why do we sometimes see persistence of aberrant conduction in multiple sequential complexes (**Figure 16-12**)?

The most widely accepted mechanism is that the blocked bundle branch undergoes retrograde depolarization from concealed trans-septal conduction, thereby making its recovery later than we might expect (**Figure 16-13**). It starts with "garden variety" phase 3 block as a premature impulse finds the right bundle branch refractory after a long-short cycle. Conduction proceeds through the unblocked left bundle branch to depolarize the ventricles and the QRS complex shows the expected RBBB morphology. But in this particular situation, the impulse transmits across the septum and then conducts retrograde to invade a portion of the right bundle branch. The blocked right bundle branch undergoes a delayed, "hidden" depolarization, thereby extending its ERP, and facilitating aberrancy of the next antegrade impulse. In simple terms, the working left bundle branch has done its job, sending the impulse on to the ventricles. But the right bundle branch has "lagged behind," depolarizing late without our knowledge (concealed), only making its presence known by influencing conduction of the next impulse. This is the proposed mechanism of persistent aberrancy in the setting of paroxysmal atrial tachyarrhythmias as well as why in acceleration-dependent BBB, the critical heart rate is at a different cycle length when the aberrancy appears versus when it resolves.

▶ PREMATURE COMPLEX CONUNDRUM: ABERRANCY VERSUS ECTOPY

In Chapter 15 we learned about the different forms of premature complexes including those originating from the atria, AV junction, and the ventricles. Supraventricular complexes with aberrant conduction have a wide QRS that resemble ventricular complexes. It's not always possible to differentiate the two, but there are ECG clues to suggest the correct diagnosis. These include (1) the presence of preceding atrial activity, (2) QRS

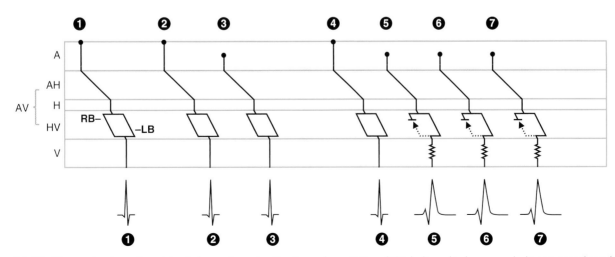

Figure 16-13. The mechanism of persistent aberrant conduction (complexes 5, 6, and 7) is believed to be concealed trans-septal conduction with retrograde depolarization of the blocked bundle branch (see text for details).

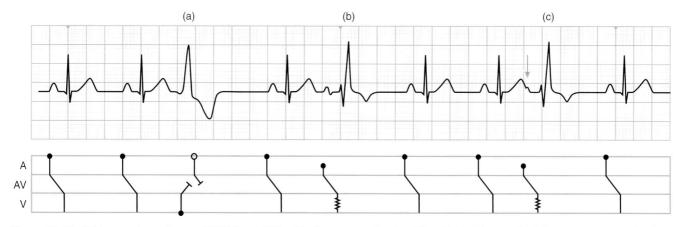

Figure 16-14. Wide complexes due to a VPC (a) and APCs with aberrant conduction (b) and (c). Evidence of atrial activity associated with an APC may be subtle, hidden in the T wave of the preceding complex (arrow).

morphology, (3) QRS duration, (4) QRS axis, and (5) cycle length variation. These criteria have the most utility when the baseline QRS complex is narrow, without fixed bundle branch block or preexcitation. Much of the information we will now review is derived from analysis of wide complex tachycardias, a topic we'll discuss in great detail in Chapter 20. The criteria used in wide complex tachycardias are useful for the analysis of the individual premature complexes. With that introduction, let's get started.

The Presence or Absence of Preceding Atrial Activity

A premature P′ wave followed by a wide QRS complex strongly suggests an atrial premature complex with aberrant conduction (**Figure 16-14**). It's important to make a careful search for a preceding P′ wave, which may be obscured in the T wave of the previous complex, particularly when heart rates are rapid. Also remember that the P′ wave of a junctional premature complex will be inverted and may appear before, after, or be hidden within the associated QRS complex (see Chapter 15, Figure 15-14).

In contrast, VPCs are wide complexes without preceding atrial activity. An exception is the P wave seen before a late (end) diastolic VPC (**Figure 16-15**), but in this situation, the P wave has normal timing and the QRS complex that follows is electrically unrelated.

Although atrial activity is present, discrete P waves are absent in the setting of atrial fibrillation and flutter and they may be hidden with supraventricular tachycardia. In these settings, other parameters reviewed in the following discussion become the primary means of differentiating ventricular ectopy from aberrant supraventricular complexes.

QRS Complex Morphology

A ventricular ectopic complex originating in the left ventricle has features of a RBBB and those arising from the right ventricle or interventricular septum resemble a LBBB. Why should that be? The reason is that in both RBBB and left ventricular ectopy, the left ventricle is activated first, followed by the right ventricle. Similarly, in both LBBB and right ventricular ectopy, the right ventricle is activated first, followed by the left ventricle. Most septal-based ventricular arrhythmias exit toward the right ventricle, so again the pattern resembles a LBBB. But there are important differences between the morphology of ectopy and aberrancy, something we can use to help distinguish the two.

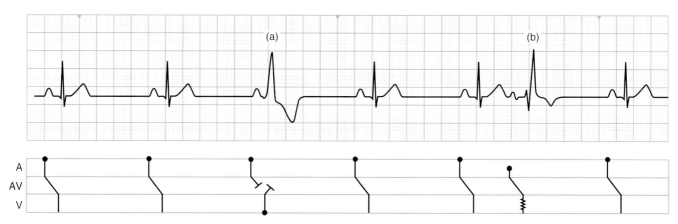

Figure 16-15. The P wave preceding a late (end) diastolic VPC (a) is electrically unrelated and occurs on time related to the native rhythm. The P′ wave of an aberrantly conducted APC (b) occurs early and relates to the following QRS complex.

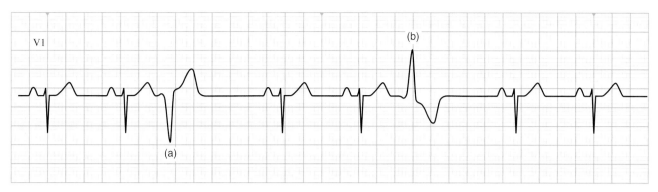

Figure 16-16. Inspect lead V1 to determine if a wide complex has the morphology of either a LBBB with an R/S ratio <1 (a) or RBBB with a R/S ratio >1 (b).

The first step in this process is to determine whether the morphology of the wide complex resembles that of a RBBB or LBBB. Thankfully, this is straightforward by looking at lead V1 (**Figure 16-16**). If the QRS complex is predominantly positive (R/S ratio >1), then it has RBBB-type morphology. If the QRS complex in lead V1 is predominantly negative (R/S ratio <1) with a negative terminal component, then it has LBBB-type morphology. That was easy! Now we can analyze the respective patterns in more detail.

 BE CAREFUL: The RBBB pattern = LV ectopy, LBBB pattern = RV ectopy and their respective morphologic patterns we will review in the following discussion are most consistent in patients without structural heart disease. VPCs arising from hearts with structural abnormalities exhibit a variety of atypical patterns that reflect prior scars due to myocardial infarction or other causes of fibrosis.

RBBB morphology complexes Let's review why the QRS pattern of a RBBB looks the way it does (**Figure 16-17**). As we learned in Chapter 8, the initial vector with RBBB is unchanged from normal, the septum depolarizing rapidly from left-to-right and anteriorly via the septal fascicle of the left bundle branch. This preserves the small and narrow initial q wave in leftward-looking leads (I, aVL, V6) and the corresponding small and narrow initial r wave in rightward and anterior-looking leads (V1, V2). Transmission proceeds via the intact left bundle branch to activate the left ventricular free wall in a normal leftward and posterior direction. Accordingly, we expect to see an R wave in leftward-looking leads and an S wave in rightward-looking leads. Depolarization now spreads via slow, myocyte-to-myocyte transmission to activate the right ventricle, producing a wide, secondary R′ in V1 or V2 and a broad, terminal S wave in lead V6. This explains the typical triphasic pattern we see in leads V1 and V2 (rSR′, rsR′, rSr′) and lead V6 (qRs).

In contrast, a VPC arising within the left ventricular myocardium originates outside of the normal conduction system. The left ventricle activates before the right ventricle, hence the RBBB-type pattern. But unlike in RBBB, the initial vector of the ectopic impulse is different from normal, slowly activating the left ventricle via myocyte-to-myocyte conduction. Eventually, the

impulse engages the specialized conduction system to more rapidly depolarize the remainder of the left and right ventricular myocardium. Because of the large mass of the left ventricle, the RBBB-type pattern is highly variable.

The above concept explains why certain RBBB-type morphologies are more likely to be aberrant whereas others suggest

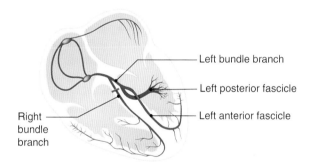

Figure 16-17. RBBB vector loop. Depolarization proceeds via the intact left bundle branch to activate the septum (vector 1) and left ventricular free wall (vector 2). The remainder of the left ventricle and right ventricle is depolarized via slow, myocyte-to-myocyte conduction (vector 3).

RBBB-Type Complexes

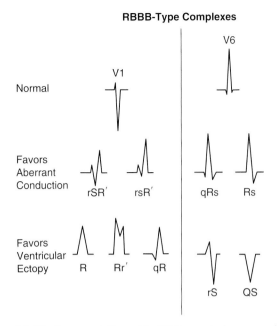

Figure 16-18. Representative wide RBBB morphology complexes. In lead V1, triphasic patterns (rSR´, rsR´, rSr´) favor aberrancy, whereas a monophasic (R), notched (Rr´), or biphasic (qR) pattern favors ventricular ectopy. In lead V6, a triphasic (qRs), or biphasic (Rs) pattern favors aberrancy, whereas a biphasic (rS) or (QS) pattern favors ventricular ectopy.

a ventricular origin (**Figure 16-18**). Rather than spend time memorizing patterns I recommend you keep some basic concepts in mind. The more the wide complex looks like a classic RBBB, the more likely there is aberrant conduction. So if you look at lead V1 and see a triphasic, (eg, rSR´, rsR´, RSR´, rSr´) pattern, especially with a small and narrow initial r wave, followed by an S wave and accompanied by a tall and wide secondary R´ deflection, the diagnosis strongly favors RBBB aberrancy. Similarly, in lead V6, a triphasic qRs complex with a wide terminal s wave favors aberrancy. The mass of the delayed right ventricular depolarization represented by the s wave is smaller than the left ventricular mass recorded as an R wave, so the R/S ratio in lead V6 with aberrant conduction is >1.

The vectors of a left ventricular ectopic complex follow a different pathway, so the wide complex should have an atypical

RBBB pattern. Looking again at lead V1, a broad, monophasic R, a notched Rr´, or biphasic qR pattern all suggest ventricular ectopy. In lead V6, a biphasic rS or monophasic QS complex favors a ventricular origin. Depolarization of both the left and right ventricles contributes to the vector directed away from V6, which leads to a deep S wave and a R/S ratio of <1.

> **BE CAREFUL:** A triphasic rsR´ or rSR´ pattern in lead V1 that favors aberrancy over ectopy resembles the biphasic rR´, RR´ morphology that cannot be used to distinguish the two diagnoses. Both have larger "right rabbit ears" with a prominent terminal R´ wave, but only the triphasic pattern with a demonstrable s (or S) wave provides a reliable clue to aberrant conduction.

> **FOR BOOKWORMS:** Ventricular ectopy originating from the base of the left ventricle or left ventricular outflow tract may show a monophasic R wave in lead V6, reflecting depolarization directed toward the lateral precordial leads.

One more clue we can use with RBBB-type complexes is to take a closer look at the initial deflection and compare this with the native complex. Because ventricular ectopic complexes originate outside the normal conduction system, there should be no reason why the initial vector would be identical to the native complex. In contrast, vector 1 with a RBBB is unchanged from baseline. So if the initial deflection of the native complex and that of the RBBB-looking wide complex are **identical**, then aberrant conduction is the more likely diagnosis (**Figure 16-19**).

LBBB morphology complexes Let's now turn to complexes with a LBBB-type morphology. We learned in Chapter 8 that with LBBB, the entire sequence of ventricular activation is altered, affecting both the initial septal and subsequent ventricular forces (**Figure 16-20**). The initial impulse conducts via the intact right bundle, rapidly depolarizing the right side of the interventricular septum and right ventricular free wall. The now right-to-left and anterior orientation of vector 1 produces a small initial positive deflection in leftward (I, V6) and anterior (V1, V2) looking leads. Vector 2 is the slow, myocyte-to-myocyte depolarization of the remainder of the left septal mass

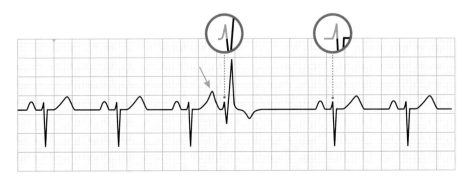

Figure 16-19. The initial portion of the wide complex, highlighted in blue, is identical to that of the native complex, supporting a supraventricular origin with aberrant conduction. Additional evidence is the presence of preceding atrial activity, seen here as a "hidden" P´ wave that deforms the T wave of the preceding complex (arrow).

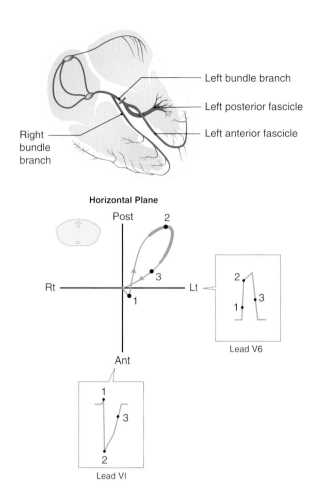

Figure 16-20. LBBB vector loop. Depolarization proceeds via the intact right bundle branch to activate the septum in a leftward and anterior direction (vector 1). The left ventricular free wall is depolarized via slow, myocyte-to-myocyte conduction (vector 2), followed by the remainder of the myocardium (vector 3).

and adjacent free wall of the left ventricle, with forces oriented to the left, posteriorly, and inferiorly. Accordingly, we see a tall, wide R wave in leads I, aVL and V6 and a deep, smooth S wave in leads V1 and V2. Vector 3 represents delayed activation of the lateral wall of the left ventricle that produces the terminal R´ in leftward-looking leads.

The QRS patterns that favor LBBB aberrancy are more subtle than those used for RBBB morphology (**Figure 16-21**). As with RBBB aberrancy, the more the complex resembles a classic LBBB, the stronger the diagnosis. And for this analysis, you should inspect *both* leads V1 and V2. In these leads, a narrow r wave and smooth, brisk S wave downstroke support LBBB-type aberrant conduction, reflecting the initial depolarization by the intact right bundle branch. Unlike RBBB aberrancy, the QRS pattern in lead V6 does not help much to favor aberrant conduction except that any q (or Q) wave is incompatible with LBBB aberration and favors ectopy (see following discussion). Other patterns containing an initial r or R wave in lead V6 are compatible with either ectopy or aberrancy.

Ectopic ventricular complexes originate outside of the normal conduction system, so we expect the initial portion of the QRS

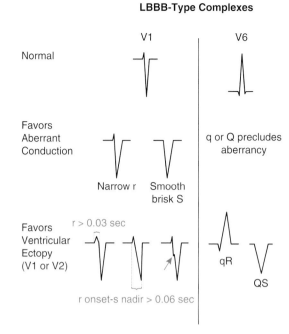

Figure 16-21. Representative wide LBBB morphology complexes. In leads V1 or V2, a wide r wave (>0.03 seconds), delayed QRS onset to S nadir (>0.06 seconds), or notched S wave (arrow) all favor ventricular ectopy. A narrow r wave and smooth, brisk S wave favor aberrant conduction. In lead V6, any q or QS wave precludes LBBB aberrancy and favors a complex of ventricular origin.

to be delayed. Therefore, findings in leads V1 or V2 that support ventricular ectopy include any of the following: (1) a wide initial R wave of >0.03 seconds, (2) a delayed R wave onset to S wave nadir of >0.06 seconds, and (3) a notch or slur on the downstroke of the S wave. Although infrequently seen, the presence of any q wave in lead V6 virtually guarantees a complex of ventricular origin. The reason is that the initial right-to-left orientation of vector 1 with LBBB *precludes* a q wave in leads I and V6.

QRS Complex Duration

When combined with bundle branch block morphology, the duration of the QRS complex can help to distinguish aberrancy from ectopy. The wider the complex, the more likely it is of ventricular origin, reflecting depolarization deep in the ventricular myocardium and away from the specialized conduction system. A QRS interval of >0.14 seconds with RBBB morphology supports ventricular ectopy as does a duration of >0.16 seconds with LBBB morphology. When analyzing QRS complex duration, remember to make your measurement in the lead that demonstrates the widest complex.

QRS axis

QRS axis does not readily differentiate ventricular complexes from those of supraventricular origin with aberrancy. However, the presence of extreme axis deviation between −90 and ±180 degrees (ie, right-superior or "northwest quadrant") is highly specific for ventricular ectopy (**Figure 16-22**). The reason is that there is no conduction abnormality, either alone or

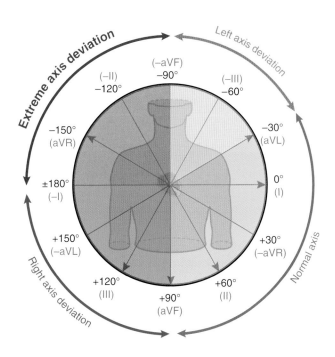

Figure 16-22. A complex with a mean frontal plane QRS axis in the right-superior (northwest) quadrant is highly likely to be ventricular ectopy.

in combination that results in this axis. Although not as specific a finding, an LBBB-type complex with right axis deviation favors ventricular ectopy. Clinical conditions typically associated with LBBB include heart failure, hypertension, and valvular heart disease, all of which are associated with left ventricular enlargement and left axis deviation. Accordingly, a LBBB-type complex with an unusual right axis likely originates from an ectopic ventricular focus.

Cycle Length Variation

A long-short sequence with sudden shortening of the cycle length (R-R interval) promotes ventricular aberrancy (Ashman phenomenon). However, this finding is not as reliable in discriminating ectopy from aberrancy when the rhythm is atrial fibrillation, something made ironic by the fact that Gouaux and Ashman's original description was in the setting of this arrhythmia. Yes, a long-short cycle seen in the presence of atrial fibrillation does promote aberrant conduction. However, a preceding long cycle also

promotes ventricular ectopy, a reentry-related phenomenon called "the rule of bigeminy." Does this mean we should forego inspection of cycle length with atrial fibrillation? No way!

There are still some cycle length clues we can apply in the setting of atrial fibrillation. Wide complexes of ventricular origin tend to exhibit fixed coupling, whereas the coupling relationship of aberrant supraventricular complexes varies over a wider range (**Figure 16-23**). Also, look for a long-short cycle where a short cycle complex is conducted normally after a particularly long cycle. If that complex conducts normally, aberrant conduction after a "less dramatic" long-short sequence should be unlikely. Finally, the pause after a ventricular premature complex tends to be longer than that of a supraventricular complex because of retrograde conduction into the AV junction, thereby rendering the region temporarily refractory to depolarization from above.

Putting Things Together

When you see a wide, premature complex on the ECG, it is often difficult and sometimes impossible to differentiate aberrant ventricular conduction from ventricular ectopy outside of the electrophysiology laboratory. Nevertheless, we learned in this chapter a number of features that can suggest (but not guarantee!) the proper diagnosis. Always use every clue at your disposal, because making the correct interpretation has important therapeutic implications. This topic will have even greater importance when we discuss wide complex tachycardias in a later chapter.

Factors favoring aberrant supraventricular conduction:

- A definite relationship between preceding atrial activity (P or P′ wave) and the anomalous complex.
- A wide complex that follows a long-short cycle (most useful when preceding atrial activity is present).
- RBBB morphology with a triphasic, rsR′ type pattern in lead V1 (particularly when the initial r wave is small and narrow, it is followed by an s wave, and the terminal R′ wave is tall and wide).
- RBBB morphology with a triphasic qRs pattern in lead V6 where the terminal s wave is wide.
- RBBB morphology where the initial vector is identical to the normal complex.
- RBBB morphology with QRS duration of ≤0.14 seconds.
- LBBB morphology with QRS duration of ≤0.16 seconds.
- Variable coupling of the wide complex with the preceding normal complex.

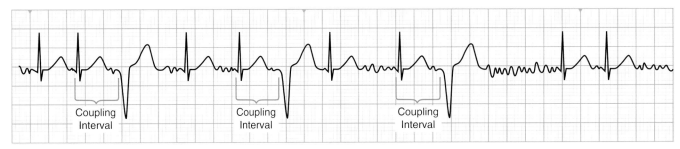

Figure 16-23. Atrial fibrillation with ventricular premature complexes. The coupling relationship of each wide complex is identical, which suggests ventricular ectopy rather than aberrant conduction. The last complex of the tracing conducts normally despite a preceding long-short sequence that might promote aberrancy, lending support that the wide complexes are VPCs.

Factors favoring ventricular ectopy:

- No definite preceding atrial activity.
- RBBB morphology with a monophasic R, notched Rr′, or biphasic qR pattern in lead V1.
- RBBB morphology with a monophasic QS or biphasic rS pattern in lead V6.
- RBBB morphology with QRS duration of >0.14 seconds.
- LBBB morphology in leads V1 or V2 with a wide r, or with a broad or notched S wave.
- LBBB morphology in lead V6 that contains a q wave.
- LBBB morphology with QRS duration of >0.16 seconds.
- Mean QRS axis between −90 and ±180 degrees (northwest quadrant).
- Fixed coupling of the wide complex with the preceding normal complex.

What's the best way to apply all these clues? Here's the approach I recommend:

- Step 1: Look for preceding, electrically related atrial activity.
- Step 2: Inspect lead V1 to determine whether RBBB or LBBB-type morphology.
- Step 3: Apply the appropriate morphology clues in leads V1 and V6.
- Step 4: Use supplementary information:
  - QRS complex duration.
  - QRS axis.
  - Coupling relationships.

Chapter 16 • SELF-TEST

1. An impulse arriving during either the absolute refractory period or the effective refractory period of the action potential will fail to propagate. True or false?
2. Phase 3 of the action potential correlates with what portion of the ECG?
3. What are the three fundamental mechanisms of phasic aberrant conduction?
4. What are the two elements responsible for phase 3 aberration?
5. At normal heart rates, which has a longer refractory period, the right bundle branch or left bundle branch?
6. Describe the relationship between heart rate (cycle length) and the refractory period.
7. What is the Ashman phenomenon?
8. List some ECG elements used to differentiate aberration from ectopy.
9. When seeing a wide complex, how do you determine whether it has a left bundle branch or right bundle branch type morphology?
10. For wide complex RBBB-type complexes, what QRS morphology in lead V1 supports aberrancy?
11. For wide complex RBBB-type complexes, what QRS morphology in lead V1 supports ventricular ectopy?
12. For wide complex LBBB-type complexes, what QRS morphology in leads V1 and V2 support ventricular ectopy?
13. For wide complex LBBB-type complexes, what QRS morphology in lead V6 supports ventricular ectopy?
14. How does QRS duration help in differentiating ectopy from aberrancy?
15. A wide complex with a mean QRS axis in which quadrant is highly specific for ventricular ectopy?
16. Which ventricular chamber is activated first in the following situations?
    - RBBB.
    - LBBB.
    - Right ventricular ectopy.
    - Left ventricular ectopy.

QUESTIONS

ANSWERS

Chapter 16 • SELF-TEST

1. True.

2. The T wave.

3. • Depolarization arriving during phase 3 of the action potential (phase 3 aberration).
   • Stimulation during phase 4 of the action potential (phase 4 aberration).
   • Concealed retrograde trans-septal conduction.

4. Unequal bundle branch refractoriness and critically timed impulses.

5. The right bundle branch.

6. The refractory period is proportional to the preceding cycle length. With higher heart rates (shorter cycle length), the refractory period shortens. With slower heart rates (longer cycle length), the refractory period lengthens.

7. The Ashman phenomenon is the eponym used to describe an aberrantly conducted complex precipitated by a long-short cycle.

8. • The presence of preceding atrial activity.
   • QRS morphology.
   • QRS duration.
   • QRS axis.
   • Cycle length variation.

9. Look at lead V1. If the complex is predominantly positive (R/S ratio >1), then it has RBBB morphology. If the complex is predominantly negative (R/S ratio <1), then the complex has LBBB morphology.

10. A triphasic complex (eg, rSR′, rsR′, RSR′, rSr′), especially with a small and narrow initial r wave, followed by an S wave, and accompanied by a tall and wide, terminal R′ deflection.

11. A monophasic R, notched Rr′, or biphasic qR pattern.

12. • A wide initial R wave of >0.03 seconds.
   • A notch or slur on the downstroke of the S wave.
   • A delayed R wave onset to S wave nadir of >0.06 seconds.

13. A q or Q wave because this is incompatible with LBBB aberrancy.

14. A QRS interval of >0.14 seconds with RBBB morphology supports ventricular ectopy as does a duration of >0.16 seconds with LBBB morphology.

15. Northwest quadrant.

16. • Left ventricle.
   • Right ventricle.
   • Right ventricle.
   • Left ventricle.

Further Reading

Akhtar M, Shenasa M, Jazayeri M, Caceres J, Tchou PJ. Wide QRS tachycardia: reappraisal of a common clinical problem. *Ann Intern med.* 1988;109:905-912.

Bagliani G, Giovanni Della Rocca D, De Ponti R, Capucci A, Padeletti M, Natale A. Ectopic beats: insights from timing and morphology. *Card Electrophysiol Clin.* 2018;10:257-275.

Denes P, Wu D, Dhingra R, Pietrs RJ, Rosen KM. The effects of cycle length on cardiac refractory periods in man. *Circulation.* 1974; 49:32-41.

De Riva M, Watanabe M, Zeppenfeld K. Twelve-lead ECG of ventricular tachycardia in structural heart disease. *Circ Arrhythm Electrophysiol.* 2015;8:951-962.

De Ponti R, Bagliani G, Padeletti L, Natale A. General approach to a wide QRS complex. *Card Electrophysiol Clin.* 2017;9:461-485.

Drew BJ, Scheinman MM. ECG criteria to distinguish between aberrantly conducted supraventricular tachycardia and ventricular tachycardia: practical aspects for the immediate care setting. *PACE.* 1995;18:2194-2208.

Fisch C. Aberration: seventy-five years after Sir Thomas Lewis. *Br Heart J.* 1983;50:297-302.

Fisch C, Zipes DP, McHenry PL. Rate dependent aberrancy. *Circulation.* 1973;48:714-724.

Gulmhusein S, Yee R, Ko PT, Klein GJ. Electrocardiographic criteria for differentiating aberrancy and ventricular extrasystole in chronic atrial fibrillation: validation by intracardiac recordings. *J Electrocardiology.* 1985;18:41-50.

Haqqani HM, Marchlinski FE. The surface electrocardiograph in ventricular arrhythmias: lessons in localization. *Heart, Lung and Circulation.* 2019;28:39-48.

Kindwall KE, Brown J, Josephson ME. Electrocardiographic criteria for ventricular tachycardia in wide complex left bundle branch morphology tachycardias. *Am J Cardiol.* 1988;61:1279-1283.

Marriott HJL, Sandler IA. Criteria old and new for differentiating between ectopic ventricular beats and aberrant ventricular conduction in the presence of atrial fibrillation. *Prog Cardiovasc Dis.* 1966;9:18-28.

Mond HG, Haqqani HM. The electrocardiographic footprints of ventricular ectopy. *Heart, Lung and Circulation.* 2020;29:988-999.

Park KM, Kim YH, Marchlinski FE. Using the surface electrocardiogram to localize the origin of idiopathic ventricular tachycardia. *PACE.* 2012;35:1516-1527.

Perez-Riera AR, Barbosa-Barros R, de Rezende Barbosa MPC, Daminello-Raimundo R, de Abreu LC, Nikus K. Left bundle branch block: epidemiology, etiology, anatomic features, electrovectorcardiography, and classification proposal. *Ann Noninvasive Electrocardiol.* 2019;24:e112572.

Sander IA, Marriott HJL. The differential morphology of anomalous ventricular complexes of RBBB-type in lead V1. *Circulation.* 1965;31:551-556.

Singer DH, Ten Eick RE. Aberrancy: electrophysiologic aspects. *Am J Cardiol.* 1971;28:381-401.

Tzeis S, Asvestas D, Ho SY, Vardas P. Electrocardiographic landmarks of idiopathic ventricular arrhythmia origins. *Heart.* 2019;105:1109-1116.

Watanabe Y, Nishimura M. Terminology and electrophysiology concepts in cardiac arrhythmias. I. Aberrant conduction. *PACE.* 1978;1:231-239.

Watanabe Y, Nishimura M. Terminology and electrophysiology concepts in cardiac arrhythmias. V. Phase 3 block and phase 4 block. Part 1. *PACE.* 1979;2:335-344.

Wellens HJJ, Bar FWH, Lie KI. The value of the electrocardiogram in the differential diagnosis of a tachycardia with a widened QRS complex. *Am J Med.* 1978;64:27-33.

Wellens HJJ, Durrer D. Supraventricular tachycardia with left aberrant conduction due to retrograde invasion into the left bundle branch. *Circulation.* 1968;38:474-479.

17

Atrioventricular Conduction Abnormalities

The term *normal sinus rhythm* indicates depolarization by the sinus pacemaker at a standard rate (60-100 bpm) followed by normal atrial depolarization and atrioventricular (AV) conduction to the ventricles. This requires perfect coordination of the entire specialized conduction system so that every P wave is accompanied by a normal PR interval and then by a QRS complex. The structures of the specialized conduction system include the SA node, interatrial and internodal bundles, the AV junction (subdivided into the AV node and the bundle of His), the bundle branches, and the Purkinje fibers. Abnormalities of AV conduction can arise anywhere along this route, which produce the ECG findings that we will review in this chapter.

► ELECTROPHYSIOLOGY OF NORMAL AV CONDUCTION

As we know, the surface ECG records most, but not all of the journey of the sinus impulse from the SA node to the ventricles. Recall that the SA nodal depolarization is too small to be visible on the surface ECG so the first evidence we have of the process is the P wave, which represents atrial depolarization. The QRS complex records ventricular depolarization as well as the early portion of repolarization. The PR interval, therefore, represents the time between the onset of atrial activation and that of the ventricular myocardium. The normal PR interval is 0.12 to 0.20 seconds, and should be measured in the lead that exhibits the longest interval from the beginning of the P wave to the beginning of the QRS complex, regardless of whether the QRS complex begins with a Q or an R wave (**Figure 17-1**).

The PR interval is actually comprised of three separate elements: (1) conduction through the atria between the SA and AV nodes, (2) passage through the AV node itself, and (3) transmission through the His-Purkinje system to the ventricular muscle.

As we will learn shortly, there are clinical implications whether a conduction abnormality resides above or below the AV node, something we cannot determine with precision on the surface ECG. To reveal these "hidden" components of AV conduction we need to utilize special techniques.

An *electrophysiologic study* with *His bundle electrocardiography* uses multipolar catheters that are inserted into the heart to record signals from multiple sites. The His bundle electrogram (HBE) records intracardiac signals from the low right atrium (A), His bundle (H), and right ventricle (V) (**Figure 17-2**). If we compare the timing of these intracardiac signals with those of the surface ECG, we can differentiate normal from abnormal AV conduction. The analysis includes an examination of the following items (**Figure 17-3**):

- **P wave**. This records atrial activation on the surface ECG. The high right atrium lies closest to the SA node and is the first atrial tissue activated. The terminal portion of the P wave reflects activation of the left atrium.
- **A wave**. This reflects activation of the low right atrium on the HBE.
- **H potential**. This is depolarization of the His bundle on the HBE. The normal range is <30 msec. Disturbances of conduction through this structure may appear as a widened, fractionated, or "split" His potential.
- **V deflection**. This records right ventricular activation on the HBE, which is concurrent with the QRS complex on the surface ECG.
- **PA interval**. This is measured from the onset of the P wave on the surface ECG to the A wave of the HBE. It approximates intra-atrial conduction from the high right atrium to the low right atrium. The normal range is 20 to 60 msec. Intra-atrial conduction is usually rapid; therefore, the PA interval normally accounts for only a small portion of the PR interval. This measurement estimates internodal conduction

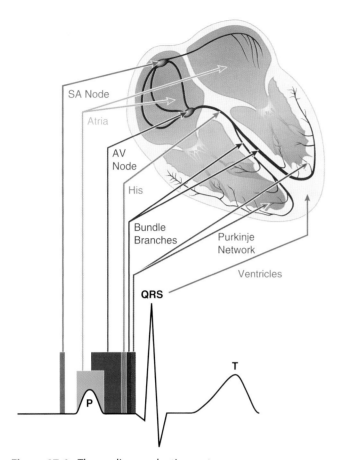

Figure 17-1. The cardiac conduction system.

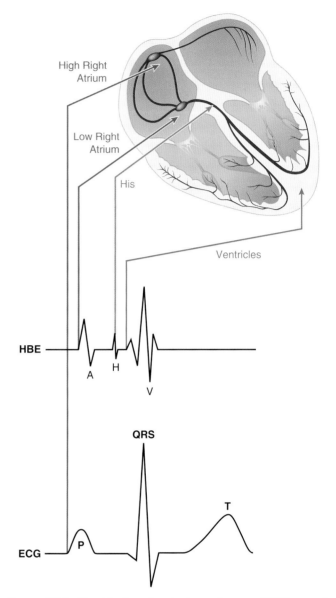

Figure 17-2. The His bundle electrocardiogram (HBE) records intracardiac signals from the low right atrium (A), His bundle (H), and the ventricles (V).

time (SA to AV node) reflecting the proximity of the high right atrium to the SA node and the low right atrium to the AV node.

- **AH interval**. This is measured from the onset of the A wave to the H deflection on the HBE. It reflects conduction through the AV node to the proximal portion of the bundle of His, which comprises the majority of the PR interval. The normal range is 50 to 120 msec and is markedly influenced by autonomic tone. Parasympathetic (vagal) influences prolong the AH interval as do medications such as beta blockers, verapamil, and digitalis, among others. Sympathetic effects shorten the AH interval.

- **HV interval**. This measurement is made from the onset of the His potential on the HBE to the first evidence of ventricular activation, whether on the surface ECG or HBE. It represents the conduction time below the AV node through the His-Purkinje system, which includes the His bundle, bundle branches, and the Purkinje network, finally reaching the ventricular myocardium. In a patient with unilateral complete bundle branch block, the HV interval measures conduction through the contralateral bundle branch or fascicle. The normal range is 35 to 55 msec, which is not appreciably affected by autonomic tone. A prolonged HV interval suggests disease in all fascicles of the distal conduction system or of the His bundle itself.

To summarize, the PR interval is the sum of the PA, AH, and HV intervals. By using His bundle electrocardiography, we can anatomically localize the site of an AV conduction abnormality that we record on the surface ECG to one or more levels. Prolongation of these measurements reflects the site of the conduction delay as follows: PA (intra-atrial), AH (AV nodal or "supraHisian"), H (intraHisian), and HV (His-Purkinje system or "infranodal").

▶ TERMINOLOGY OF AV CONDUCTION ABNORMALITIES

Before we proceed, let's review some of the terms used to describe AV conduction abnormalities. **AV conduction delay** refers to *prolongation* of the time for the atrial depolarization to conduct to the ventricles. **AV block** implies *failure* to conduct

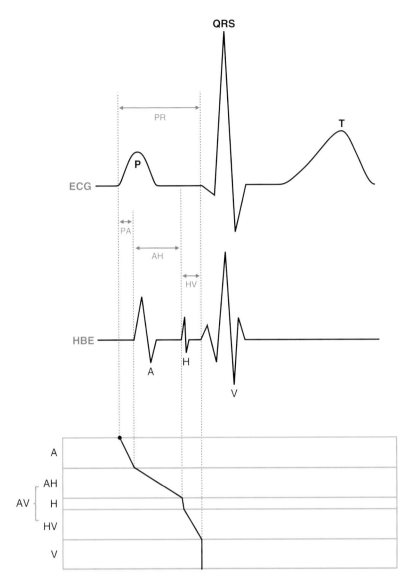

Figure 17-3. Representative timing of the ECG, HBE, and HBE laddergram. The PR interval records the time between atrial activation and the ventricular myocardium. The HBE records intervals that represent conduction between the SA and AV nodes (PA), through the AV node (AH), His bundle (H), and the His-Purkinje system (HV). On the laddergram, the AH, H, and HV intervals comprise the AV conduction tier.

the atrial impulse further through the conduction system. Furthermore, use of the term *block* implies an abnormal pathological process rather than normal physiological behavior caused by refractoriness.

Based on ECG patterns, AV conduction abnormalities are broadly categorized into **first, second, and third (complete) degree AV block**. Although some categories actually involve only conduction delay, the terms mentioned earlier share the common designation of "AV block." All the various forms of AV block may be either transient or permanent. Let's review each in turn now.

 FOR BOOKWORMS: You will encounter textbooks that divide AV block into two major categories, incomplete and complete. Incomplete AV block indicates that at least *some* supraventricular impulses successfully depolarize

the ventricles. This term includes first-degree, second-degree, and other forms of advanced or high-grade AV block that are not absolute. Complete AV block implies that *none* of the supraventricular impulses transmit to the ventricles. Not surprisingly, this is called complete or third-degree AV block.

▶ FIRST-DEGREE AV BLOCK

A diagnosis of first-degree AV block is made when every sinus impulse conducts to the ventricles, but with a **prolonged PR interval** >0.2 seconds (**Figure 17-4**). The finding represents not a true failure of conduction, but rather denotes a conduction delay; therefore, the term is a misnomer. First-degree AV block is caused by a delay in any portion of the conduction sequence from the SA node through the His-Purkinje system

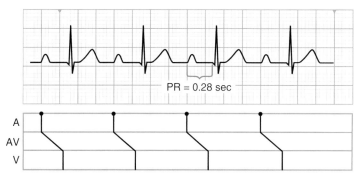

Figure 17-4. First-degree AV block. The prolonged PR interval in this example is 0.28 seconds.

(**Figure 17-5**). Most commonly the delay is at the level of the AV node, proximal to the bundle of His. The His bundle electrocardiogram records this as prolongation of the A-H interval. Less frequently, the abnormality is in the His-Purkinje system, which will then demonstrate prolongation of the H-V interval. In this circumstance, the underlying etiology is either slowed conduction within the His bundle itself, or a slight, but equal delay in both bundle branches (the synchronous activation maintaining the narrow complex). On occasion, the cause of first-degree AV block is widening of the P waves due to

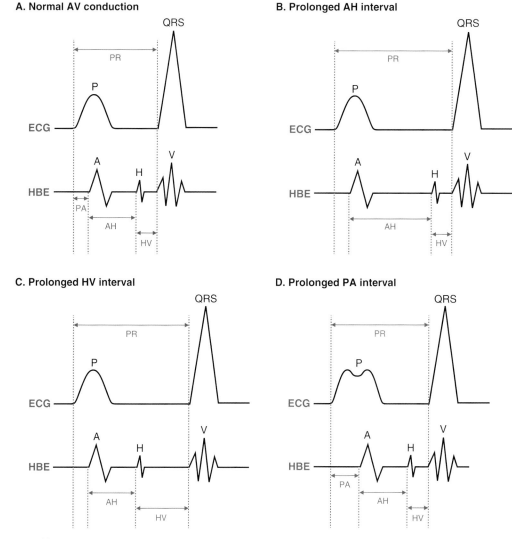

Figure 17-5. Causes of first-degree AV block. Abnormalities of normal AV conduction (a) may result in first-degree AV block. The conduction delay may be located at the level of the AV node with AH prolongation (b), in the His-Purkinje system with HV delay (c), or due to intra-atrial block with PA widening (d).

intra-atrial block, which is recorded on the His bundle electrogram as a prolonged PA interval.

Criteria for First-Degree AV Block
- Sinus rhythm in which every P wave is followed by a QRS.
- The PR interval is prolonged >0.2 seconds.

 CLINICAL TIP: First-degree AV block is almost always benign. It is seen in the setting of enhanced vagal tone, highly trained athletes, acute rheumatic fever, and due to medications such as verapamil, diltiazem, beta blockers, and digitalis.

▶ SECOND-DEGREE AV BLOCK

Second-degree AV block is defined by an *intermittent* failure of AV conduction. This category encompasses a number of electrocardiographic patterns that we will review in the following discussion. All represent a situation where *at least one* of the P waves that would be expected to conduct to the ventricles, fails to do so; therefore, a P wave appears without a QRS complex. The missing QRS complex is often called a "dropped beat," but it's better to describe this as a *nonconducted* or *blocked* P wave. The relationship between the number of P waves in a sequence and the conducted QRS complexes is termed the **conduction ratio**. During normal sinus rhythm, the P to QRS relationship is 1:1. In second-degree AV block, the conduction ratio of a sequence may be 3:2, 5:4, 2:1, 4:1, or another combination where the number of P waves must be greater than the number of QRS complexes.

Second-degree AV block is subdivided into two major electrocardiographic patterns, type I and type II, which are determined by the behavior of the PR intervals before and after the nonconducted P wave. To differentiate type I from type II, at least **two consecutively conducted P waves** must be evident prior to the failure of conduction. This allows evaluation of the behavior of the PR interval before the missing QRS complex.

Other forms of second-degree AV block are 2:1 AV block and high-grade/advanced AV block.

 FOR HISTORY BUFFS: In 1899, Karl Wenckebach first described delayed AV conduction from the atria to the ventricles without the benefit of the electrocardiogram, which had yet to be invented. By observing the jugular venous pulse waves, he identified gradual lengthening of the intervals representing atrial and ventricular contraction, eventually followed by an absent pulse. In 1906, Wenckebach and John Hay simultaneously described a second form of AV block, one that occurred without progressive lengthening of the conduction time between the atria and the ventricles. By 1924, Woldemar Mobitz was able to use the electrocardiogram to correlate the clinical findings previously described, suggesting that the first form of AV block with progressive PR prolongation be called "type I" and the second form with constant PR intervals, "type II." Today we commonly refer to the two types of second-degree AV block as Mobitz I (Wenckebach) and Mobitz II block.

Second-Degree AV Block, Type I (Mobitz I, Wenckebach)

The "classic" form of type I second-degree AV block is typified by the **Wenckebach phenomenon** (**Figure 17-6**). The features of this distinctive electrocardiographic pattern include (1) The PR intervals of successive complexes progressively lengthen until one P wave fails to conduct; (2) the PR interval of the first conducted P wave after the blocked impulse is the shortest of the sequence; (3) the greatest increment of PR prolongation is between the first and second conducted complexes; (4) the PR intervals continue to lengthen until conduction fails, but do so in progressively smaller increments; (5) the R-R intervals shorten progressively until one is missing; (6) the R-R interval containing the nonconducted P wave is less than the sum of two P-P intervals; and (7) the dropped complexes make the R-R intervals appear arranged together, a pattern described as "group beating." Classic Wenckebach sequences are most commonly seen with a conduction ratio of 3:2, 4:3, or occasionally 5:4.

I find the Wenckebach phenomenon one of the most fascinating aspects of electrocardiography, but it's sometimes a source of confusion. Let's review this behavior in more detail.

Figure 17-6 shows an idealized classic AV Wenckebach sequence. Beginning with the first complex, there are five P waves for the four QRS complexes, so the conduction

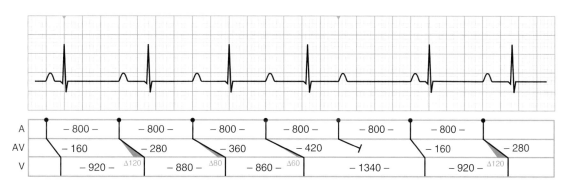

Figure 17-6. Type I second-degree AV block—classic Wenckebach. There is progressive PR prolongation until failure of conduction. The incremental increase of the PR interval (Δ) is less with each successive complex, which explains the progressively shorter R-R intervals. The R-R interval containing the nonconducted P wave (1340 msec) is less than twice the baseline P-P interval (1600 msec). Note the mathematical relationship between this interval and the Δ measurement, 1340 = 1600 − (120 + 80 + 60).

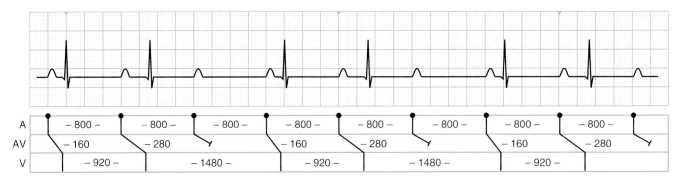

Figure 17-7. Type I second-degree AV block with a 3:2 conduction ratio demonstrating "group beating."

ratio is 5:4. The first P wave in the sequence, as well as the one after the pause, has the shortest PR interval (0.16 seconds). This represents baseline, unimpaired AV conduction. The PR interval of the second complex in the series is prolonged (0.28 seconds). The sequence continues with the third complex having a PR interval of 0.36 seconds and the fourth with one of 0.42 seconds, following which a P wave fails to conduct. Notice that each conducted P wave has a **successively longer PR interval**. But as the PR interval lengthens, the *incremental increase* (Δ) is less than the complex before. The seemingly paradoxical result is that the R-R intervals become shorter and the ventricular rate modestly *accelerates*.

Figure 17-7 shows another classic Wenckebach series, this time with a 3:2 conduction ratio. Here you can see another of the "footprints" of Wenckebach, namely group beating.

 FOR BOOKWORMS: The underlying electrophysiological mechanism of Wenckebach-type behavior can be explained by an impulse encountering tissue during its relative refractory period. Normally, the sinus impulse travels through the AV node without delay. In type I second-degree AV block, the AV node has an abnormally long relative refractory period. The rate of conduction through the AV node (and the duration of the PR interval) depends on when the impulse arrives; the earlier the impulse, the greater the delay. With Wenckebach periodicity, each successive atrial impulse arrives slightly earlier in the relative refractory period until it reaches the effective refractory period, whereupon conduction fails. After the pause, the sinus impulse encounters the recovered AV node when it is

no longer refractory and conducts normally. That explains the shorter PR interval in the first conducted complex compared with the one before the pause.

The Wenckebach phenomenon is not limited to the AV node and can be seen virtually anywhere in the cardiac conduction system. Recall that we first encountered this behavior when we discussed SA block in Chapter 14.

OK, if you thought that understanding the classic Wenckebach phenomenon was all you needed to know about type I second-degree AV block, think again! It turns out that most cases **do not** exhibit the classic Wenckebach pattern. Now what?

The "common" form of type I second-degree AV block involves changes in the PR interval that do not follow the mathematical rules of classic Wenckebach. **Figure 17-8** shows such an example. The long 8:7 sequence begins with conducted complexes in which the PR intervals gradually prolong. But note that the complex with the longest PR interval (arrow) is not at the end of the sequence. This complex is then followed by two more with a slightly shorter and constant PR interval before the nonconducted P wave. Unlike in classic Wenckebach, the longest PR interval in the common form is unpredictable, often present in the middle of a series, so it's essential that you inspect the entire sequence. The R-R intervals follow the pattern of PR prolongation, so they too will deviate from the classic accelerating pattern described in the preceding discussion. Importantly, in *both* the classic and common forms, the PR interval of the *first* conducted complex in a sequence is the *shortest*, as the speed of conduction is always facilitated after a pause.

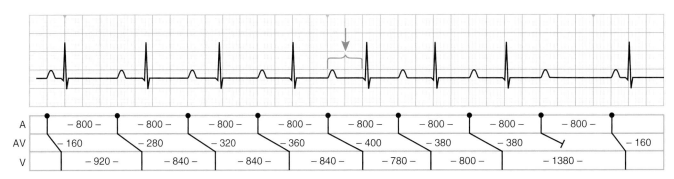

Figure 17-8. The "common" form of type I second-degree AV block does not exhibit all the findings of the classic Wenckebach pattern. The longest PR interval (400 msec) occurs in the middle of the sequence (arrow) followed by slightly shorter and constant PR intervals before conduction fails. In both the classic and common forms, the PR interval of the first conducted complex after the pause is the shortest of the sequence.

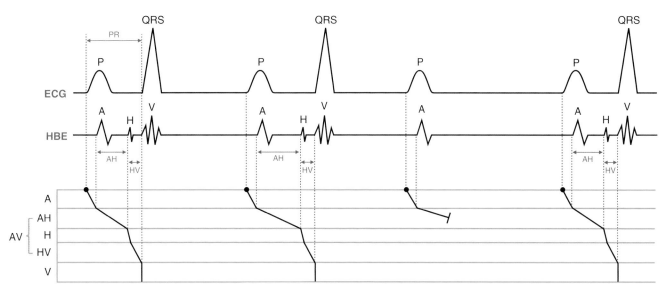

Figure 17-9. The site of the conduction abnormality of type I second-degree AV block is at the level of the AV node. On the HBE, note the progressive lengthening of the AH interval until the missing H deflection. The laddergram depicts that the conduction defect is in the AV node above the bundle of His (supraHisian).

To summarize, the defining characteristics of both the classic and common forms of type I second-degree AV block is that a single P wave fails to conduct to the ventricles, preceded by *variable* PR prolongation relative to the first conducted complex of a sequence. In classic Wenckebach, we see *progressive* PR prolongation before the blocked P wave. In the more common form, the degree of PR interval prolongation *varies* within the sequence.

Criteria for Second-Degree AV Block, Type I
- Sinus rhythm with at least two consecutively conducted complexes.
- Intermittent failure of AV conduction when expected.
  - A single P wave is not followed by a QRS complex.
- A nonconducted P wave that ends the sequence is preceded by at least one or more sinus complexes with a prolonged PR interval relative to the first conducted complex.
  - Classic form:
    - Progressive PR prolongation exhibiting the Wenckebach phenomenon.
    - The shortest PR interval is the first in a sequence.
    - The maximal prolongation of the PR intervals occurs between the first and second conducted complexes in a sequence.
    - The incremental change in PR prolongation decreases with each conducted complex. This results in progressively shorter R-R intervals.
    - The R-R interval containing the nonconducted P wave is less than the sum of two P-P intervals.
  - Common form:
    - Variable PR prolongation without a progressive pattern.
    - The shortest PR interval is the first in a sequence.
- Supporting features:
  - The conducted QRS complexes are usually narrow.

Electrophysiologic and clinical correlation Type I second-degree AV block is usually associated with a narrow QRS

complex. If so, the anatomical site of the conduction abnormality is at the level of the AV node, proximal to the bundle of His (supraHisian). The His bundle electrogram shows prolongation of the AH interval, with a normal HV interval (**Figure 17-9**). The conduction abnormality may be seen in otherwise healthy individuals and is often transient, becoming evident during vagal stimulation. It may result from medications affecting the AV node including beta blockers, diltiazem, verapamil, or digitalis. It may also be seen transiently in inferior wall myocardial infarction with AV nodal ischemia. This typically resolves with time and permanent pacemaker insertion is usually not indicated.

Less frequently, type I second-degree AV block is seen with a wide (≥0.12 seconds) QRS complex. In this situation the site of the conduction abnormality remains more likely in the AV node, but disease more distal in the His-Purkinje system (infranodal) cannot be excluded. An electrophysiologic study can determine if HV prolongation and infranodal block is present.

Second-Degree AV Block, Type II (Mobitz II)

Type II second-degree AV block is characterized by a **constant PR interval** both before and after the nonconducted P wave. The baseline PR interval may be either normal or prolonged. The pause encompassing the nonconducted P wave is **exactly twice** that of the baseline P-P interval (**Figure 17-10**).

Criteria for Second-Degree AV Block, Type II
- Sinus rhythm with at least two consecutively conducted complexes.
- Intermittent failure of AV conduction when expected.
  - A single P wave is not followed by a QRS complex.
- The PR interval is constant in the complexes before and after the nonconducted P wave.
- The R-R intervals are constant, with those straddling the nonconducted P wave equal to the sum of two P-P intervals.
- Supporting features:
  - The QRS complex is usually wide (≥0.12 seconds).

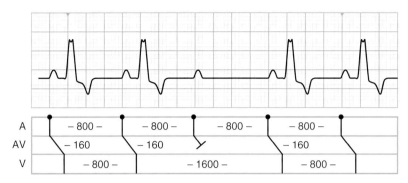

Figure 17-10. Type II second-degree AV block. Constant PR intervals (160 msec) are seen in the complexes both before and after the nonconducted P wave. The R-R interval containing the blocked P wave is exactly twice that of the baseline P-P interval. The QRS complex is typically wide.

Electrophysiologic and clinical correlation The conduction abnormality of type II second-degree AV block is located in the His-Purkinje system, below the AV node. On the HBE, the non-conducted P wave is associated with an H deflection that is not followed by a V deflection (absent HV interval) (**Figure 17-11**). The conducted complexes are typically wide QRS complexes (≥0.12 seconds) with prolongation of the HV interval, which indicates disease in all fascicles of the bundle branches. I find it helpful to think that type II block occurs when one diseased bundle branch is nonfunctional, and the remaining injured bundle branch fails intermittently, resulting in sudden interruption of AV conduction. Type II block is characteristically associated with structural heart disease with potential progression to complete AV block, for which pacemaker implantation is required.

Much less frequently, type II block presents with a narrow complex. But even in this situation the conduction defect remains infranodal, located within the His bundle itself. The QRS complex remains narrow because any impulse conducting below the His bundle proceeds in a normal, synchronous fashion through both bundle branches. The prognosis of type II AV block with a narrow QRS is equivalent to that associated with a wide complex.

 BE CAREFUL: Type II second-degree AV block and type I block can sometimes be mistaken. This is particularly true with long type I sequences where there may be no perceptible increase in the PR interval before the block. The clue to type I block is that the first post-block sinus complex will always have a PR interval that is shorter than before the pause. With type II block, the PR intervals are constant before and after the blocked P wave.

2:1 Second-Degree AV Block

In this form of second-degree AV block, nonconducted P waves alternate with those that do conduct (2:1 conduction ratio). It *cannot* be further categorized as either type I or type II and should be characterized only as 2:1 second-degree AV block. The reason is that you need *at least two consecutively conducted P waves* to determine the behavior of the PR intervals before the

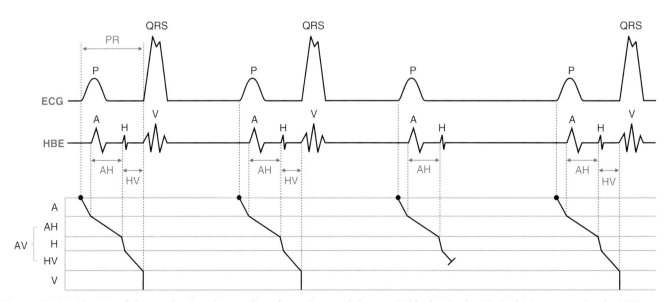

Figure 17-11. The site of the conduction abnormality of type II second-degree AV block is in the His-Purkinje system. On the HBE, note the constant AH intervals and His deflection with sudden absence of a V deflection, resulting in a nonconducted P wave. This identifies the defect as infranodal, as illustrated in the laddergram. The QRS complex is typically wide with a prolonged HV interval in the conducted complexes.

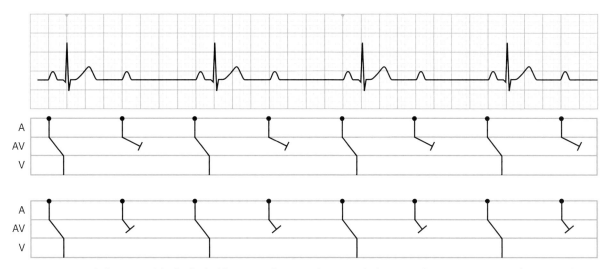

Figure 17-12. 2:1 second-degree AV block. The laddergrams illustrate that type I behavior with progressive PR prolongation (top) and type II behavior with constant PR intervals (bottom) appear the same on the surface ECG. Two consecutively conducted P waves are required to differentiate the two processes, something not present with 2:1 AV block.

pause. This can be a confusing concept, but I'm going to clear it up for you now.

Figure 17-12 shows an example of 2:1 AV block, where every other P wave fails to conduct. In the top laddergram, type I behavior is present, with progressive delay in AV conduction that results in a nonconducted P wave. If that complex had been conducted, the PR interval would have been prolonged. The bottom laddergram demonstrates type II behavior, where the rate of AV conduction of the nonconducted P waves is exactly the same as those that are conducted. How can you tell the difference between these two scenarios in the setting of 2:1 AV block? Outside of the electrophysiology laboratory, you can't! That's why 2:1, second-degree AV block is called just that, with no further distinction into type I or type II.

CLINICAL TIP: Differentiating type I and type II behavior in the setting of 2:1 AV block has important clinical implications. Type I behavior implicates conduction delay in the AV node, which carries a low likelihood of complete heart block. Type II behavior is more ominous, implying infranodal disease and the potential need for a pacemaker. You can often determine the underlying mechanism of 2:1 AV block by using prolonged electrocardiographic monitoring. This frequently provides the opportunity to see at least two consecutively conducted complexes before the blocked P wave that is not apparent on the ECG you have before you. You may also see periods of typical type I or type II behavior that reveals the diagnosis. It is very unusual

to see both type I and type II block in the same patient, so you can make an assumption of the fundamental conduction abnormality of 2:1 AV block "by the company it keeps."

An understanding of the conduction system's response to autonomic nervous system manipulation can also help you make the correct diagnosis. The SA and AV nodes are sensitive to both sympathetic and parasympathetic (vagal) stimulation. Below the AV node, sympathetic effects predominate. Parasympathetic inhibition with atropine or sympathetic stimulation with exercise typically improves AV nodal conduction and type I second-degree AV block. In contrast, the increase in heart rate from these maneuvers will either aggravate type II block, or have no effect. Carotid sinus pressure increases the vagal effect at the SA and AV node and worsens type I block. In type II block, this maneuver will either improve conduction or have no effect as the heart rate slows.

Criteria for 2:1 Second-Degree AV block
- Sinus rhythm is present.
- Conducted P waves alternate with those that are nonconducted.

High-Grade/Advanced Second-Degree AV Block

When two more P waves fail to conduct to the ventricles, the degree of AV block is termed **high grade** or **advanced** (**Figure 17-13**). By definition, the conduction ratio is 3:1 or greater, but generally presents with even numbers (4:1, 6:1, 8:1, etc.).

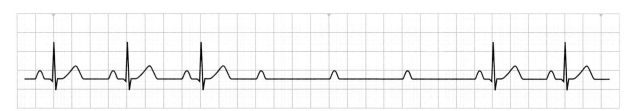

Figure 17-13. High-grade AV block. The conduction ratio of the blocked sequence is defined as 4:1 with one conducted P wave followed by three that are blocked.

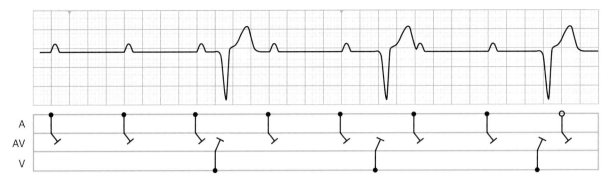

Figure 17-14. Complete (third-degree) AV block. Sinus rhythm is present, but none of the P waves conducts to the ventricles. A ventricular escape rhythm is present.

In the presence of high conduction ratios the abnormality may resemble complete AV block, but evidence of *any* conducted complexes indicates the block is high grade, rather than complete. Escape complexes may be present as a subsidiary pacemaker emerges in response to the impaired conduction.

Criteria for High-Grade/Advanced Second-Degree AV Block
- Sinus rhythm is present.
- The atrial rate must be greater than the ventricular rate.
- Two or more P waves fail to conduct to the ventricles.

Electrophysiologic and clinical correlation The abnormality in high-grade, second-degree AV block may be located either at the level of the AV node (type I behavior) or in the His-Purkinje system (type II behavior). Despite use of the ominous sounding terms "high grade" or "advanced," the prognosis of the conduction impairment may not be unfavorable. This is particularly true when the QRS complex is narrow or the abnormality appears related to vagal influences (see following discussion). Conversely, high-grade AV block associated with a wide complex and structural heart disease may progress to complete AV block.

► COMPLETE (THIRD-DEGREE) AV BLOCK

Complete AV block is a complete failure of any atrial impulses to reach the ventricles. The atrial rate must be greater than the ventricular rate. An escape rhythm either in the AV junction or the ventricles may be present, but the P waves bear no electrophysiologic relationship to the QRS complexes (**Figure 17-14**). With underlying sinus rhythm, ventriculophasic sinus arrhythmia may be seen (see chapter 14, Figure 14-7). Complete AV block may also be associated with atrial fibrillation and flutter. In this setting, clues to the diagnosis are slow, regularized escape complexes from either the AV junction or the ventricles (**Figure 17-15**).

Criteria for Complete (Third-Degree) AV Block
- There is an absence of AV conduction with P waves and QRS complexes completely dissociated.
  - Comment: An escape rhythm may originate either in the AV junction or ventricles.
- The atrial rate must be greater than the ventricular rate.
  - Comment: The rhythm may be a supraventricular rhythm other than sinus, such as atrial fibrillation, atrial flutter, or another supraventricular arrhythmia.

Electrophysiologic and clinical correlation Complete AV block may be localized to anywhere in the cardiac conduction system. The site is the AV node in cases of congenital complete AV block, or in the setting of acute inferior wall myocardial infarction with excessive vagal tone. The AV node is also the most likely site when complete AV block is due to medications such as beta blockers, diltiazem, verapamil, and digitalis. In most of these cases, a narrow complex escape rhythm will be present and the prognosis is favorable.

In contrast, complete AV block due to major structural heart disease such as anterior myocardial infarction or aortic valve disease most likely resides within the His-Purkinje system and is associated with a wide complex escape rhythm. If an adequate escape rhythm fails to emerge, ventricular asystole will result in syncope or cardiac arrest. Pacemaker implantation is required.

 CLINICAL TIP: A unique reversible cause of complete AV block is Lyme carditis. Infection with this tick-borne spirochete (*Borrelia burgdorferi*) causes progressive inflammation of the cardiac conduction system, progressing through first-degree, second-degree, and potentially complete AV block. The site of the conduction abnormality is the AV node and responds to antibiotic therapy.

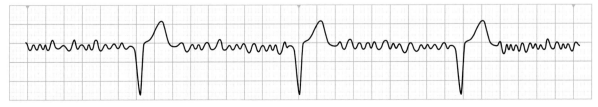

Figure 17-15. Atrial fibrillation with complete AV block and a ventricular escape rhythm. The clue to complete AV block is the slow, regularized ventricular complexes. Normally, atrial fibrillation would be associated with rapid, irregular AV conduction.

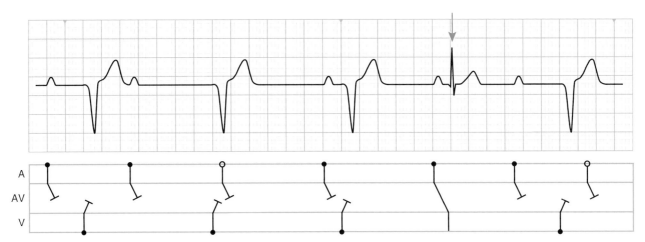

Figure 17-16. High-grade AV block with a capture complex. The native rhythm is sinus arrhythmia with high-grade AV block with a ventricular escape rhythm. Most of the P waves fail to conduct, but the presence of a capture complex (arrow) indicates the degree of AV block is high grade rather than complete.

 FOR HISTORY BUFFS: The sudden, transient loss of consciousness caused by complete AV block or other major bradyarrhythmia has been termed an Adams-Stokes (or Stokes-Adams) attack, named after Robert Adams and Williams Stokes, two Irish physicians who described the phenomenon in 1827 and 1846, respectively.

Complete Versus High-Grade AV block

Differentiating high grade from complete AV block is an important distinction. In both circumstances, you will find multiple P waves that fail to conduct with a QRS complex. The presence of **capture complexes** provides evidence that even though the degree of block is high grade, it is not complete. **Figure 17-16** shows just such a scenario. The basic rhythm is sinus with multiple nonconducted P waves and a ventricular escape rhythm. At first glance one might invoke complete AV block as the mechanism. But note the early, narrow QRS complex indicated by the arrow. This results from a sinus impulse that arrived when the AV node and ventricles were no longer refractory and able to *capture* the ventricles. The presence of *any* conducted P wave rules out a diagnosis of complete AV block.

Vagally Mediated AV Block

Vagal influences can transiently produce all of the forms of AV block reviewed in the preceding discussion, from first-degree through complete. As we have learned, parasympathetic influence depresses *both* sinus node and AV node function. Therefore, the clue to vagally mediated AV block is the concomitant **slowing of** the sinus rate either just prior to or simultaneous with the AV conduction block (**Figure 17-17**). This form of AV block may be seen in highly trained athletes, during deep sleep, and associated with nausea, coughing or even hiccups. Because the site of the conduction delay is in the AV node, the prognosis is favorable even with higher forms of AV block.

 BE CAREFUL: Subjects with vagally mediated second-degree AV block may show constant PR intervals both before and after the nonconducted P wave. Failure to recognize simultaneous slowing of the sinus rate may lead you to erroneously interpret this as Mobitz type II second-degree AV block due to infranodal block, which has a very different prognosis. The presence of a narrow complex also makes second-degree type II AV block unlikely.

Is It Block or Behavior?

Vital to understanding AV conduction abnormalities is the ability to differentiate normal physiology (behavior) from abnormal pathology (block). You can think of the AV node as the heart's "gatekeeper," designed to allow time for the ventricles to fill during rapid stimulation from supraventricular impulses. Although variable and depending on autonomic tone, there is a progressive physiologic delay in resting AV conduction with increasing supraventricular rates, a phenomenon called *decremental conduction*. Normal 1:1 conduction of sinus impulses is expected up to a heart rate of approximately 130 bpm. In the electrophysiology laboratory with atrial pacing rates >150 to 160 bpm, Mobitz type I AV block becomes evident. When atrial rates exceed

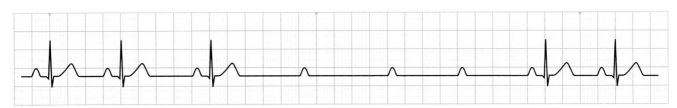

Figure 17-17. Vagally induced AV block. Slowing of the sinus rate occurs concomitantly with the development of high-grade AV block.

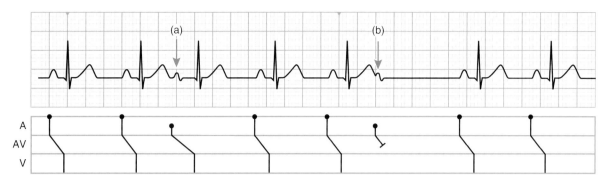

Figure 17-18. Physiological conduction delay and block of atrial premature complexes. The PR interval of APC (a) is prolonged because the complex arrives during the relative refractory period of the AV node, thereby conducting with a delay. APC (b) fails to conduct because it arrives earlier, when the AV node is completely refractory. Both findings represent expected physiological behavior and not AV block.

200 bpm, such as present in atrial flutter or atrial tachycardia, uniform 2:1 AV conduction is the norm. All of these represent normal, physiologic behavior and not AV block.

 FOR BOOKWORMS: In contrast to the situation at rest, 1:1 AV conduction is maintained as the sinus rate rises during exercise. Release of catecholamines during adrenergic stimulation enhances AV conduction so that the type I response does not occur, even at heart rates approaching 200 bpm.

Other physiologic findings often confused with AV block are related to premature complexes that encounter normally refractory tissue. We know that after being depolarized, every cardiac cell enters a period when it is either completely or partially refractory to further stimulation. A *premature* impulse that arrives during the AV node's effective refractory period will fail to conduct (**Figure 17-18**). One arriving early during the relative refractory may conduct, but with a delay. Again this represents normal physiology and not pathology. In contrast, AV block is present when the impulse fails to conduct despite arriving *on time* and with the expectation of normal conduction.

Concealed conduction is also frequently mistaken for AV block. For example, we learned in Chapter 15 that the sinus

impulse following an interpolated ventricular premature complex (VPC) often conducts with a prolonged PR interval (**Figure 17-19**). This does not reflect first-degree AV block and is a physiologic consequence of the "hidden" retrograde depolarization of the AV node from the VPC. Similarly, a junctional premature complex (JPC) that lacks *both* antegrade and retrograde conduction is electrocardiographically hidden, but interferes with transmission of the next sinus impulse, imitating AV block (**Figure 17-20**).

AV Dissociation

One of the most commonly misunderstood terms in electrocardiography is AV dissociation. It is not the same as AV block! AV dissociation is a general term that describes any situation where the atria and ventricles are activated *independently* of one another, the atria governed by one pacemaker and the ventricles by another. It is never a primary disturbance and is always a consequence of another rhythm disorder. AV dissociation is caused by three basic mechanisms (1) a slowing or default of the sinus impulse with the emergence of a subsidiary pacemaker; (2) abnormal acceleration of a normally latent pacemaker that usurps control; (3) AV block that prevents transmission of the atrial impulse from reaching the ventricles. All of the above may

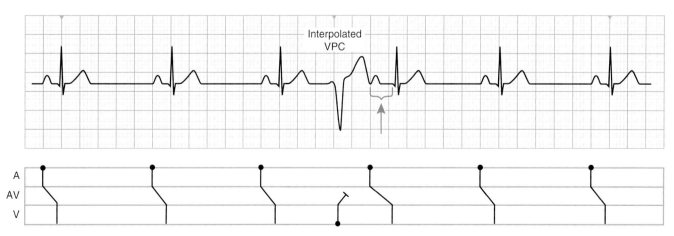

Figure 17-19. Interpolated VPC with concealed retrograde conduction. The ventricular depolarization demonstrates retrograde conduction into the AV node. The following sinus impulse encounters partially refractory tissue in the AV node, which physiologically prolongs the PR interval (arrow).

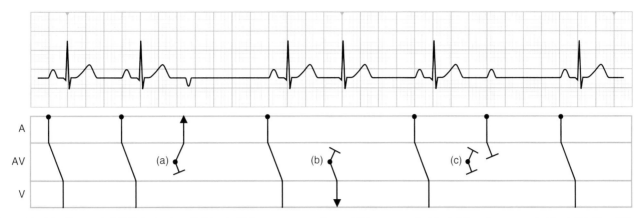

Figure 17-20. Concealed JPCs imitating AV block. JPCs are present that exhibit antegrade block (a) and retrograde block (b). The JPC with both antegrade and retrograde block (c) is concealed on the surface ECG, but gives the erroneous appearance of block of the normal sinus impulse. The presence of concealed JPCs can be suspected when other junctional complexes are evident.

be present alone or in combination. Let's now review some examples of each mechanism.

AV dissociation due to slowing of the sinus impulse **Figure 17-21** shows marked sinus arrhythmia with emergence of a junctional escape rhythm as the sinus rate slows. With the acceleration of the sinus rate, normal AV conduction resumes. Another example of this process is shown in **Figure 17-22**. Here a ventricular premature complex interrupts sinus bradycardia, conducting retrograde and suppressing the normal recovery of the sinus node. Junctional escape complexes emerge with a brief period of AV dissociation.

AV dissociation due to acceleration of a subsidiary pacemaker In **Figure 17-23**, an abnormally rapid AV junctional rhythm "hijacks" the ventricular depolarization at the third complex from the sinus node. Impulses from the sinus node remain, but cannot penetrate the AV node because the junctional depolarization has rendered the region refractory to further stimulation. The P waves and QRS complexes appear in close proximity, but remain electrically unrelated, a pattern termed *isorhythmic AV dissociation*. The independent subsidiary pacemaker producing AV dissociation may also be located in the ventricles such as might occur with accelerated idioventricular rhythm or ventricular parasystole.

Ventricular tachycardia induces AV dissociation by the same mechanism, except here the abnormal depolarization originates in the ventricles rather than the AV junction (**Figure 17-24**). Note the capture and fusion complexes, which confirm that there are two independent sites of depolarization, one ventricular and one atrial.

 FOR BOOKWORMS: A term you may encounter in describing the mechanism of AV dissociation unrelated to AV block is *interference*. This reflects the fact that cardiac tissue depolarized from one source will, for a period of time, normally become refractory to further stimulation by another pacemaker. For example, if the AV junction depolarizes the ventricles, a sinus impulse occurring close in time will be prevented from capturing the same tissue. Simply put, one depolarization *interferes* with that of another. This term has been fraught with multiple definitions, confusion, and misuse and I discourage its use.

AV dissociation due to complete AV block Complete AV block accompanied by an escape rhythm is perhaps the "purest" and easiest to understand mechanism of AV dissociation (see Figures 17-14 and 17-15). None of the atrial impulses transmits to the ventricles, which results in completely independent and unrelated atrial and ventricular depolarizations.

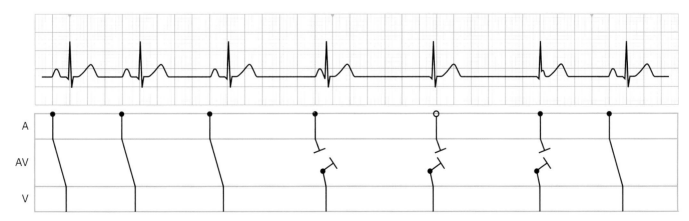

Figure 17-21. AV dissociation due to slowing of the sinus impulse. The native rhythm is marked sinus arrhythmia with a junctional escape rhythm.

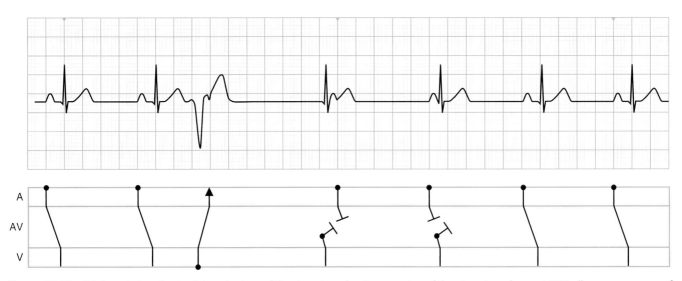

Figure 17-22. AV dissociation due to delayed return of the sinus impulse. Suppression of the sinus impulse post-VPC allows emergence of a junctional escape rhythm.

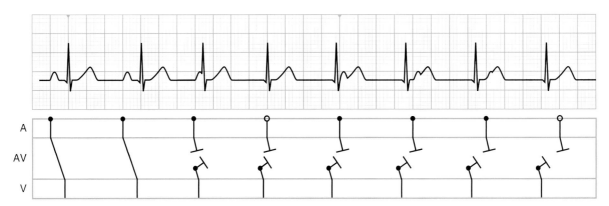

Figure 17-23. AV dissociation due to usurpation of the sinus impulse. An accelerated AV junctional rhythm seizes control of ventricular depolarization from the sinus node. The depolarization rates of the AV junctional rhythm and that of the sinus node are nearly identical, resulting in a period of isorhythmic dissociation.

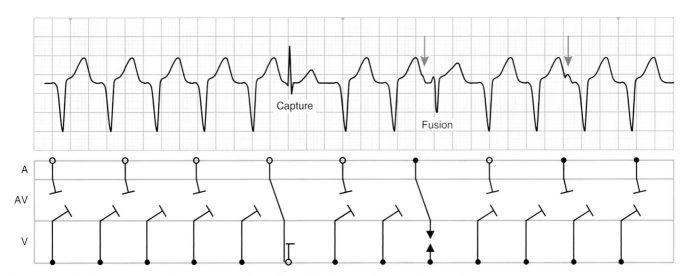

Figure 17-24. AV dissociation due to ventricular tachycardia. The rapid ventricular depolarization usurps control as the dominant pacemaker. The sinus node continues to depolarize and periodically conduct to the ventricles, evidenced by capture and fusions complexes. P waves, whether conducted or nonconducted, are sometimes visible (arrows).

Chapter 17 • SELF-TEST

1. The PR interval records conduction through which three elements of the specialized conduction system?

2. The following items measured during His bundle electrocardiography (HBE) represent what aspects of cardiac conduction?
   - A wave.
   - PA interval.
   - H deflection.
   - AH interval.
   - V deflection.
   - HV interval.

3. Define first-degree AV block.

4. List the characteristic findings of the classic Wenckebach pattern of type I second-degree AV block.

5. The conduction abnormality of type I second-degree AV block is typically located in what portion of the specialized conduction system and how does this manifest on the HBE?

6. In type II second-degree AV block, describe the behavior of the PR intervals before and after the nonconducted P wave.

7. The conduction abnormality of type II second-degree AV block is typically located in what portion of the specialized conduction system and how does this manifest on the HBE?

8. The distinction between type I and type II second-degree AV block requires at least two consecutively conducted complexes. True or false?

9. What ECG finding provides a clue to vagally induced AV block?

10. What are the three primary mechanisms of AV dissociation?

ANSWERS

Chapter 17 • SELF-TEST

1. • Conduction through the atria between the SA and AV nodes.
   • Passage through the AV node itself.
   • Transmission through the His-Purkinje system to the ventricular muscle.

2. • A wave: Right atrial depolarization.
   • PA interval: Intra-atrial conduction between the SA and AV nodes.
   • H deflection: His bundle depolarization.
   • AH interval: AV nodal conduction.
   • V deflection: Initial depolarization of the ventricles.
   • HV interval: Transmission through the His-Purkinje system.

3. Sinus rhythm with 1:1 AV conduction with a PR interval >0.20 seconds.

4. • The PR intervals of successive complexes progressively lengthen until one P wave fails to conduct.
   • The PR interval of the first conducted P wave after the blocked impulse is the shortest of the sequence.
   • The greatest increment of PR prolongation is between the first and second conducted complexes.
   • The PR intervals continue to lengthen until conduction fails, but do so in progressively smaller increments.
   • The R-R intervals shorten progressively until one is missing.
   • The R-R interval containing the nonconducted P wave is less than the sum of two P-P intervals.
   • The dropped complexes make the R-R intervals appear arranged together, a pattern described as "group beating."

5. The abnormality is at the level of the AV node which results in prolongation of the AH interval on the HBE. The blocked P wave is associated with an absent H deflection.

6. The PR intervals are constant in the conducted complexes both before and after the blocked P wave.

7. The abnormality is in the His-Purkinje system, below the AV node. The HBE of the blocked P wave records a normal AH interval, followed by an H deflection with an absent V deflection. A wide complex QRS is typical with prolongation of the HV interval in the conducted complexes.

8. True.

9. Concomitant slowing of the sinus rate either just prior to or simultaneous with the AV conduction block.

10. • Slowing or default of the sinus impulse with the emergence of a subsidiary pacemaker.
    • Abnormal acceleration of a normally latent pacemaker that usurps control.
    • AV block that prevents transmission of the atrial impulse from reaching the ventricles.

Further Reading

Alboni P, Holz A, Brignole M. Vagally mediated atrioventricular block: pathophysiology and diagnosis. *Heart*. 2013;99:904-908.

Bagliani G, Della Rocca, DG, DiBiase L, Padeletti L. PR interval and junctional zone. *Card Electrophysiol Clin*. 2017;9:411-433.

Bagliani G, Leonelli FM, DePonti R, Mesolella E, Padeletti L. Atrioventricular nodal conduction disease. *Card Electrophysiol Clin*. 2018;10:197-209.

Barold SS. Type I Wenckebach second-degree AV block: a matter of definition. *Clin Cardiol*. 2018;41:282-284.

Barold SS, Friedberg HD. Second-degree atrioventricular block: a matter of definition. *Am J Cardiol*. 1974;33:311-315.

Barold SS, Hayes DL. Second-degree atrioventricular block: a reappraisal. *May Clin Proc*. 2001;76:44-57.

Barold SS, Stroobandt RX, Sinnaeve AF, Andries E, Herweg B. Reappraisal of the traditional Wenckebach phenomenon with a modified ladder diagram. *Ann Noninvasive Electrocardiol*. 2012;17:3-7.

Childers R. The AV node: normal and abnormal physiology. *Prog Cardiovasc Dis*. 1977:19:361-384.

Hecht HH, Kossmann CE, Childers RW, et al. Atrioventricular and intraventricular conduction. *Am J Cardiol*. 1973;31:232-244.

Markowitz SM, Lerman BB. A contemporary view of atrioventricular nodal physiology. *J Interv Card Electrophysiol*. 2018;52:271-279.

Marriott HJL, Menendez MM. A-V dissociation revisited. *Prog Cardiovasc Dis*. 1966;8:522-235.

Scheinman MM. Atrioventricular nodal conduction and refractoriness. *PACE*. 1993;16:592-598.

Wang K, Benditt DG. AV dissociation, an inevitable response. *Ann Noninvasive Electrocardiol*. 2011;16:227-231.

Zipes DP. Second-degree atrioventricular block. *Circulation*. 1979;60: 465-472.

Supraventricular Arrhythmias

▶ INTRODUCTION

A supraventricular arrhythmia is one that originates from the His bundle or above. The source of the arrhythmia may be the AV junction, atrium, or within the sinus node itself (**Figure 18-1**). This category encompasses ectopic complexes both premature and late and as well as a variety of tachyarrhythmias. We'll first review isolated ectopic supraventricular complexes and rhythms, a subject we introduced in Chapter 15. Then we'll move on to the broad topic of supraventricular tachycardia (SVT), finishing up with atrial flutter and fibrillation. For the purpose of this discussion, we will consider ventricular conduction as normal, which will result in a narrow QRS complex. We reviewed aberrant conduction in Chapter 16 and we'll cover the topic of wide complex tachycardia in Chapter 20.

Atrial Premature Complex

Origin and morphology An atrial premature complex (APC) originates anywhere in the atrial myocardium outside of the sinus node. The morphology of the P′ wave is either unchanged or different from the normal P wave, which reflects its ectopic location. If the depolarization arises near the sinus node, the configuration will be nearly normal. If originating near the AV node, it will be inverted reflecting retrograde depolarization of the atria. The morphology of the P′ wave in different leads may be notched, biphasic or isoelectric, depending on its source located in either atrium (**Figure 18-2**). The impulse is transmitted through the AV node and His-Purkinje system as usual, producing a P′R interval that is either normal, or slightly shorter depending on its proximity to the AV node. At times, the premature impulse may find the AV node partially refractory whereupon the associated P′R interval will be prolonged over baseline.

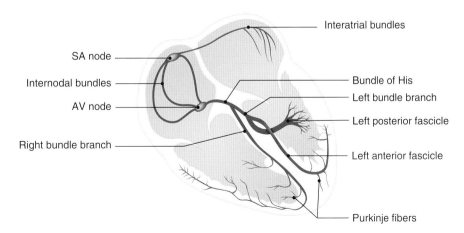

Figure 18-1. A supraventricular arrhythmia is one whose origin is above the bifurcation of the bundle of His.

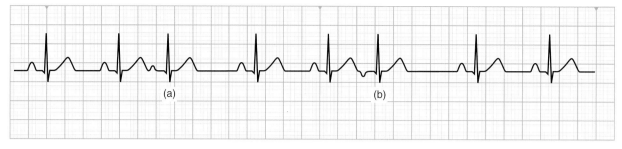

Figure 18-2. Atrial premature complexes with different P′ wave morphologies, upright (a) and inverted (b).

Timing APCs appear early in relation to the cycle length of the native sinus rhythm. The ectopic atrial depolarization typically depolarizes the SA node, resetting the native rhythm. This produces a post-ectopic pause that is *not fully compensatory (noncompensatory)* (**Figure 18-3**). However, if the impulse happens *not* to reset the sinus node, the post-ectopic pause will be fully compensatory.

Repetitive APCs, or occurring in a pattern APCs may occur alone (*isolated*), grouped repetitively, or present in a pattern related to the native sinus complex. Two APCs in a row are termed an atrial *couplet* or *pair*. A group of three rapid APCs in a row at a rate >100 bpm defines *supraventricular tachycardia*. Atrial *bigeminy* describes APCs that alternate with each sinus complex. Atrial *trigeminy* refers to when the APC appears every third complex.

Conduction The fate of the APC depends on the state of the conduction system distal to the premature depolarization. To reach the ventricular myocardium, the impulse must conduct through the AV junction, the bundle branches, and the Purkinje fibers. We know that after depolarization, there is a period of time when each myocyte becomes either partially or completely refractory to further stimulation. Accordingly, a premature impulse may find these cells either partially or completely inhibited to further conduction (**Figure 18-4**). Therefore, the APC may conduct with an AV delay, be completely blocked, or exhibit aberrant ventricular conduction.

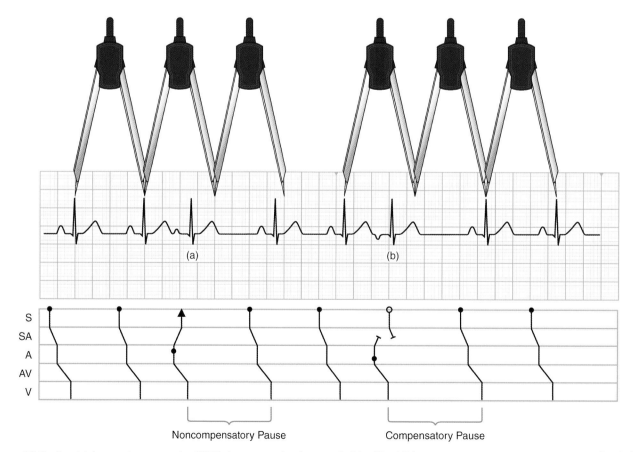

Figure 18-3. An atrial premature complex (APC) that resets the sinus node (a) will exhibit a noncompensatory pause. An APC that fails to reset the sinus node (b) will result in a fully compensatory pause.

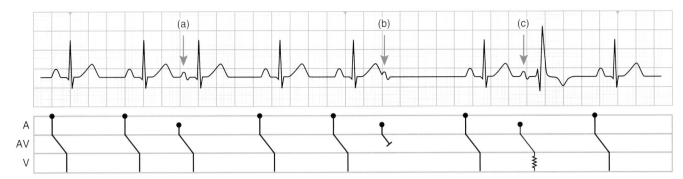

Figure 18-4. An atrial premature complex may conduct normally (a), blocked (b), or exhibit aberrant conduction (c).

Criteria for Atrial Premature Complex
- The complex appears early relative to the native rhythm.
- A nearly normal P′ wave is present, but may be biphasic or inverted.
- The P′R interval is typically within the normal range (0.12-0.20 seconds), but may be shorter or longer than that of the baseline sinus complex.
- The P′ wave is followed by a QRS complex identical to the native rhythm.
- Supporting criteria:
  - The complex is followed by a noncompensatory pause.
- Exceptions and modifiers.
  - Nonconducted (blocked) APC.
  - APC with aberrant conduction.

AV Junctional Premature Complex

Origin and morphology JPCs originate in the AV node or bundle of His. Retrograde conduction to the atrium typically results in an inverted P′ wave, seen best in leads II, III, and aVF. The retrograde P′ wave may appear before, after, or hidden within the QRS complex, depending on the relative speeds of both antegrade and retrograde conduction (**Figure 18-5**). When the P′ wave appears prior to the QRS, the P′R interval is short (<0.12 seconds), which differentiates a JPC from an APC.

Timing JPCs appear early relative to the normal sinus rhythm. The post-ectopic pause is highly variable. Retrograde depolarization of the SA node may occur, resetting the native rhythm and resulting in a post-ectopic pause that is not fully compensatory (noncompensatory). If the JPC and the normal sinus depolarization occur nearly simultaneously, the complexes may fuse and a fully compensatory pause will be evident. Alternatively, retrograde block may prohibit reset of the sinus node by the junctional depolarization.

Conduction The fate of the JPC depends on the refractory state of tissue *both* proximal and distal to the depolarization (**Figure 18-6**). With blocked antegrade conduction, an inverted P′ wave is present, but without a following QRS complex. With blocked retrograde conduction, a normal complex QRS is present, but without a retrograde P′ wave. Rarely a JPC occurs with both blocked antegrade and retrograde conduction. If so, the depolarization is not evident on the ECG (concealed) and is inferred by the effect on another complex such as a delay or failure of expected conduction.

Criteria for AV Junctional Premature Complex
- The complex appears early relative to the native rhythm.
- An inverted, retrograde P′ wave is present that may appear before, within, or after the QRS complex.
- When present before the QRS complex, the P′R interval is short (<0.12 seconds).
- The P′ wave is followed by a QRS complex identical to the native rhythm (unless aberrant conduction).
- Exceptions and modifiers.
  - Abnormalities of both antegrade and retrograde conduction may be present.

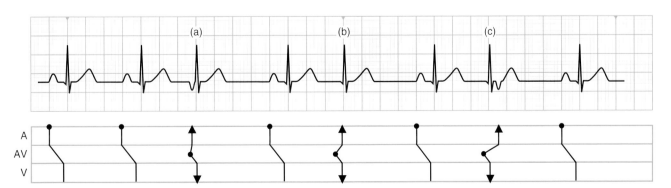

Figure 18-5. Depending the relative speeds of antegrade and retrograde conduction, the P′ wave of a junctional premature complex can appear either before (a), within (b), or after (c) the QRS complex. In this example, the sinus node is not reset and the pause after the premature complex is fully compensatory.

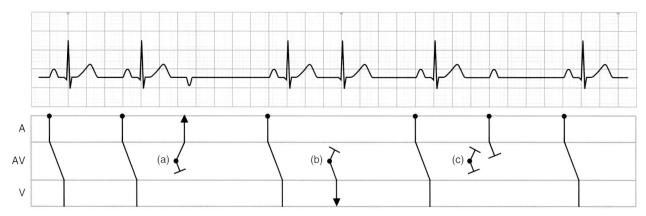

Figure 18-6. Junctional premature complexes may exhibit conduction block in an antegrade (a), retrograde (b), or both antegrade and retrograde direction (c).

Supraventricular Escape Complexes

Escape complexes are those that arise from a subsidiary pacemaker following a pause in the native rhythm that is *longer* than the normal cycle length. They have all the same morphologic characteristics as premature complexes, but emerge only when a faster, more dominant pacemaker has failed. Escape complexes are most often of AV junctional origin (**Figure 18-7**), but they can arise from regions of the atria. In the absence of aberrant conduction, the QRS complex is identical to the native rhythm.

Criteria for Atrial Escape Complex
- The complex appears late relative to the cycle of the normal rhythm, emerging due to a failure of a normally faster physiologic pacemaker.
- The P′ wave is nearly normal relative to the native P wave, but may be inverted.
- The P′R interval usually remains within the normal range (0.12-0.20 seconds).
- The QRS complex is identical to the native rhythm.

Criteria for AV Junctional Escape Complex
- The complex appears late relative to the cycle of the normal rhythm, emerging due to a failure of a normally faster physiologic pacemaker.

- P′ waves are commonly absent.
- If present, an inverted, retrograde P′ wave may appear before, within, or after the QRS complex.
- The P′R interval is short (<0.12 seconds), when present before the QRS.
- The QRS complex is identical to the native rhythm.

Escape, Wandering, and Ectopic Supraventricular Rhythms

Supraventricular escape rhythm A pattern of two or more escape complexes is termed an **escape rhythm**. The escape rhythm may arise from cells in the atrium, but most commonly originates from the AV junction, which serves as the primary "backup" pacemaker to the sinus node (**Figure 18-8**).

Wandering pacemaker At times, the focus of the impulse gradually shifts from the sinus node to another site, either within the atrium or to the AV junction. This gradual, cyclic shift in depolarization is termed a *wandering pacemaker*. If the stimulus remains within the atrium the rhythm is termed a **wandering atrial pacemaker**, characterized by a nearly normal P′ wave and P′R interval. If the focus migrates distally into the AV junction, the rhythm is called a **wandering pacemaker to the AV junction** (**Figure 18-9**). Rarely,

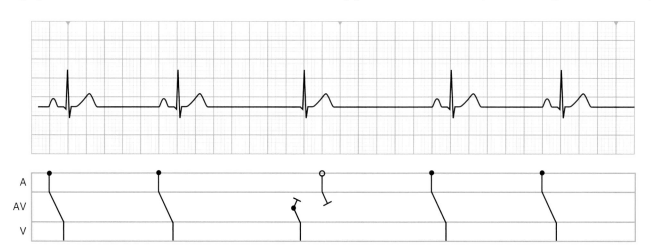

Figure 18-7. Sinus pause with emergence of a junctional escape complex. Here the junctional complex conducts only antegrade.

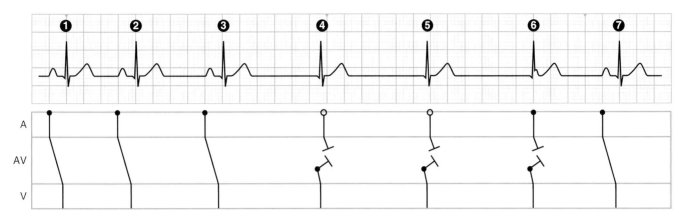

Figure 18-8. Junctional escape rhythm. The baseline rhythm is sinus arrhythmia. The pause after complex 3 allows for a junctional escape rhythm to emerge (complexes 4-6). The sinus rate is sufficient to resume control with complex 7.

a wandering pacemaker remains within the sinus node (see Chapter 14).

Criteria for Wandering Atrial Pacemaker

- Normal sinus rhythm that exhibits gradual, cyclic alteration in P (P′) wave configuration and PR (P′R) interval until two or more sequential atrial complexes appear.
- The P′ wave is nearly normal relative to the native P wave, but may be biphasic or inverted.
- The PR (P′R) interval may have slight variation, but usually remains within the normal range (0.12-0.20 seconds).
- The heart rate is typically either slow (<60 bpm) or at the lower limits of normal.

Criteria for Wandering Pacemaker to the AV Junction.

- Normal sinus rhythm that exhibits gradual, cyclic alteration in P (P′) wave configuration and PR (P′R) interval until two or more sequential AV junctional complexes appear.
- The junctional complexes display an inverted, retrograde P′ wave that may appear before, within, or after the QRS complex.
- When present before the QRS complex, the P′R interval of the junctional complex is short (<0.12 seconds).
- The heart rate of the junctional rhythm is typically 40-60 bpm.

Ectopic supraventricular rhythms It is not uncommon to see an independent ectopic rhythm without a preceding sinus mechanism. An atrial or AV junctional rhythm present without evidence of a pause or gradual change in focus is termed an **ectopic atrial rhythm** or **AV junctional rhythm**, respectively (**Figure 18-10**).

Criteria for Ectopic Atrial Rhythm

- A rhythm whose origin is an atrial pacemaker other than the sinus node.
- The P′ wave may be nearly normal, biphasic, or inverted.
  - When inverted P′ waves are present, the rhythm may be termed a "low" atrial rhythm (reflecting the proximity to the AV node).
- The P′R interval may have slight variation, but usually remains within the normal range (0.12-0.20 seconds).
- The heart rate is typically within the normal range.
  - If the HR is <60 bpm, the rhythm is described as a "slow" ectopic atrial rhythm (or ectopic atrial bradycardia).

Criteria for AV Junctional Rhythm

- A rhythm whose origin is the AV junction.
- An inverted, retrograde P′ wave is present that may appear before, within, or after the QRS complex.
- When present before QRS complex, the P′R interval is short (<0.12 seconds).
- The heart rate is typically 40-60 bpm.

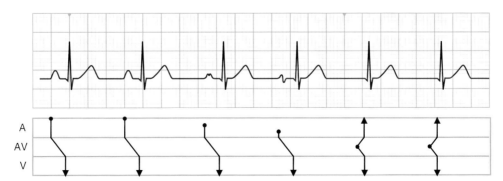

Figure 18-9. Wandering atrial pacemaker to the AV junction. Note the gradual change in P′ wave morphology and P′R interval until it becomes hidden within the QRS complex.

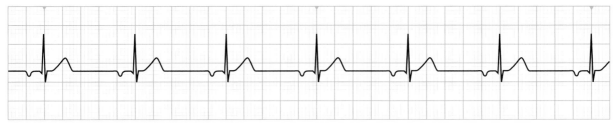

Figure 18-10. Ectopic (low) atrial rhythm. The P′R interval is in the normal range distinguishing this rhythm from one of AV junctional origin.

 CLINICAL TIP: Isolated, ectopic and wandering pacemaker rhythms are rarely clinically significant and are usually the result of enhanced vagal tone.

Accelerated AV junctional rhythm The normal intrinsic rate of the AV junction is 40-60 bpm. In the setting of hyperautomaticity, the depolarization rate of the AV junction rises (61-130 bpm), producing an **accelerated AV junctional rhythm** (**Figure 18-11**). When the HR is >100 bpm, I prefer to characterize the rhythm as an *accelerated AV junctional tachycardia*. The onset and termination of this arrhythmia is gradual, which is the basis for an older term you will encounter, *nonparoxysmal junctional tachycardia*. Another rare form of paroxysmal junctional tachycardia, *focal junctional tachycardia*, is better categorized as a form of SVT and is discussed later in this chapter.

Criteria for Accelerated AV Junctional Rhythm
- An AV junctional rhythm with a rate higher than the normal intrinsic rate of the AV junction (>60 bpm).
- Gradual onset and termination.
- Comment: Also called *nonparoxysmal junctional tachycardia*. When the HR is >100 bpm, it may be termed *accelerated AV junctional tachycardia*.

 CLINICAL TIP: Accelerated AV junctional rhythm is a hyper-automatic disorder of impulse formation that may emerge due to acute myocarditis, rheumatic fever, myocardial infarction, or with the infusion of catecholamines. When associated with digitalis toxicity, the mechanism is triggered activity with late afterdepolarizations.

▶ INTRODUCTION TO SUPRAVENTRICULAR TACHYCARDIA

Supraventricular tachycardia (SVT) is defined as a series of ≥3 consecutive ectopic supraventricular complexes at a heart rate >100 bpm. SVT encompasses a variety of rapid rhythms whose origin ranges from the sinus node through the AV junction. *Paroxysmal* SVT has an abrupt onset and termination and frequently results in symptoms of palpitation. In clinical practice, the most common form of paroxysmal SVT is AV nodal reentrant tachycardia (AVNRT), which involves dual AV nodal physiology. This is followed by atrioventricular reentrant tachycardia (AVRT), which utilizes an AV bypass connection. Atrial tachycardia (AT) is the least common form of paroxysmal SVT. Unusual or rare forms of SVT include sinus node reentrant tachycardia (SNRT) and junctional tachycardia (JT). Along with atrial flutter and atrial fibrillation, SVT falls within the category of **narrow complex tachycardias**.

Multiple mechanisms may be involved in generating the different forms of SVT, including disordered automaticity, triggered activity, and reentry. A thorough understanding of these mechanisms helps us to understand what we observe on the ECG. With that in mind, let's do a quick review of the electrophysiology of arrhythmias, something we covered in detail in Chapter 13.

SVT Mechanism

Disordered automaticity Automaticity associated SVT is most often due to accelerated normal automaticity (hyperautomaticity) (**Figure 18-12**). This is a disorder of impulse formation resulting from the alteration of an *ionically normal* pacemaker mechanism that increases the normal rate

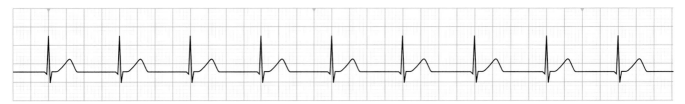

Figure 18-11. Accelerated AV junctional rhythm. The rhythm is *accelerated*, because the rate is greater than the normal intrinsic depolarization rate of the AV junction.

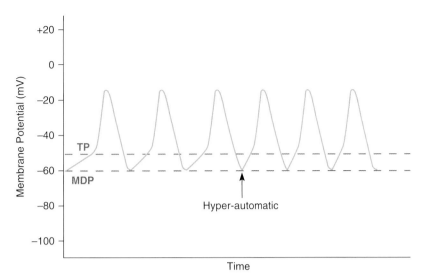

Figure 18-12. Hyper-automaticity. Think of this mechanism as disordered automaticity that involves acceleration of an otherwise normal automatic mechanism. Abbreviations: TP = threshold potential, MDP = maximum diastolic potential.

of depolarization. Abnormal automaticity, where the action potential is *ionically abnormal* due to cellular injury, is not implicated as a cause of SVT.

Triggered activity Unlike automatic rhythms that arise *de novo* in the absence of prior electrical activity, arrhythmias related to triggered activity occur in response to a preceding impulse (the trigger). Triggered activity results from *afterdepolarizations*, which are oscillations of membrane voltage consequent to a preceding action potential (**Figure 18-13**). These occur either during repolarization (early afterdepolarizations) or shortly after full repolarization (late afterdepolarizations). The afterdepolarizations may then trigger further impulses that may be either isolated or sustained.

Reentry The majority of SVTs are due to reentry. Recall that after each depolarization, the cell is temporarily rendered refractory to further stimulation. But under the proper circumstances, the initial depolarization can return and reexcite the original tissue, producing a sustained tachyarrhythmia. For reentry to occur, an initiating stimulus must encounter *all* of the following factors.

1. The presence of at least two functionally or anatomically distinct pathways that are connected to form a circuit.

2. Unidirectional block in one of the pathways.

3. An area of slow conduction.

Figure 18-14 illustrates the processes required for reentry. Panel (a) shows a cardiac fiber that divides into two limbs, labeled (α) and (β), which connect distally. If both pathways have identical properties, any impulse reaching the branch point (x) will travel down both limbs, conducting both distally and toward each other, meeting simultaneously at the connection, as shown in panel (b). Each stimulus extinguishes at the connection, unable to proceed as it meets depolarized refractory tissue from the other direction. But if the pathways have

different properties, the setting is ripe for reentry. Panel (c) shows a fiber where each limb has different properties, an α pathway that conducts slowly and has a short refractory period and a β pathway that conducts rapidly and has a long refractory period. With fortuitous timing, a premature impulse may find the β pathway refractory, blocking the impulse and allowing conduction only through the slower α pathway. And with enough antegrade delay in the α pathway, the now recovered β pathway permits retrograde conduction of the impulse. The returning stimulus finds the α pathway repolarized and reexcitable, which perpetuates the cycle.

 CLINICAL TIP: Here's a way you can remember the electrophysiologic properties of the two limbs of the circuit necessary for reentry. We just reviewed that one arm of the circuit conducts rapidly and has a long refractory period and the other conducts slowly and has a short refractory period. This will make sense if you think of each limb as two members of a track team, one a sprinter and the other a jogger. The sprinter runs with maximum effort, but the intensity requires an extended recovery before the next race (rapid conduction/long refractory period). The jogger plods along slowly, but the easy pace allows for a quick recovery (slow conduction/short refractory period).

SVT Analysis and Classification

A maddening array of options exists for characterizing SVT. No one classification serves all purposes and each has value depending on whether your focus is electrocardiography, electrophysiology, or clinical care. Before we discuss each individual arrhythmia, let's review the elements and terminology contained in our SVT "toolbox."

Anatomical chamber of origin By definition, SVT originates above the bifurcation of the bundle of His. This includes the sinus node, atrium, and AV junction (AV node and His bundle).

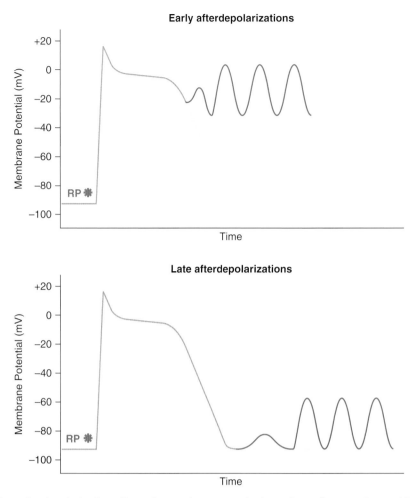

Figure 18-13. Early and late afterdepolarizations. Some forms of supraventricular tachycardias are triggered by late afterdepolarizations. Abbreviations: RP = resting potential, (*) = stimulus.

Mechanism SVT can be broadly categorized into those involving reentry versus nonreentry. This has significant implications regarding options for treatment, as reentrant SVT may be particularly amenable to ablation.

Paroxysmal versus nonparoxysmal The term paroxysmal is the clinical description of a sudden, intermittent presentation of the tachycardia. Nonparoxysmal implies a more gradual onset, chronic, or sustained arrhythmia. Leading to confusion is that the terms have been used inconsistently and can be misleading. For example, some forms of SVT that have been historically called *paroxysmal* can be long-lasting, whereas others termed *nonparoxysmal* present as a series of recurrent brief events. In general, paroxysmal SVT is caused by reentry, whereas nonparoxysmal SVT is a disorder of either hyper-automaticity or triggered activity.

AV node dependency AV node-dependent SVT requires the active participation of the AV node in the genesis and maintenance of the arrhythmia. The typical mechanism is reentry, where the AV node is a necessary part of the circuit. Any intervention that produces AV block will normally terminate the reentrant arrhythmia. In AV node-independent SVT, the AV node serves only as a passive conduit of AV conduction from another stimulus. SVT that is AV node independent will persist in the presence of AV block.

Regularity Multifocal atrial tachycardia (MAT) and atrial fibrillation are characteristically irregular arrhythmias. Focal AT, macroreentrant AT and atrial flutter are typically regular arrhythmias that become irregular when there is variable AV conduction.

Onset and termination Sudden onset and termination is characteristic of SVT with a reentry mechanism. Gradual acceleration (warm-up) followed by deceleration (cool down) is typical of an automatic mechanism. An SVT that ends with a nonconducted, retrograde P′ wave implicates a mechanism based on reentry that requires the AV node as part of the circuit.

Identification of atrial activity The rhythm should be analyzed for P (P′), flutter, or fibrillatory waves. Identification may be difficult in the presence of rapid heart rates and certain forms of SVT where atrial depolarization is obscured by the QRS complex or T wave. Methods to uncover discrete atrial activity include the Valsalva maneuver, carotid sinus massage, and the use of AV-blocking agents such as adenosine.

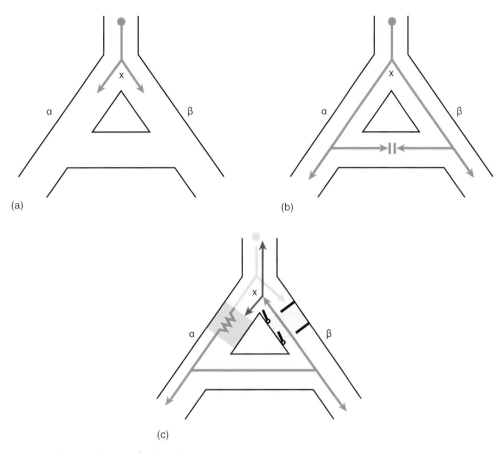

Figure 18-14. Reentry mechanism. See text for details.

 CLINICAL TIP: The Valsalva maneuver is performed by asking the patient to perform forced exhalation against a closed glottis. The patient can also be asked to "push up" against a hand pressed on the abdomen. The resulting increase in intrathoracic pressure stimulates baroreceptors that augment vagal tone and promote AV block. Carotid sinus massage stimulates carotid baroreceptors in the carotid sinus that induce a reflex increase in vagal tone. It is performed by placing the patient in a supine position with the neck extended and applying pressure over one carotid artery for 5 to 10 seconds. If no response is obtained, repeat on the contralateral side (never both simultaneously). Carotid sinus massage should be performed with continuous cardiac monitoring and should be avoided in subjects with carotid artery disease.

   Another useful tool is to record the ECG at double speed (50 mm/sec), which can allow identification of atrial activity otherwise made difficult by a rapid atrial rate.

Atrial rate   There is considerable overlap between the various forms of SVT, so atrial rate alone is rarely diagnostic. An exception is when the atrial rate is >240 bpm, which usually indicates atrial flutter. On occasion, these atrial rates are seen with AT and AVRT.

Atrial morphology   The morphology of the P (P′) wave provides clues as to the site of origin. In the frontal plane, the normal P wave is usually upright in leads I, II, III, aVL, and aVF and negative in lead aVR. In the horizontal plane, it may be upright, inverted, or biphasic (upright followed by inverted) in lead V1. Inspect the P′ wave to determine whether its morphology resembles normal sinus, is abnormal from an ectopic atrial focus, or is depolarized retrograde from the AV junction.

   Abnormal P′ waves exhibit a variety of deviations from the normal P wave morphology depending on whether the origin is the right atrium, left atrium, or related structures such as the pulmonary veins.

 FOR BOOKWORMS: Analysis of the P′ wave in lead V1 and aVL can help discriminate left from right-sided atrial depolarization. An origin from the posteriorly situated left atrium will proceed anteriorly, typically resulting in a P′ wave that is upright in lead V1 and negative or flat in lead aVL. Conversely, the anteriorly positioned right atrium directs the impulse posteriorly, typically producing a P′ wave that is inverted in lead V1, and upright or biphasic in lead aVL. Further variation depends on whether the impulse derives from a superior or inferior origin. In either atrium, a superior origin will proceed inferiorly, resulting in an upright P′ wave in leads II, III, and aVF. Conversely, an inferior focus produces an inverted P′ wave in those leads as the depolarization advances in a superior direction.

A retrograde P′ wave originating from the AV junction is characteristically inverted in leads II, III, and aVF, reflecting

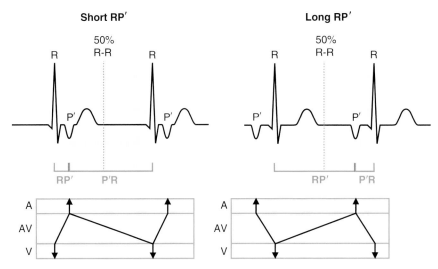

Short RP′

R   50%   R
           R-R

              P′   P′

         RP′   P′R

A
AV
V

Long RP′

R   50%   R
           R-R

  P′   P′

              RP′   P′R

A
AV
V

Figure 18-15. The RP′ interval reflects the difference in time between antegrade activation of the ventricle and retrograde activation of the atrium. A short RP′ interval is <50% of the R-R interval (left). A long RP′ interval is >50% of the R-R interval (right).

the inferior-to-superior atrial depolarization. In lead V1, the retrograde, posterior-to-anterior activation typically produces a small, upright P′ wave.

P′ wave timing (RP′-P′R relationship)   Analysis of the position of the P′ wave relative to the QRS complex provides insight as to the mechanism of some forms of SVT. We are accustomed to considering the atrial-ventricular relationship as the PR interval, which is a measure of antegrade AV conduction. Here our focus is the RP′ interval. Why on earth should that be? The reason is that the most common forms of SVT are reentry-based, AV node-dependent tachyarrhythmias that involve retrograde atrial depolarization. The RP′ interval reflects the difference in time between antegrade activation of the ventricle and retrograde activation of the atrium (**Figure 18-15**). In SVT with rapid retrograde conduction, the P′ wave appears just after the QRS complex, producing a short RP′ interval. When rapid retrograde conduction matches that of antegrade conduction, the P′ wave falls within the QRS complex and the RP′ interval is undetectable. With slower retrograde conduction, the inverted P′ wave will be separated after the QRS complex. Does this sound familiar? It should because it's the same concept we discussed earlier in this chapter regarding isolated junctional complexes (see Figure 18-5). The position of the inverted P′ wave in relation to the QRS complex depends on the relative speeds of antegrade and retrograde conduction. Here we apply the same concept to repetitive depolarizations rather than a single junctional complex.

 FOR BOOKWORMS: Electrophysiologists often divide SVT into short RP′ and long RP′ interval categories, determined by whether the RP′ interval is less than or greater than half the R-R interval (see Figure 18-15). Short RP′ interval SVT is typically AVNRT, AVRT, and sometimes AT. More detailed measurements of the short RP′ interval can help discriminate between these three diagnoses (see selections for further reading). Long RP′ interval SVT is purely descriptive and further analysis does not readily differentiate between the various forms of SVT that fall within this category.

▶ TYPES OF SUPRAVENTRICULAR TACHYCARDIA

It's now time to discuss the various types of SVT. It's important to realize that despite our best efforts, the ECG does not always allow us to determine a definite diagnosis. In these circumstances, it's perfectly reasonable to interpret the rhythm simply as a supraventricular or narrow complex tachycardia.

Sinus Node Reentrant Tachycardia

We discussed basic sinus rhythm abnormalities in Chapter 14. A relatively rare and unique form of SVT is *sinus node reentrant tachycardia* (**Figure 18-16**). Here, an atrial premature depolarization initiates a reentry circuit within the sinus node and contiguous atrial tissue. The P (P′) wave is identical to that of normal sinus, making the arrhythmia difficult to distinguish from sinus tachycardia. Unlike sinus tachycardia, which starts

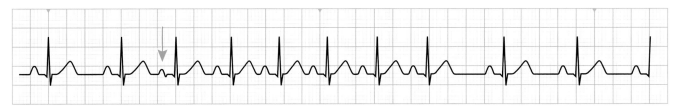

Figure 18-16. Sinus node reentrant tachycardia is usually initiated by an APC (arrow).

and stops gradually, SNRT is paroxysmal, typically initiated by and terminated with an APC.

Criteria for Sinus Node Reentrant Tachycardia
- P (P′) wave of sinus origin.
  - Normal P (P′) wave configuration (upright in leads I, II, and aVF, and inverted in aVR).
  - Normal mean axis (between 0 and +75 degrees).
- Normal PR (P′R) interval (0.12-0.20 seconds).
- HR >100 bpm.
- Typically paroxysmal onset.
- Usually initiated by and terminated with an APC.

 FOR BOOKWORMS: You may encounter SNRT categorized as a form of AT because the reentry circuit utilizes portions of atrial tissue.

Atrial Tachycardia

The classical ECG definition of atrial tachycardia is a series of discrete, monomorphic atrial complexes at a rate >100 bpm (usually 150-240 bpm). The rhythm is regular with 1:1 AV conduction with P′ waves separated by an isoelectric baseline (**Figure 18-17**, top). At higher heart rates (>150 bpm), physiologic AV conduction delay is common (see Figure 18-17, bottom).

Advances in electrophysiology have demonstrated the limitations of the classical ECG criteria for AT. Whereas P′ waves separated by an isoelectric baseline are typical of AT, it has been shown that neither atrial rate nor the presence of an isoelectric baseline excludes atrial flutter. This has led to a new classification based on electrophysiologic mechanism, dividing AT into *focal* and *macroreentrant*. Importantly, the ECG alone cannot differentiate focal from macroreentrant AT, so the classical criteria remain valid for routine ECG interpretation.

Focal atrial tachycardia This form of AT is characterized by regular atrial activation from a small, localized point source that spreads out centrifugally. Multiple mechanisms are possible, including hyper-automaticity, triggered activity, or microreentry within a small anatomical region. Analysis of P′ wave morphology can point to the origin of the focus, which is most commonly the right atrium. Left atrial focal AT frequently originates from the region of the pulmonary veins.

 CLINICAL TIP: Short episodes of focal AT are common during cardiac monitoring in patients with no overt heart disease. Paroxysmal AT may also occur in patients with acute myocardial infarction, pulmonary disease, electrolyte abnormalities, excessive alcohol, theophylline, cocaine, and other stimulants. Here the mechanism is typically hyper-automaticity. A rare form of incessant, hyper-automatic AT may lead to a tachycardia-induced cardiomyopathy. Focal AT may also occur in patients with a history of ablation for atrial fibrillation or cardiac surgery as local areas of fibrosis create the potential for microreentry. The different forms of focal AT cannot be distinguished by the ECG alone and require electrophysiologic study to determine those based on disordered automaticity from reentry.

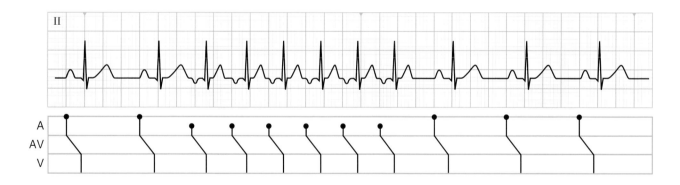
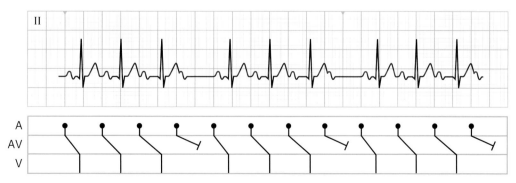

Figure 18-17. Focal atrial tachycardia. Note the subtle increase in tachycardia rate ("warm up" phenomenon) often seen with this arrhythmia (top). Functional, Mobitz type I conduction delay may be seen at rapid atrial rates (bottom).

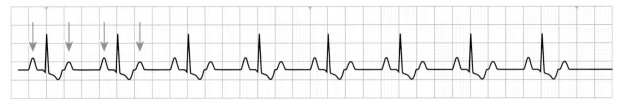

Figure 18-18. Atrial tachycardia with 2:1 AV block. Every other P′ wave (arrow) is blocked in a patient with digitalis toxicity.

Classical Criteria for Atrial Tachycardia

- Series of ≥3 monomorphic atrial complexes (P′ waves).
- P′ wave of atrial origin.
  - Morphology and axis are variable, depending on atrial origin.
- Atrial rate >100 bpm (usually 150-240 bpm).
- Regular, 1:1 AV conduction.
  - Physiologic AV conduction delay is common at higher atrial rates.
- Normal P′R interval (0.12-0.20 seconds).
- P′ waves separated by an isoelectric line.

A unique form of focal AT is **atrial tachycardia with block** (**Figure 18-18**). Typically (but not always) associated with digitalis toxicity, the arrhythmia mechanism is triggered activity with late afterdepolarizations. One clue to this form of focal AT is the presence of 2:1 AV conduction with a relatively slower atrial rate (<200 bpm), where physiologic conduction delay would not be expected.

Criteria for Atrial Tachycardia with Block

- Repetitive monomorphic atrial complexes (P′ waves).
- Atrial rate >100-240 bpm (usually <200 bpm).
- 2:1 or higher degree of AV conduction block.
- P′ waves separated by an isoelectric line.
- Comment: This arrhythmia often historically carries the mechanistically inaccurate name of *paroxysmal* atrial tachycardia (PAT) with block.

Macroreentrant atrial tachycardia The underlying mechanism of macroreentrant AT involves regular atrial activation around a "large" central obstacle. In most cases, the circuit propagates around a scar in the right or left atrium that results from either surgery for congenital heart disease or after surgical or catheter-based interventions for atrial fibrillation.

 BE CAREFUL: You may encounter the term *intra-atrial reentry tachycardia* (IART). This can be confusing because intra-atrial reentry usually refers to a macroreentrant AT, but could also be used to describe a focal microreentrant AT. This imprecision is why I discourage use of the term IART.

Another confusing item is that macroreentrant AT is now the preferred term for rhythms previously called *atypical atrial flutter*. Tradition compels us to discuss atrial flutter as a separate entity, but the primary mechanisms of all forms of atrial flutter and macroreentrant AT are the same. As we will discuss shortly, the difference lies in the specifics of the central obstacle around which the reentry circuit propagates.

Multifocal Atrial Tachycardia

This is an AT characterized by multiple P′ wave morphologies (**Figure 18-19**) and varying P′R intervals. The rhythm is irregular with at least three P′ waves of varying sizes and shapes. A dominant pacemaker is absent with the varying R-R intervals separated by an isoelectric baseline. Some of the P′ waves may be nonconducted or conducted aberrantly. The term *multifocal (chaotic) atrial rhythm* is utilized when the HR is ≤100 bpm.

The mechanism of MAT is hyper-automaticity with multiple ectopic foci that depolarize within the atria. Severe pulmonary disease is the clinical condition most often associated with MAT, but the rhythm may also be present in patients with metabolic abnormalities and congestive heart failure.

 BE CAREFUL: Both MAT and atrial fibrillation are irregular rhythms than can easily be confused for each other. MAT has discrete P′ waves, whereas atrial fibrillation does not. MAT must also be distinguished from sinus tachycardia with frequent multiform APCs. In sinus rhythm, one dominant pacemaker can be identified, whereas in MAT this is absent.

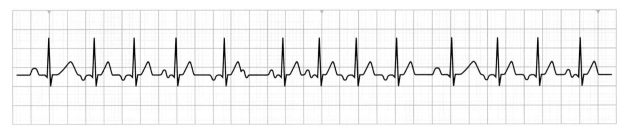

Figure 18-19. Multifocal atrial tachycardia. At least three different P′ wave morphologies are present without a dominant atrial focus. Some of the atrial complexes may fail to conduct.

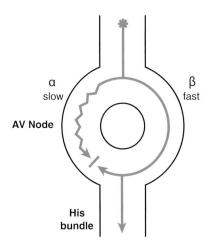

Criteria for Multifocal Atrial Tachycardia
- Rapid atrial rhythm with ≥3 consecutive P′ waves of different morphologies.
- Atrial rate >100 bpm.
  - When rate ≤100 bpm the rhythm is termed "multifocal or chaotic atrial rhythm."
- Absence of a single, dominant atrial pacemaker.
- Variable P′-P′, P′R, and R-R intervals.
- P′ waves separated by an isoelectric line.

Junctional Tachycardia

There are two forms of junctional tachycardia. We previously discussed accelerated (nonparoxysmal) AV junctional tachycardia, which is the term used when the rate of accelerated AV junctional rhythm exceeds 100 bpm. Another, more unusual form of JT is *focal junctional tachycardia.* Other names for this rhythm are *automatic junctional tachycardia* or *paroxysmal (ectopic) junctional tachycardia.*

Focal junctional tachycardia is a rare clinical entity. The ectopic, hyper-automatic rhythm is usually seen in pediatric patients with congenital heart disease. In adults JT can occur after ablation for AVNRT. JT is typically paroxysmal with a HR ranging from 110-250 bpm. As with other junctional rhythms, the retrograde P′ wave may appear before, within, or after the QRS complex.

Criteria for Focal Junctional Tachycardia
- A rapid rhythm whose origin is the AV junction.
- Junctional rate >100 bpm (typically 110-250 bpm).
- Inverted, retrograde P′ waves that may be present before, within, or after the QRS complex.
- When present before the QRS complex, the P′R interval is short (<0.12 seconds), when present before the QRS.
- Typically has a paroxysmal onset.

AV Nodal Reentrant Tachycardia

This common form of paroxysmal SVT involves **dual AV nodal pathways**, each with different conduction properties that set the stage for classic reentry (**Figure 18-20**). Remember the key to reentry is the presence of one pathway with fast conduction and a long refractory period and another with slow conduction and a short refractory period that meet in a final common pathway. **Figure 18-21** illustrates the typical mechanism that initiates AVNRT. In sinus rhythm the impulse conducts normally, preferentially utilizing the fast limb to depolarize the ventricles (complexes 1-2). The impulse proceeds simultaneously down the slow limb, but meets oncoming retrograde depolarization from the fast pathway, neither impulse able to advance. However, if an atrial premature depolarization (APD) fortuitously arrives while the fast pathway is still refractory, the impulse is directed antegrade solely down the slow pathway, conducting with a prolonged P′R interval (complex 3). With sufficient delay, the impulse travels retrograde up the now recovered fast pathway to reexcite the atrium and begin a new cycle (complexes 4-7). If AV conduction is interrupted (after complex 7) the reentry cycle terminates, allowing a return to sinus rhythm (complexes 8-9).

Figure 18-20. Dual AV nodal pathways. The sinus depolarization (*) simultaneously travels down two separate pathways; an α limb that exhibits slow conduction with a short refractory period, and a β limb that exhibits rapid conduction with a long refractory period. The impulse transmits rapidly via the fast pathway toward the His bundle, also conducting retrograde where it collides with the impulse passing via the slow pathway, thereby preventing reentry.

This typical form of AVNRT is called "slow-fast," so named for the initial antegrade conduction via the slow pathway followed by retrograde conduction via the fast pathway.

 CLINICAL TIP: AVNRT, and other forms of SVT that utilize reentry can be terminated by medications that produce AV nodal block. As seen in Figure 18-21, the AV node is a mandatory part of the reentry circuit. By interrupting AV conduction, the cycle will cease. Adenosine is a rapidly acting intravenous medication that is particularly useful to produce transient AV block and convert this form of SVT to sinus rhythm.

The ECG findings of slow-fast AVNRT reflect the electrophysiologic mechanism of the arrhythmia. The initial, slowly conducting APD exhibits a prolonged P′R interval. The inverted P′ waves that follow are usually buried within the QRS complex, owing to the rapid retrograde conduction. When visible, they may appear either as a pseudo s wave in leads II, III, and aVF, or a pseudo r′ wave in lead V1, neither of which was present during sinus rhythm (**Figure 18-22**). The rapid retrograde conduction with a visible P′ wave that appears just after the QRS complex places this form of AVNRT in the category of a short RP′ interval SVT.

An uncommon, atypical form of AVNRT (fast-slow) is one where the fast pathway serves as the antegrade limb of the circuit and the retrograde limb the slow pathway (**Figure 18-23**). In sinus rhythm, antegrade conduction is as usual via the fast pathway (complexes 1-2). But in this atypical form of AVNRT, a fortuitously timed ventricular premature depolarization (VPD) finds the fast pathway refractory, preferentially conducting the impulse retrograde via the slow pathway to depolarize the atria (complex 3). If sufficient delay allows recovery of the fast pathway, the impulse conducts antegrade back to the ventricles and

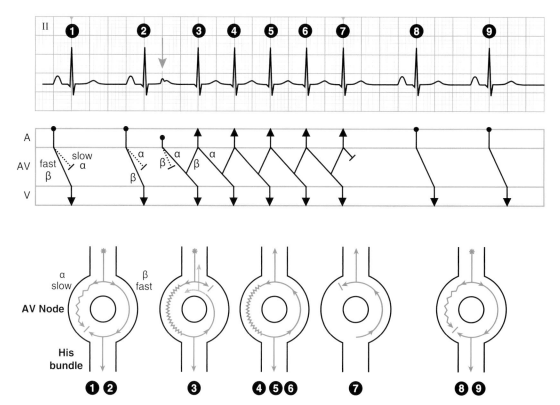

Figure 18-21. Slow-fast AVNRT. An APD (arrow) blocks in the fast pathway (β) and conducts with a delay down the slow pathway (α). The impulse returns to reexcite previously depolarized and now recovered tissue (orange) and initiates reentry (see text for details).

perpetuates the cycle (complexes 4-6). AV block terminates the cycle (after complex 6), allowing a return to sinus rhythm (complexes 7-8). The ECG findings of fast-slow AVNRT are similar to the typical slow-fast form except that the slower retrograde conduction allows the inverted P′ wave to become visible well beyond the QRS complex. Accordingly, this represents a long RP′ interval SVT.

 CLINICAL TIP: AVNRT is particularly amenable to catheter-based ablation. Empirically ablating the slow pathway area eliminates the substrate for reentry. You can remember which pathway to ablate by referring back to our track team analogy. The slower runner (slow pathway) is the one most likely to be cut (ablated) from the team.

Atrioventricular Reentrant Tachycardia

This form of SVT incorporates an **accessory pathway** (AP) as one limb of the reentry circuit along with the AV node as the other. As discussed in Chapter 9, accessory pathways include a variety of anomalous electrical conduits between the atrium and the ventricle that bypass the normal route via the AV node (AVN) and His-Purkinje system (HPS). The most clinically important pathway is an **atrioventricular bypass connection**. Depending on the properties of the AP, conduction may occur antegrade only, retrograde only, or most commonly in both directions. Unlike the AVN where the speed of transmission can vary, bypass pathways usually conduct in an all or none fashion. The AP may be *manifest*, where antegrade conduction

produces the typical ECG findings of preexcitation that include a delta wave, short PR interval, wide QRS complex, accompanied by ST segment and T wave abnormalities (WPW pattern) (**Figure 18-24**). Alternatively the AP may be *concealed*, where the pathway conducts only retrograde and is not evident during normal sinus rhythm. Preexcitation may be *intermittent*, defined as the presence and absence of preexcitation on the same tracing. *Inapparent or latent preexcitation* refers to preexcitation that is absent during sinus rhythm, but evident either during atrial arrhythmias or with atrial stimulation in the electrophysiology laboratory.

AVRT is classified as *orthodromic* if antegrade conduction during the arrhythmia occurs via the AVN-HPS and *antidromic* if antegrade conduction occurs via the AP (**Figure 18-25**). Accordingly, orthodromic AVRT displays a narrow complex tachycardia and antidromic AVRT exhibits a wide, preexcited complex. In most forms of AVRT, the AP serves as the limb with rapid conduction and a longer refractory period and the AVN-HPS as the limb with slower conduction and a shorter refractory period, regardless of whether conduction via each limb is antegrade or retrograde. The initiating trigger for both orthodromic and antidromic AVRT is typically an APD, with a triggering VPD less common.

 CLINICAL TIP: If you struggle with the terms orthodromic and antidromic AVRT, you are not alone. Orthodromic is derived from the Greek *orthos* (straight) and *dromos* (passage, walkway, or race course). That's why orthodromic is used to describe the normal (straight) antegrade

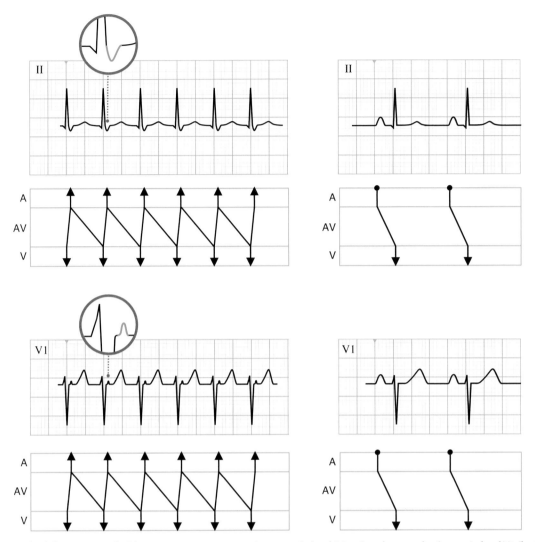

Figure 18-22. On the left, a retrograde P′ wave appears as a pseudo s wave in lead II (top) and a pseudo r′ wave in lead V1 (bottom), neither of which are present during normal sinus rhythm as seen on the right.

conduction (passage) through the AV node. Antidromic is the opposite, or *anti*, of normal orthodromic conduction. An easy reminder that antidromic AVRT conducts antegrade through the accessory pathway is to remember "triple A" (AAA), which is "antidromic-antegrade-accessory pathway."

Orthodromic (narrow complex) AVRT   Most AVRT is orthodromic, found in approximately 95% of cases. Here the antegrade limb of the circuit is the AVN-HPS and the AP serves as the retrograde limb. Orthodromic, narrow complex AVRT can be triggered by either an APD or VPD and may occur either when the baseline ECG is normal or shows manifest preexcitation. Let's take a look how this might occur.

Figure 18-26 shows AVRT in the presence of a manifest accessory pathway. Preexcitation is present at baseline, showing the typical wide QRS complex, delta wave, and short PR interval that results from simultaneous conduction via the normal AVN-HPS and the AP (complexes 1-2). An APD (complex 3) finds the AP completely refractory and now

conducts only through the AVN-HPS, resulting in a narrow QRS complex that is no longer preexcited. AV conduction is delayed with a prolonged P′R interval, either because the AVN is found relatively refractory or due to conduction via the slow pathway of a dual AV nodal system. The AV delay provides time for the AP to recover and conduct the impulse retrograde, reexciting the atrium, and starting another cycle (complex 4). The QRS complexes that follow are all narrow because depolarization proceeds antegrade only through the AVN-HPS (complexes 5-9).

Orthodromic AVRT also occurs when the accessory pathway is concealed and capable only of retrograde conduction (**Figure 18-27**). The mechanisms of induction of orthodromic AVRT in patients with manifest and concealed pathways are identical, except that in patients with concealed pathways antegrade block in the AP is present at baseline. The baseline normal sinus impulse proceeds only via the AVN so the complex is narrow. The AP is penetrated retrograde, but the impulse cannot produce reentry because the atrial tissue it meets is still refractory. However, if an APD conducts through

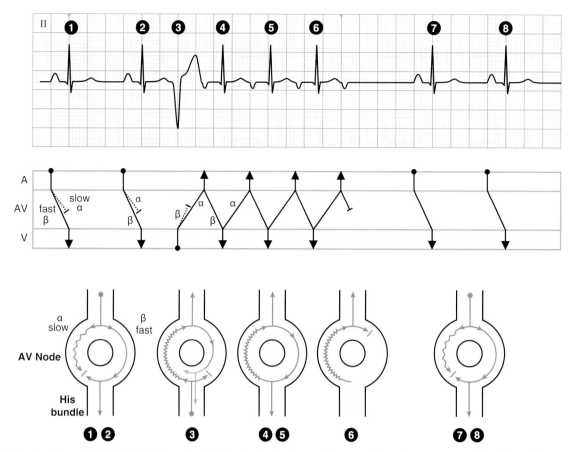

Figure 18-23. Fast-slow AVNRT. A VPD (complex 3) blocks in the fast pathway and conducts retrograde with a delay via the slow pathway. The impulse returns to reexcite previously depolarized and now recovered tissue (orange) and initiates reentry (see text for details).

the AVN with sufficient delay, retrograde conduction via the AP now finds atrial tissue that is reexcitable, thereby initiating reentry.

A VPD can also initiate orthodromic AVRT in patients with both overt and concealed bypass connections. Here the mechanism is slightly different, but remains based on the differential conduction properties of the AVN-HPS and AP. In the uncommon situation where the AP has a retrograde refractory period that is shorter than that of the HPS, a VPD can block in the HPS and conduct retrograde via the AP. The retrograde impulse can reach the atrium, enter the AVN-HPS, and with adequate delay, conduct antegrade to reexcite the ventricles.

> FOR BOOKWORMS: A rare form of orthodromic AVRT involves retrograde conduction via a concealed AP with the unusual properties of slow and decremental conduction. It usually presents in children and has the unfortunate and inaccurate name of *permanent* or *incessant junctional tachycardia.* The name is a misnomer because the focus is not specifically junctional and although frequently long-lasting, is not permanent.

Antidromic (wide complex) AVRT The focus of this section is narrow complex SVT. Antidromic AVRT is a **wide complex**

SVT, but it is prudent to discuss this topic here because of the reentry concepts involved. Preexcited AVRT is rare, occurring in approximately 5% of cases. Here the antegrade limb of the circuit is the AP and the AVN-HPS serves as the retrograde limb. **Figure 18-28** shows the process. The baseline ECG typically shows preexcitation (complexes 1-2), but it may be narrow if conduction over the AP is intermittent or inapparent. As we noted in the preceding discussion, an APD usually initiates orthodromic AVRT because it blocks in the AP, which typically has a longer refractory period than the AVN. With antidromic AVRT, the APD blocks in the AVN and conducts preferentially antegrade via the AP (complex 3). Why the difference? The reason is either because the refractory period of the AP is unusually short or the ectopic atrial depolarization occurs so close to the AP that it facilitates entry. The impulse returns retrograde via the AVN-HPS, and with sufficient delay in the circuit, finds the atrium and AP recovered, allowing reentry to occur (complexes 4-9). Note that antegrade conduction is now *entirely* over the AP, producing a very wide and bizarre QRS complex.

A VPD can also initiate antidromic AVRT by blocking retrograde in the AP and conducting with a retrograde delay via the AVN-HPS. The impulse then returns antegrade via the AP to perpetuate the cycle.

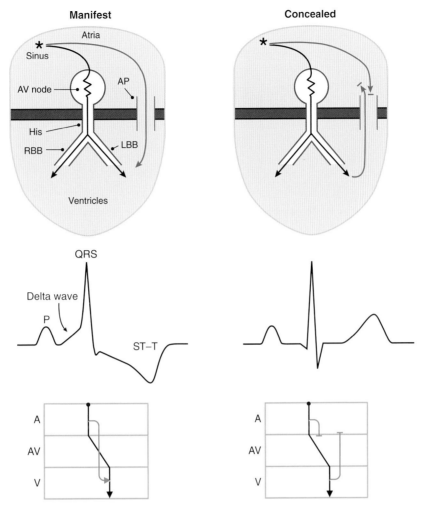

Figure 18-24. Atrioventricular bypass connection (WPW pattern). A manifest pathway (left) shows ECG evidence of preexcitation that includes a short PR interval, delta wave, and wide QRS complex, along with ST segment and T wave abnormalities. The laddergram illustrates concurrent transmission through both the normal conduction system (black) and the accessory pathway (blue). The characteristic WPW pattern represents the fusion of the transmitted impulses via the different routes. A concealed pathway (right) allows only retrograde conduction so the complex has a normal appearance. Conduction can proceed retrograde, but is blocked during normal sinus rhythm when reaching still refractory atrial tissue. Abbreviations: AP = accessory pathway, His = bundle of His, RBB = right bundle branch, LBB = left bundle branch.

 BE CAREFUL: With antidromic AVRT, the QRS complex morphology reflects conduction entirely over the AP and will be even wider and more bizarre than the fusion complex typical of the baseline WPW pattern. Ventricular depolarization proceeds entirely via slow, myocyte-to-myocyte conduction that resembles ventricular tachycardia. The retrograde P′ wave may not be discernable, buried within the wide QRS complex, ST segment, or T wave.

 CLINICAL TIP: Atrial fibrillation is the most serious arrhythmia associated with the WPW syndrome. Rapid transmission of the atrial impulses antegrade over the AP removes the normally protective conduction delay of the AVN. The AV node has the property of decremental conduction, meaning that the velocity of impulse conduction diminishes with increasing rate of stimulation. The AP usually lacks the AV node's property of decremental conduction, which means the refractory period of the AP shortens as the heart rate increases. This allows rapid

ventricular conduction that may degenerate into ventricular fibrillation and sudden death.

▶ ATRIAL FLUTTER

Introduction

Let's now turn our attention to atrial flutter. **Typical atrial flutter** is defined as an atrial rhythm with an atrial rate of 240 to 350 bpm that has a continuously undulating "sawtooth" appearance in leads II, III, and aVF (**Figure 18-29**). This has been used to distinguish atrial flutter from **atrial tachycardia**, classically defined as an atrial rhythm with an atrial rate of <240 bpm that contains an isoelectric line between the P′ waves. **Atypical atrial flutter** has been used to describe any other continuous atrial rhythm with an atrial rate of 240 to 350 bpm with a pattern different from typical atrial flutter. We now know this strict categorization is incompatible with our understanding of the electrophysiologic mechanism of

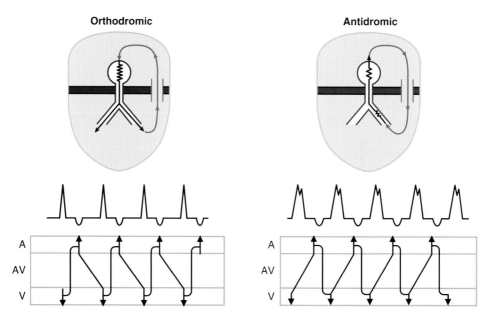

Figure 18-25. AVRT is classified as orthodromic (left) if antegrade conduction during the arrhythmia occurs via the AVN-HPS and antidromic (right) if antegrade conduction occurs via the AP.

these arrhythmias. Neither the atrial rate nor identification of an isoelectric line allows us to distinguish these entities. That's why all forms of atrial flutter now fall under the electrophysiologic category of *macroreentrant atrial tachycardias*. Confounding the issue is that the ECG does not reliably distinguish the mechanisms of focal from macroreentrant atrial tachycardia. No, we're not going to abandon the terms atrial flutter and atrial tachycardia. Macroreentrant atrial tachycardia is an electrophysiologic, not an ECG diagnosis. So it's

perfectly reasonable for us to utilize the terms atrial flutter and atrial tachycardia for ECG interpretation, as long as we appreciate that the diagnoses and underlying mechanisms overlap. It helps to have an understanding of the rationale behind the modern categorization, so let's start with a little anatomy lesson.

We learned earlier in this chapter that the underlying mechanism of all forms of macroreentrant AT involves regular atrial activation around a large central obstacle. With typical

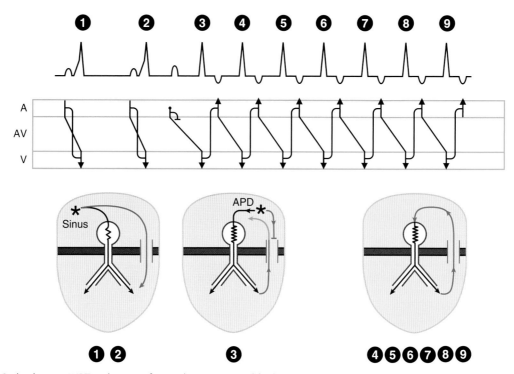

Figure 18-26. Orthodromic AVRT with a manifest pathway. An APD blocks in the AP and conducts antegrade via the AVN-HPS (complex 3). AV nodal delay allows the impulse to return retrograde via the AP and reexcite previously depolarized atrial tissue (orange). Note the loss of preexcitation during the arrhythmia.

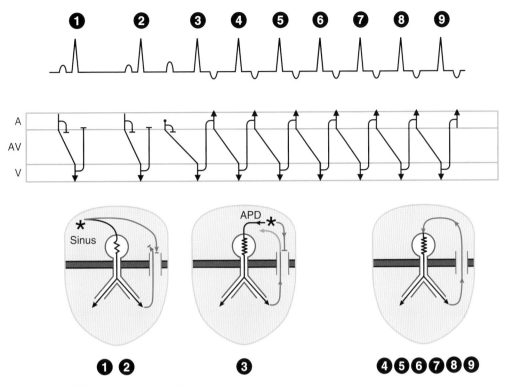

Figure 18-27. Orthodromic AVRT with a concealed AP.

atrial flutter that obstacle is the **cavo-tricuspid isthmus** (CTI) (**Figure 18-30**). The CTI is a segment of right atrial myocardium bounded posteriorly by the inferior vena cava and anteriorly by the tricuspid annulus. Also involved is the **crista terminalis**, a muscular ridge in the right atrium that serves as an area of conduction block. These components provide the

protected area of slow conduction we know is necessary for all reentrant circuits. An APD is usually the trigger, precipitating a reentrant circuit that circles around the right atrium. The left atrium is activated passively from the right atrium and is not involved in the genesis of the reentrant circuit. Typical atrial flutter is called *isthmus-dependent*, because of the integral role

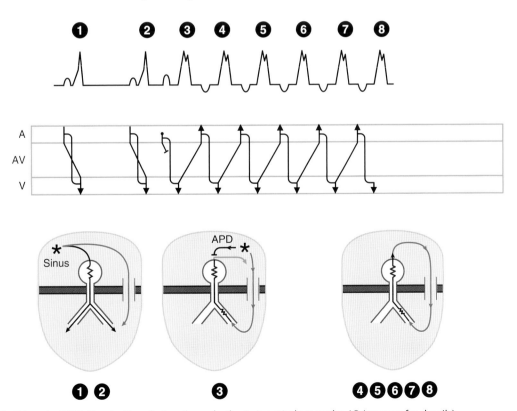

Figure 18-28. Antidromic AVRT. Conduction during the arrhythmia is entirely over the AP (see text for details).

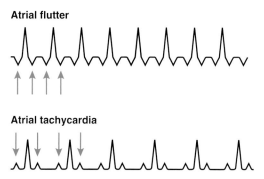

Figure 18-29. Atrial flutter with 2:1 AV conduction (top) with typical sawtooth flutter waves (arrows). Atrial tachycardia with 2:1 AV conduction (bottom) with discrete P′ waves (arrows) separated by an isoelectric baseline.

of the CTI in the reentry circuit. What has been considered as atypical atrial flutter involves a central obstacle other than the CTI, whether another atrial region or areas of scar related to previous cardiac surgery or catheter-based interventions. Accordingly, these forms of macroreentrant atrial tachycardia are considered *nonisthmus-dependent*.

Typical atrial flutter Typical atrial flutter is subdivided according to the rotational direction of the circuit as viewed in the LAO projection (**Figure 18-31**). In the large majority of cases the rotation is **counterclockwise**, the net effect of which is a highly recognizable, negative deflection (flutter or "F" wave) in leads II, III, and aVF, and a positive deflection in lead V1 (**Figure 18-32**). Rarely the circuit rotates **clockwise**, which reverses the polarity of the flutter waves.

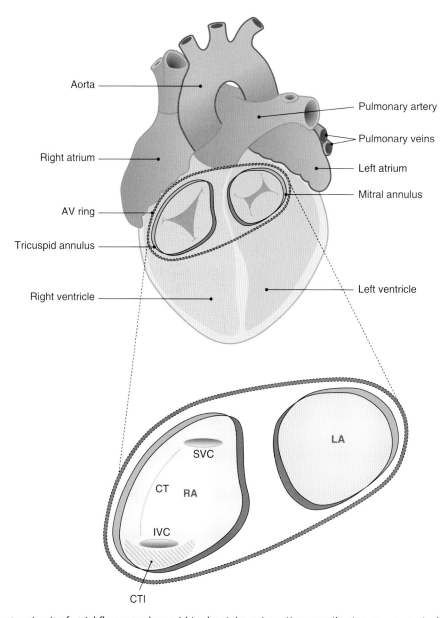

Figure 18-30. The reentry circuit of atrial flutter evolves within the right atrium. Key contributing structures include the crista terminalis (CT), which provides an area of block and the cavo-tricuspid isthmus (CTI), which provides an area of slow conduction. Cardiac structures are shown in the LAO view. Abbreviations: RA= right atrium, LA = left atrium, IVC = inferior vena cava, SVC = superior vena cava.

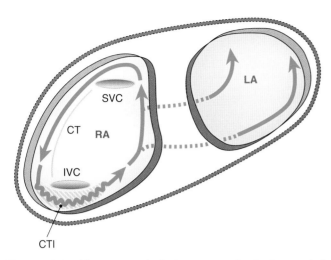

Figure 18-31. The counterclockwise reentry circuit characteristic of the common form of typical atrial flutter.

FOR BOOKWORMS: The ECG diagnosis of typical atrial flutter is defined by the presence of flutter (F) waves. Instead of discrete P′ waves, the reentrant depolarization of the atria produces continuously undulating baseline deflections. Even though the reentry circuit originates in the right atrium, the direction of left atrial activation is the prime determinant of the morphology of the flutter wave. With counterclockwise atrial flutter, the left atrium depolarizes in a predominantly inferior to superior direction, which generates negative flutter waves in the inferior leads. With clockwise atrial flutter, the orientation is reversed, leading to positive flutter waves in those leads.

The atrial rate in atrial flutter is characteristically >240 bpm. Not every atrial depolarization is conducted to the ventricles, limited by the physiologic properties of the AV node. That's a good thing because 1:1 AV conduction of atrial flutter would result in extremely high ventricular rates that could lead to hemodynamic collapse. The conduction ratio of atrial flutter is typically 2:1, which represents a normal physiologic response. The conduction ratio may be higher in the presence of AV nodal disease or treatment with AV-blocking agents (**Figure 18-33**). When interpreting an ECG with atrial flutter, report the physiologic 2:1 conduction ratio as atrial *conduction*, rather than *block*, which implies pathology. Use the term block to describe a conduction ratio >2:1 because it represents abnormal physiology. Variable conduction is used to describe the presence of multiple conduction ratios within a single tracing.

CLINICAL TIP: The second F wave of atrial flutter with 2:1 AV conduction is frequently hidden within the QRS complex. If you encounter a narrow complex tachycardia at a rate of ~150 bpm, always suspect atrial flutter with 2:1 AV conduction. Make a search for hidden flutter waves and consider means to uncover them such as the Valsalva maneuver, carotid massage, or the use of short-acting AV blocking agents such as adenosine.

Criteria for Typical Atrial Flutter

- An atrial rhythm with an atrial rate between 240 and 350 bpm.
- Flutter waves with a continuously undulating "sawtooth" morphology.
  - The polarity of the flutter waves in leads II, III, aVF, V1 depends on the direction of rotation, but is usually negative in the inferior leads and positive in lead V1.
- Conduction ratio is typically 2:1.
- Comment: There are atypical forms of atrial flutter that overlap with forms of atrial tachycardia (see text for details).

Atypical atrial flutter versus atrial tachycardia—a classification conundrum Considerable confusion surrounds the use of the term atypical atrial flutter, which has had different definitions over time. Like typical atrial flutter, atypical atrial flutter is a form of macroreentrant atrial tachycardia. But remember, macroreentrant atrial tachycardia is an electrophysiologic, not an ECG diagnosis. Since there's no universal agreement, let's keep it simple. Use the term atypical atrial flutter for regular atrial rhythms with an atrial rate 240 to 350 bpm, but with a pattern different from the classic sawtooth flutter waves of typical atrial flutter (**Figure 18-34**). Diagnose atrial tachycardia when you see discrete P′ waves with an atrial rate <240 bpm (**Figure 18-35**). Remember that neither the P′ wave morphology nor the atrial rate can reliably distinguish a focal from any form of reentrant atrial tachycardia, something that can be determined only in the electrophysiology lab. That is why you use the ECG diagnosis of atrial tachycardia, without modifying it with "focal," "macroreentrant," or "microreentrant" for that matter. This less than perfect approach for atypical atrial flutter and atrial tachycardia works fine, as long as you understand you are describing the ECG findings, which have overlapping diagnoses and do not predict the underlying mechanism.

▶ ATRIAL FIBRILLATION

Introduction

Other than isolated premature complexes, atrial fibrillation is the most common cardiac arrhythmia. The mechanism is multifactorial and incompletely understood, but ultimately results in multiple foci of disorganized atrial activity (**Figure 18-36**). Atrial fibrillation may be precipitated by rapidly firing myocardial cells in the pulmonary veins that propagate into the atrial myocardium. According to a prevailing theory, this initiates multiple reentrant wavelets that sustain the arrhythmia. Other atrial arrhythmias may promote the development of atrial fibrillation, including atrial flutter, SVT, and frequent atrial premature complexes.

A number of clinical conditions are associated with atrial fibrillation. These include hypertension, heart failure, valvular heart disease, coronary artery disease, obesity, sleep apnea, diabetes, and hyperthyroidism, as well as older age. Atrial remodeling and fibrosis play a role in both the propensity to develop atrial fibrillation and the maintenance of the arrhythmia once it occurs.

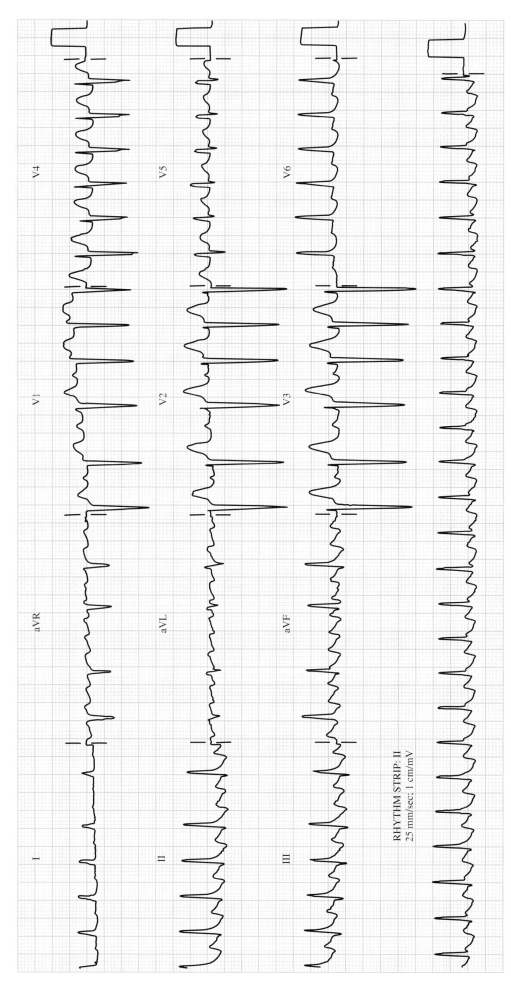

Figure 18-32. Typical atrial flutter. Note the typical sawtooth pattern prominent in leads II, III, and aVF. The conduction ratio is predominantly 2:1 with the second flutter wave obscured by the QRS complex. The brief period of a 4:1 AV conduction ratio after the fourth QRS complex allows clear visualization of the flutter waves.

RHYTHM STRIP: II
25 mm/sec; 1 cm/mV

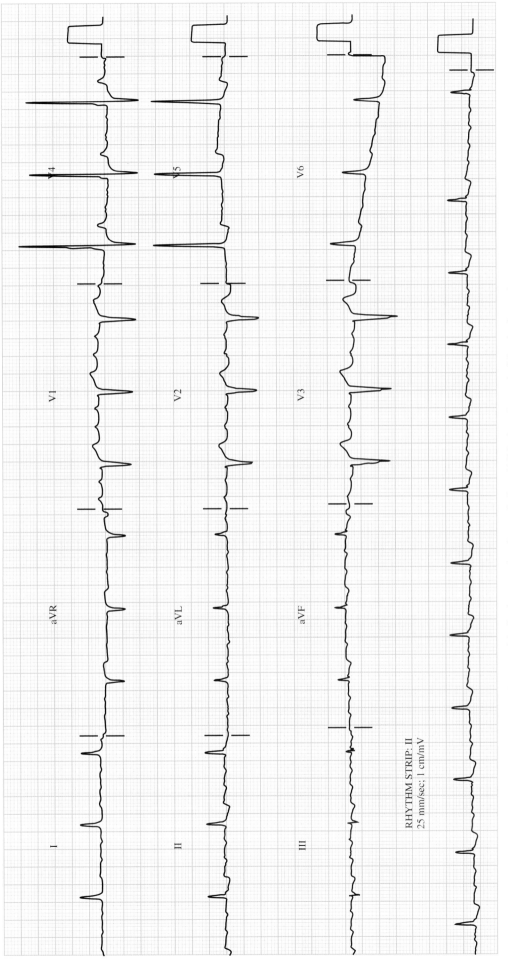

Figure 18-33. Typical atrial flutter with predominantly 4:1 AV block. There is a brief period of 6:1 AV block at the end of the rhythm strip.

RHYTHM STRIP: II
25 mm/sec; 1 cm/mV

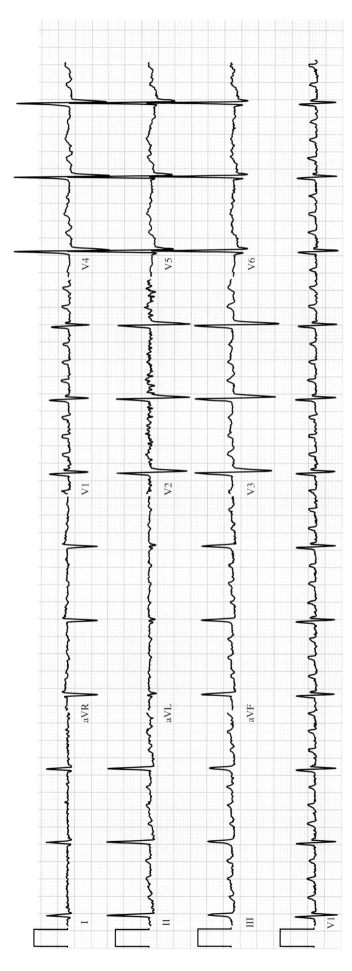

Figure 18-34. Atypical atrial flutter with 4:1 AV block. The atrial rate is 280 bpm but lacks a typical sawtooth pattern. Atrial tachycardia is an alternative diagnosis.

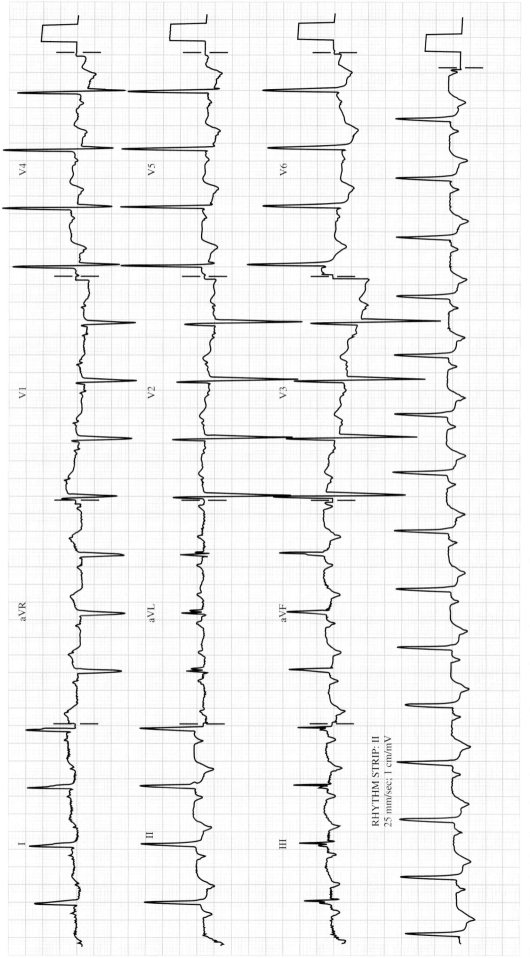

Figure 18-35. Atrial tachycardia with 2:1 AV conduction. The atrial rate is ~180 bpm. Atypical atrial flutter is an alternative diagnosis.

RHYTHM STRIP: II
25 mm/sec; 1 cm/mV

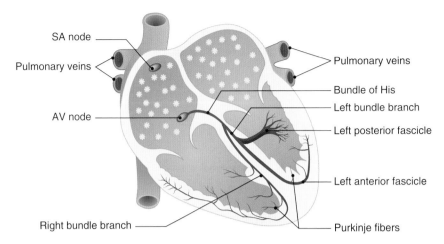

Figure 18-36. Atrial fibrillation with multiple reentrant wavelets.

Atrial fibrillation is customarily categorized with a temporal-based system. It is classified as *first-detected* in patients with no known history of the arrhythmia, regardless of its potential duration. Any occurrence after resolution of the first detected episode is termed *recurrent*. After termination, a recurrent episode is classified as either *paroxysmal* or *persistent*. Paroxysmal atrial fibrillation is characterized by self-terminating episodes that last less than 7 days. Episodes lasting longer than 7 days or are not self-terminating are termed persistent. *Longstanding persistent* atrial fibrillation refers to an arrhythmia that lasts longer than 1 year. *Permanent* atrial fibrillation is the designation after failed cardioversion or when further attempts to terminate the arrhythmia are abandoned. As new techniques emerge, patients with ostensibly permanent atrial fibrillation may undergo attempts to restore sinus rhythm. In this situation, it is appropriate to rename the previously considered "permanent" arrhythmia as "longstanding persistent" atrial fibrillation.

 CLINICAL TIP: Atrial fibrillation predisposes to the formation of thrombi, most commonly located in the left atrial appendage. This may lead to emboli that may circulate to the brain and cause a stroke. Anticoagulant medications can markedly lower this risk.

Electrocardiographic Findings

P waves are absent in atrial fibrillation, replaced by small, irregular deflections called fibrillatory (f) waves that oscillate at a rate between 350 and 600 bpm (**Figure 18-37**). The morphology of the f waves continuously varies and may be coarse such that they resemble flutter waves, or so fine as to be barely discernable.

The ventricular response is variable, leading to the characterization of atrial fibrillation as "irregularly irregular." The AV node is bombarded by the rapid atrial impulses, but because the AV node has the property of decremental conduction, not every atrial impulse reaches the ventricles. The ventricular rate is usually in the range of 90 to 170 bpm. Because the rhythm is irregular, you should use the 6-second method to estimate the average ventricular rate (**Figure 18-38**). The ventricular rate of atrial fibrillation is characterized as either being controlled (60-100 bpm), rapid (>100 bpm), or slow (<60 bpm) (**Figure 18-39**). The rate is typically higher in younger individuals and with sympathetic stimulation. Lower ventricular rates are seen with older age, parasympathetic stimulation, and with the use of AV-blocking medications.

 CLINICAL TIP: Do not fall into the habit of describing a patient as having "rapid afib." Atrial fibrillation is always rapid, the depolarizations occurring at a rate >350 bpm. The correct description of the arrhythmia is atrial fibrillation with a *rapid ventricular response*.

At times, atrial fibrillation is associated with an unusual ventricular response. In the setting of advanced conduction disease or excessive AV blocking agents, atrial fibrillation may become "regularized," which is a manifestation of high grade or complete AV block (**Figure 18-40**). In this situation, none of the fibrillatory impulses transmits to the ventricles and the visualized QRS complexes represent an escape rhythm from the AV junction or below. At the opposite end of the spectrum, an extremely rapid ventricular response may be present when conduction occurs over an accessory bypass pathway. Finally, the irregular ventricular response is likely to include "long-short" sequences, which we know raises the potential for aberrant conduction (Ashman phenomenon), a topic we reviewed in detail in Chapter 16 (**Figure 18-41**).

 BE CAREFUL: A number of other irregular atrial arrhythmias may be mistaken for atrial fibrillation. This includes sinus rhythm with frequent APCs, MAT, and when atrial flutter or atrial tachycardia has variable AV conduction. Artifacts from electrical interference or patient motion are also sources of error.

Criteria for Atrial Fibrillation

- P waves are replaced by fibrillatory waves with an atrial rate of 350 to 600 bpm.
- The ventricular response is normally irregularly irregular.

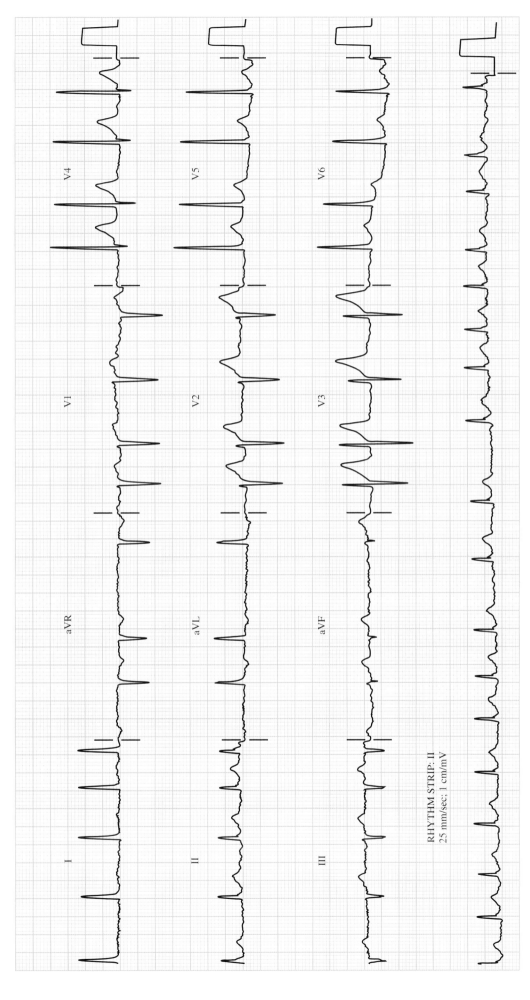

Figure 18-37. Atrial fibrillation is characterized as an irregularly irregular rhythm. P waves are replaced with fibrillatory (f) waves.

RHYTHM STRIP: II
25 mm/sec; 1 cm/mV

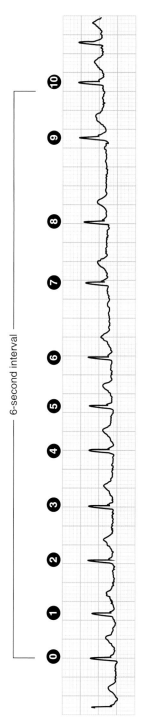

Figure 18-38. Using the 6-second method to calculate the average heart rate, which is estimated here as 98 bpm.

Rapid

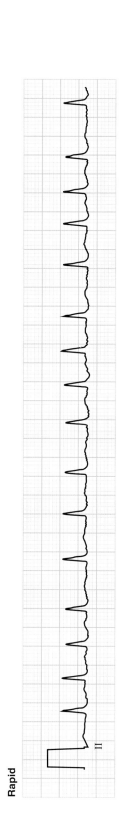

Slow

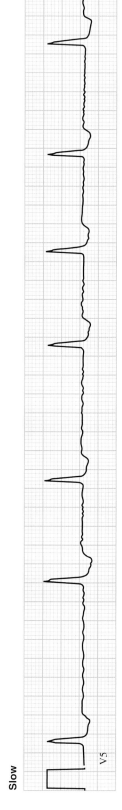

Figure 18-39. Ventricular response in atrial fibrillation. Rapid (top), seen here with an average heart rate of 140 bpm. Slow (bottom), seen here with an average heart rate of 46 bpm.

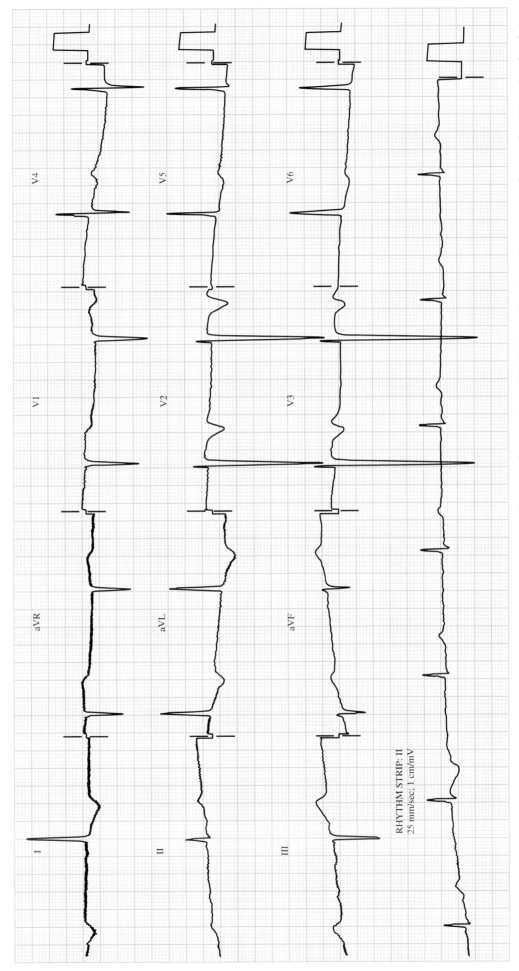

Figure 18-40. Atrial fibrillation with complete heart block and a junctional escape rhythm. The normally irregular atrial fibrillation is "regularized" as an escape focus in the AV junction depolarizes the ventricles at a rate of 42 bpm.

RHYTHM STRIP: II
25 mm/sec; 1 cm/mV

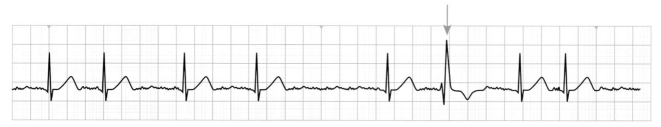

Figure 18-41. Ashman phenomenon. An aberrantly conducted complex (arrow) is seen after a long-short sequence.

Chapter 18 · SELF-TEST

QUESTIONS

1. An atrial premature complex that resets the sinus node will produce what type of post-ectopic pause?

2. What is the term for a complex emerging from a subsidiary pacemaker that appears after a pause in the native rhythm?

3. The inverted, retrograde P wave of a junctional complex can appear before, within, or after the QRS complex. True or false?

4. Define supraventricular tachycardia.

5. What form of supraventricular tachycardia is most commonly seen in clinical practice?

6. The majority of supraventricular tachycardia is due to what electrophysiologic mechanism?

7. Name the key three factors required for reentry.

8. What are two bedside maneuvers that can help uncover "hidden" P′ waves?

9. How can you differentiate sinus node reentrant tachycardia from sinus tachycardia?

10. Describe the classical criteria for atrial tachycardia.

11. Atrial tachycardia with block is commonly associated with what drug toxicity?

12. Define multifocal atrial tachycardia.

13. In typical slow-fast AV node reentrant tachycardia (AVNRT), which pathway is the antegrade limb and which is the retrograde limb?

14. In atypical AVNRT the fast pathway serves as the antegrade limb and the slow pathway serves as the retrograde limb. True or false?

15. Which pathway is the target of ablation of AV node reentrant tachycardia (AVNRT)?

16. Atrioventricular reentrant tachycardia (AVRT) that utilizes retrograde conduction via an accessory pathway will result in what type of complex (narrow or wide)?

17. A tachyarrhythmia with an atrial rate >240 bpm that has a sawtooth configuration in the inferior limb leads is characteristic of what rhythm disorder?

18. With typical atrial flutter and an atrial rate >240 bpm, what is the expected atrial-ventricular conduction ratio?

19. Define atrial fibrillation.

20. What is the preferred method for estimating the heart rate with atrial fibrillation?

ANSWERS

Chapter 18 • SELF-TEST

1. Noncompensatory.

2. Escape complex.

3. True.

4. SVT is defined as a series of ≥3 consecutive ectopic supraventricular complexes at a heart rate >100 bpm.

5. AV node reentrant tachycardia (AVNRT).

6. Reentry.

7. For reentry to occur an initiating stimulus must encounter:
   • The presence of at least two functionally or anatomically distinct pathways that are connected to form a circuit.
   • Unidirectional block in one of the pathways.
   • An area of slow conduction.

8. Carotid sinus massage and the Valsalva maneuver.

9. Sinus node reentrant tachycardia is paroxysmal and is typically initiated by and terminated with an atrial premature complex. Sinus tachycardia starts and stops gradually.

10. The classical criteria for atrial tachycardia are:
    • Series of ≥3 monomorphic atrial complexes.
    • Atrial rate 100 bpm (usually 150-240 bpm).
    • Regular, 1:1 AV conduction.
    • Normal P′R interval.
    • P′ waves separated by an isoelectric line.

11. Digoxin.

12. Criteria for multifocal atrial tachycardia are:
    • Rapid atrial rhythm with ≥3 consecutive P′ waves of different morphologies.
    • Atrial rate >100 bpm.
    • Absence of a single dominant atrial pacemaker.
    • Variable P′-P′ and R-R intervals.
    • P′ waves separated by an isoelectric line.

13. The slow pathway is the antegrade limb and the fast pathway is the retrograde limb.

14. True.

15. Slow pathway.

16. Narrow.

17. Typical atrial flutter.

18. 2:1.

19. P waves are absent in atrial fibrillation, replaced by small, irregular fibrillatory (f) waves of continuously varying morphology. The ventricular response is characterized as irregularly irregular.

20. 6-second method.

Further Reading

Bagliani G, DePonti R, Sciarra L, Zingarini G, Leonelli FM. Accessory pathway-mediated tachycardias. *Card Electrophysiol Clin*. 2020:12:475-493.

Bagliani G, Leonelli F, Padeletti L. P wave and the substrates of arrhythmias originating in the atria. *Card Electrophysiol Clin*. 2017;9:365-382.

Bhatia A, Sra J, Akhtar Masood. Preexcitation syndromes. *Curr Probl Cardiol*. 2016;41:99-137.

Brugada J, Katritsis DG, Arbelo E, et al. 2019 ESC guidelines for the management of patients with supraventricular tachycardia. *Eur Heart J*. 2020;41:655-720.

Butta C, Tuttolomondo A, Giarrusso L, Pinto A. Electrocardiographic diagnosis of atrial tachycardia: Classification, P-wave morphology, and differential diagnosis with other supraventricular tachycardias. *Ann Noninvasive Electrocardiol*. 2015;20:314-327.

Cossu AF, Steinberg JS. Supraventricular tachyarrhythmias involving the sinus node: clinical and electrophysiologic characteristics. *Prog Cardiovasc Dis*. 1998;41:51-63.

DiBiase, L, Gianni C, Bagliani G, Padeletti L. Arrhythmias involving the atrioventricular junction. *Card Electrophysiol Clin*. 2017;9:435-452.

Fisch C. Sinoatrial nodal reentrant tachycardia: a clinically important but rarely recognized entity. *ACC Curr J Rev*. 1995;4:61-63.

Fox DJ, Tischenko A, Krahn AD, et al. Supraventricular tachycardia: diagnosis and management. *Mayo Clin Proc*. 2008;83:1400-1411.

Garcia-Cosio, F, Fuentes AP, Angulo AN. Clinical approach to atrial tachycardia and atrial flutter from an understanding of the mechanisms, electrophysiology based on anatomy. *Rev Esp Cardiol*. 2012;65:363-375.

Kastor JA. Multifocal atrial tachycardia. *N Engl J Med*. 1990;322:1713-1717.

Kou WH, Morady F, Dick M, Nelson SD, Baerman JM. Concealed anterograde accessory pathway conduction during the induction of orthodromic reciprocating tachycardia. *J Am Coll Cardiol*. 1989;13:391-398.

Leonelli F, Bagliani G, Boriani G, Padeletti L. Arrhythmias originating in the atria. *Card Electrophysiol Clin*. 2017;9:383-409.

Link MS. Evaluation and initial treatment of supraventricular tachycardia. *N Engl J Med*. 2012;367:1438-1348.

Letsas KP, Weber R, Herrera-Siklody C, et al. Electrocardiographic differentiation of common type atrioventricular nodal reentrant tachycardia for atrioventricular reciprocating tachycardia via a concealed accessory pathway. *Acta Cardiol*. 2010;65:171-176.

Mahtani AU, Nair DG. Supraventricular tachycardia. *Med Clin N Am*. 2019;103:863-879.

Roberts-Thompson KC, Kistler PM, Kalman JM. Focal atrial tachycardia I: clinical features, diagnosis, mechanisms and anatomic location. *PACE*. 2006;29:643-652.

Saoudi N, Cosio F, Walso A, et al. A classification of atrial flutter and regular atrial tachycardia according to electrophysiological mechanisms and anatomical bases. *Eur Heart J*. 2001;22:1162-1182.

Shah RL, Badhwar N. Approach to narrow complex tachycardia: noninvasive guide to interpretation and management. *Heart*. 2020;106:772-783.

Wellens HJJ. 25 years of insights into the mechanisms of supraventricular arrhythmias. *PACE*. 2003;26:1916-1922.

Ventricular Arrhythmias

▶ VENTRICULAR PREMATURE COMPLEXES

A premature depolarization that originates in the ventricular myocardium or terminal Purkinje fibers is termed a *ventricular premature complex* (VPC). The impulse is initiated outside of the specialized conduction system, activating the nearby myocardium via slow, myocyte-to-myocyte transmission. The impulse then engages the His-Purkinje system to depolarize the remaining myocardium. We know that this type of transmission produces a wide QRS complex (≥0.12 seconds) with secondary T wave abnormalities that are directed opposite to that of the dominant R wave (**Figure 19-1**).

VPC Timing

VPCs occur early relative to the cycle length of the normal sinus rhythm. One of the defining characteristics of VPCs is that they arise independently of the sinus mechanism; therefore, they are electrically unrelated to any preceding P wave. The *coupling interval* refers to the time between the onset of the VPC and the QRS of the preceding complex. Ectopic complexes from one focus tend to have the same coupling interval, whereas those from multiple locations have different coupling intervals (**Figure 19-2**).

In most circumstances, the VPC does not conduct retrograde to depolarize and reset the SA node, so the sinus mechanism continues without interruption. You usually can't see the P wave because it is hidden in the ventricular complex, so we depict the missing P wave on our laddergram as a "virtual" or "hidden" depolarization. The VPC renders the ventricles (and likely the AV junction) refractory, so the sinus depolarization cannot generate a QRS complex. After the VPC, the next P wave and related QRS complex appear as expected. This *fully compensatory pause* between the VPC and the normal sinus complex is another of the characteristic features of ventricular ectopy (**Figure 19-3**). Remember that you can check for a fully compensatory pause by using your calipers to confirm that the R-R (or P-P) interval containing the VPC is exactly twice that of the normal cycle length. If so, the post-ectopic pause is fully compensatory.

On occasion, the ventricular depolarization can "reverse course" through the specialized conduction system to depolarize the atria. If so, a retrograde inverted P wave (P′) may be seen in leads II, III, and aVF. Alternatively, the P′ wave may be hidden within the ST segment or T wave of the VPC. If the retrograde impulse travels through the atria to depolarize the SA node, the normal sinus rhythm will be reset, resulting in a pause that is not fully compensatory (noncompensatory). Depending on the recovery time of the sinus node, the noncompensatory post-ectopic pause may be either shorter or longer than the native sinus cycle (**Figure 19-4**).

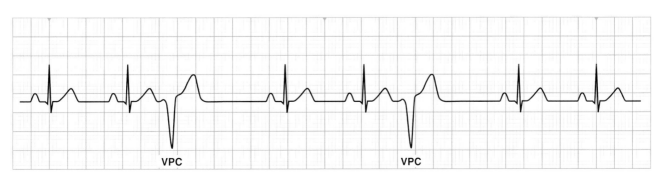

Figure 19-1. Ventricular premature complexes.

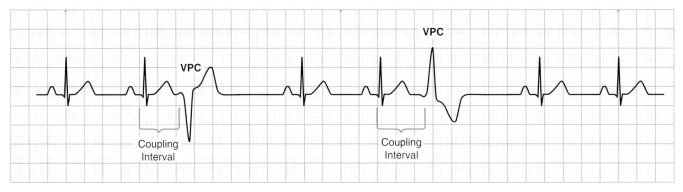

Figure 19-2. Ventricular premature complexes with two different morphologies and coupling intervals.

An *interpolated* VPC is one that appears interposed between two normal sinus impulses (**Figure 19-5**). A typical finding of an interpolated VPC is prolongation of the PR interval of the following sinus complex due to *concealed retrograde conduction* of the ventricular depolarization into the AV junction. This causes partial refractoriness and a delay in antegrade conduction of the next sinus impulse. The retrograde conduction is considered "concealed" because it is not visible on the surface ECG, revealed only by its effect on the following complex. Interpolated VPCs are more common when the native sinus rhythm is relatively slow.

Late (end) diastolic VPC Sometimes the VPC has a coupling interval late in the cardiac cycle such that it fortuitously occurs just after the P wave. This is called a *late or end diastolic* VPC (**Figure 19-6**). Importantly, even though you see a P wave, it is **electrically unrelated** to the following QRS complex. A *fusion complex* may be seen if there is just enough time for the sinus impulse to travel through the specialized conduction system to merge with the VPC. This complex is wider than the normal QRS, but narrower than that of the VPC, reflecting the blending of the two waves of depolarization, one supraventricular and the other ventricular.

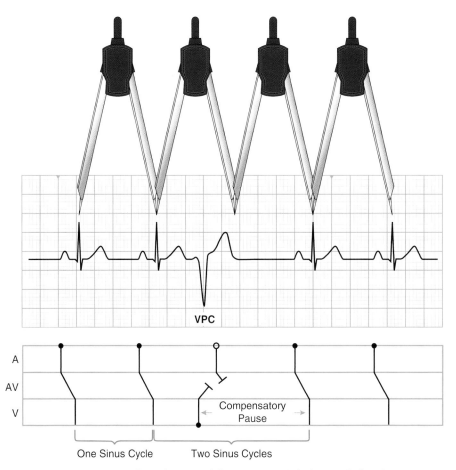

Figure 19-3. A fully compensatory pause is one where the sum of the R-R intervals before and after the premature complex equals twice that of the native sinus cycle.

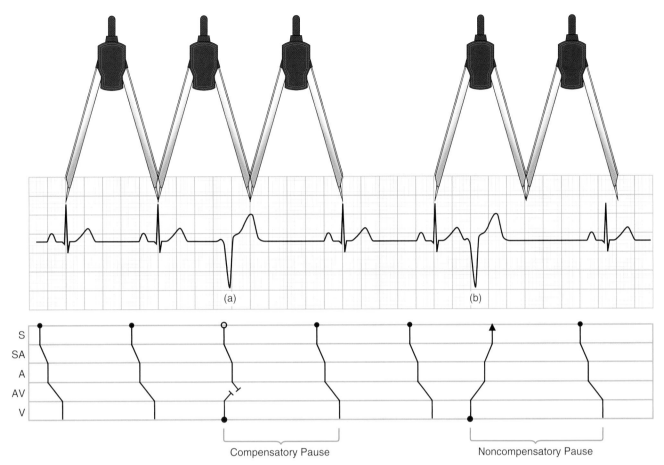

Figure 19-4. The VPC on the left (a) does not disturb the sinus cycle and the post-ectopic pause is fully compensatory. The VPC on the right (b) demonstrates retrograde activation through the atria. The SA node resets early, resulting in a noncompensatory pause. Depending on the time it takes for SA nodal recovery, the post-ectopic pause may be either shorter or longer than the native sinus cycle.

R on T phenomenon A VPC with a short coupling interval may fall on or near the T wave of the preceding complex (**Figure 19**-7). This is during the repolarization phase of the action potential, which historically has been considered a *vulnerable period* that could precipitate ventricular tachycardia. Clinical experience suggests this risk is small.

Repetitive VPCs, or occurring in a pattern VPCs may occur alone (*isolated*), grouped repetitively, or present in a pattern related to the native sinus complex (**Figure 19-8**). Two VPCs in a row are termed a ventricular *couplet* or *pair*. The morphology of the two complexes may either be uniform or multiform. A group of three rapid VPCs in a row defines *ventricular*

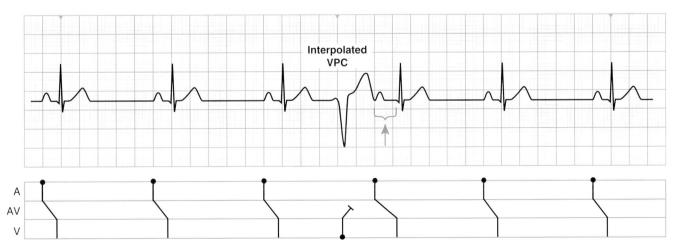

Figure 19-5. Interpolated VPC. The PR interval of the first sinus complex after the VPC is prolonged (arrow) due to concealed retrograde conduction into the AV junction, which renders the region partially refractory.

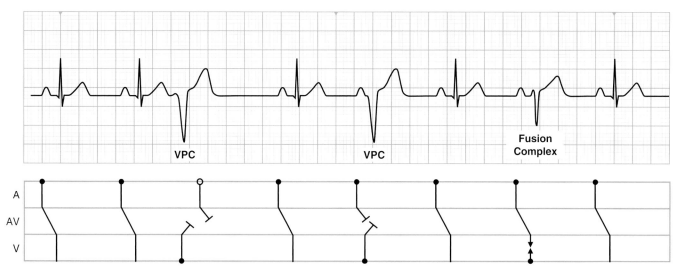

Figure 19-6. Late (end) diastolic VPC and fusion complex. The middle VPC occurs late in diastole, electrically unrelated to, but appearing just after inscription of the P wave. The VPC on the right occurs slightly later, producing a fusion complex that represents merging of the ventricular and normal sinus depolarizations.

tachycardia. Ventricular *bigeminy* describes VPCs that alternate with each sinus complex. Ventricular *trigeminy* is used if the VPC appears every third complex.

Parasystole Ventricular parasystole is a unique form of ventricular ectopy (**Figure 19-9**). In classic parasystole, an automatic ventricular focus fires completely independent of the sinus mechanism. A zone of unidirectional *entrance block* "protects" the abnormal site from outside depolarization while allowing the impulse to exit and capture the ventricles when they are not refractory. Think of the parasystolic focus as akin to an electronic fixed-rate pacemaker, unable to sense the native rhythm and firing at set intervals. The clues to ventricular parasystole are premature complexes that vary in relationship to the sinus mechanism (variable coupling intervals), longer interectopic intervals that are multiples of the shortest interectopic interval, and the presence of interpolated and fusion complexes.

Morphology and Origin

VPCs with the same QRS morphology are termed *uniform*, and typically arise from one ventricular site (unifocal). Those with

different morphologies are termed *multiform*, typically arising from multiple sites (multifocal).

The morphology of the VPC provides clues as to its origin. An ectopic complex originating in the left ventricle has features of a RBBB and those arising from the right ventricle or interventricular septum resemble a LBBB (**Figure 19-10**). Why should that be? The reason is that in both left ventricular ectopy and RBBB, the left ventricle is activated first, followed by the right ventricle. Similarly, in both right ventricular ectopy and LBBB, the right ventricle is activated first, followed by the left ventricle. Most septal-based ventricular arrhythmias preferentially exit toward the right ventricle, depolarizing the LV free wall afterwards, so again the pattern resembles a LBBB. One way to remember the similarity is that in both bundle branch block and ventricular ectopy, the average QRS forces are directed toward the last ventricular chamber activated.

We can further localize the origin of ventricular ectopic complexes using our knowledge of vectors. Why do we care about localizing a VPC? Isn't it enough to identify the complex correctly and move on? For routine ECG interpretation this is generally true. But the origin of a VPC has clinical implications, so a more detailed analysis has value (and makes you a master

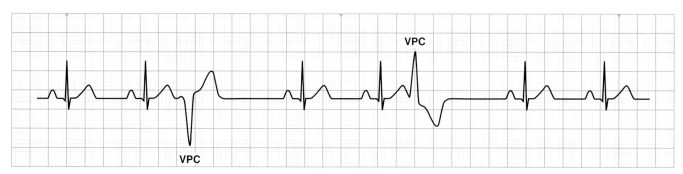

Figure 19-7. R on T phenomenon. The VPC on the right has a short coupling interval such that the R wave of the premature complex falls on the downslope of the T wave of the preceding sinus complex.

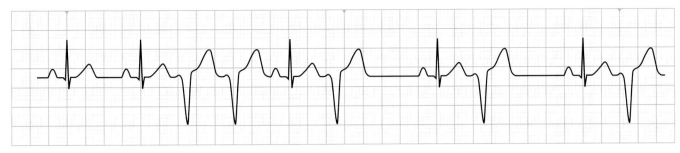

Figure 19-8. The first two repetitive VPCs are paired (couplet), followed by those that alternate with normal complexes in a pattern of bigeminy.

electrocardiographer). The concepts used to localize an isolated ventricular complex also apply to the analysis of ventricular tachycardia that we will discuss shortly. So with that introduction, let's take a deep dive into pinpointing the origin of a VPC.

Electrophysiologic Anatomy

Our first step is to review the relevant cardiac anatomy, something that is vital to localizing the ectopic ventricular focus. This can be a source of confusion due to considerable inconsistencies in the nomenclature, use of a "valentine" depiction, and a lack of standardization. The best anatomical approach is based on the *in situ* position of the heart in the chest, using what is called an *attitudinally correct* orientation (**Figure 19-11**). Using the proper convention you can understand two basic "rules" of normal cardiac anatomy (1) the left-sided chambers (eg, left atrium and left ventricle) lie **posterior** to their right-sided counterparts; and (2) the atrial chambers are positioned predominantly **rightward** of their corresponding ventricles.

The internal cavities of both the right and left ventricles can be divided broadly into three components (**Figure 19-12**). These are (1) an inlet (inflow tract), (2) a muscular, apical trabecular portion, and (3) an outlet (outflow tract). Although

functionally different, there are no discrete borders between the adjacent portions. The inlet portion of each ventricle surrounds and supports its respective AV valve, the tricuspid valve for the right ventricle and mitral valve for the left ventricle. The muscular apical component comprises the familiar "pumping" portion of the ventricles. The outlet portion of each ventricle leads to its corresponding semilunar valve, the pulmonary valve for the right ventricle and the aortic valve for the left ventricle. Note the unique geometry of the outflow tracts, both of which lie superior to their respective ventricles. The right ventricular outflow tract (RVOT) begins anterior and rightward of the left ventricular outflow tract (LVOT). During the twisting process of embryogenesis, the RVOT wraps around the LVOT and aortic root such that the pulmonary valve ends up leftward, anterior, and superior to the aortic valve (see Figure 19-11).

> **FOR BOOKWORMS:** The right and left ventricular outflow tracts are complex structures with various valvular components that are oriented relatively anterior, posterior, left, and right to each other. Crescents of ventricular myocardial cells extend into these elements, providing a substrate for arrhythmias.

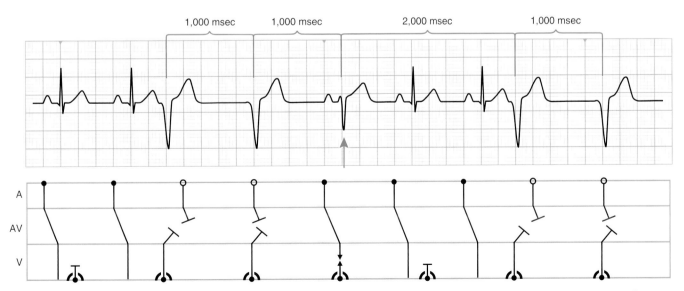

Figure 19-9. Ventricular parasystole. A parasystolic focus, protected by entrance block, depolarizes the ventricles when not refractory. The longest interectopic interval (2000 msec) is a multiple of the shortest interectopic interval (1000 msec). The fusion complex (arrow) results from the merging of the sinus and ventricular impulses.

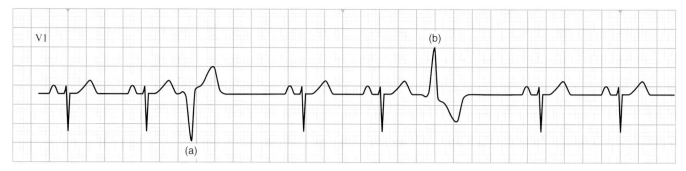

Figure 19-10. Inspect lead V1 to determine if a wide complex has the morphology resembling either a LBBB with an R/S ratio <1 (a) or a RBBB with a R/S ratio >1 (b).

There are other terms used to describe regions of the left and right ventricles that serve as foci for arrhythmias. The **apex** is the tip of each cone-like ventricular chamber. The **base** of the heart is roughly defined by a plane that separates the atria from the ventricles (**Figure 19-13**). It includes the AV rings, portions of the atria, and the ventricular outlets. The **interventricular septum** divides the right and left ventricles. The **free wall** of each ventricle is that portion of the ventricular myocardium which is not in contact with either the interventricular septum or apex.

The left ventricle is divided further into regional segments. We first encountered this topic when we learned about myocardial infarction. Recall that for the interpretation of myocardial infarction, we elected to continue using a number of older, commonly used terms that are not easily abandoned (eg, posterior MI). For the modern field of electrophysiology, we can use contemporary definitions of the left ventricular segments that help us to more accurately describe the direction of the vectors derived from these

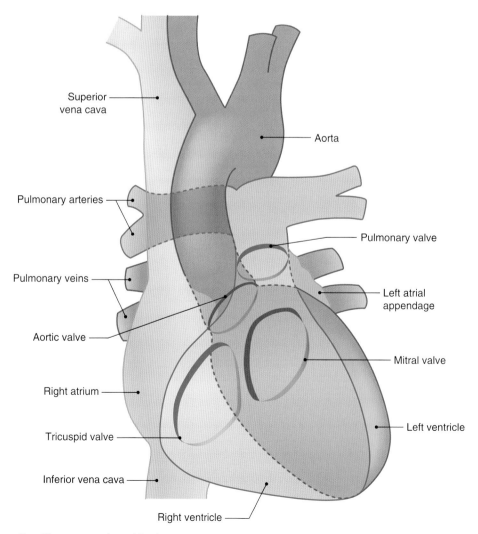

Figure 19-11. The cardiac silhouette as viewed *in-situ*.

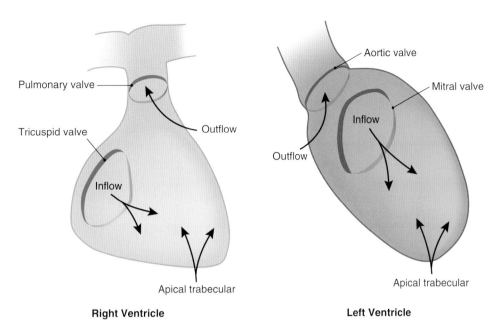

Right Ventricle   **Left Ventricle**

Figure 19-12. The right and left ventricles can be broadly separated into an inlet (inflow), an apical trabecular portion, and an outlet (outflow).

regions. Using this updated classification, the left ventricle is divided in the short axis into four walls: **septal**, **anterior**, **inferior**, and **lateral**, each with further subdivisions in the long axis according to whether the segment is **apical**, **midcavity**, or **basal** for a total of 17 segments (**Figure 19-14**).

Again note the elimination of the term "posterior," which is included within the lateral region.

 BE CAREFUL: Even the "modern" electrophysiologic nomenclature has been found somewhat wanting and imprecise when describing myocardial anatomy. One key reason is that segments that are referred to as *anterior* are actually anatomically *superior*. Look again at the bull's-eye plot of Figure 19-14 and you can understand that the opposite of inferior is really superior. By mentally translating anterior into superior, you may better understand some of the patterns you find on the ECG.

FOR BOOKWORMS: Most ventricular ectopy derives from the ventricular endocardium. Rarely, an epicardial region is the source. Two such areas are the *crux* and left ventricular *summit*. The crux is an area formed by the junction of the AV groove and posterior interventricular groove, which form a cross at the base of the heart at the point where the four cardiac chambers intersect. The summit is a triangular region on the superior surface of the heart demarcated by the left anterior descending and the left circumflex coronary arteries.

Putting Things Together

OK, now that we understand the anatomy, let's get to work to determine the origin of the ectopic ventricular impulse. It's important to realize that the concepts we will now review are most reliable in the absence of structural heart disease. In an otherwise normal heart, the focus of these *idiopathic ventricular arrhythmias* is localized and the associated vectors predictable.

Figure 19-13. The planes of the cardiac apex and base.

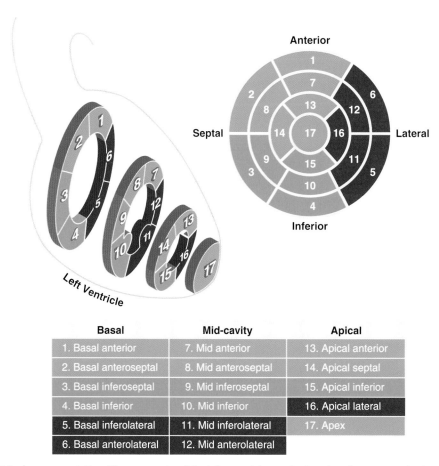

Figure 19-14. Left ventricular segmentation. The segments of the left ventricle are depicted as they appear *in situ* and as a polar "bulls eye" plot (see text for details). The table lists the segments using revised nomenclature.

The situation is very different in the presence of *structural heart disease* as myocardial scar interferes with transmission of the impulse, altering the propagation and direction of the vectors.

Regardless of the underlying substrate, we can apply some useful principles to locate a ventricular focus. These include analysis of (1) bundle branch block pattern, (2) QRS width, (3) frontal plane QRS axis, and (4) precordial lead pattern.

Bundle branch block pattern   If the VPC in **lead V1** is predominantly positive with a "dominant R wave" (R/S ratio >1), then it has RBBB-type morphology and originates from the left ventricle (**Figure 19-15**). If a complex in lead V1 is predominantly negative having a "dominant S wave" (R/S ratio <1) with a negative terminal component, then it has LBBB-type morphology. If so, it arises from either the right ventricle or the interventricular septum.

QRS width   An impulse that originates deep within the myocardium of the left ventricular free wall will produce a wider QRS complex with a more bizarre morphology. In contrast, a VPC located in the interventricular septum will be comparatively narrow, due to its proximity to the specialized conduction system. A note of caution is that complex width is affected by factors other than location, such as the presence of underlying myocardial disease or treatment with antiarrhythmic agents, both of which may widen the QRS.

Frontal plane axis   Leads II, III, and aVF are used to determine a superior versus inferior location (**Figure 19-16**). From a superior location, the depolarization vector will proceed inferiorly so we will see dominant R waves in those leads. Conversely, if the VPC arises from an inferior site, leads II, III, and aVF will have dominant S waves, resulting from a vector directed away from those leads.

Precordial lead pattern   The precordial leads are useful to distinguish an apical versus basal site within the LV (**Figure 19-17**). Impulses originating at the apex are directed posteriorly, generating predominantly negative QRS complexes. Conversely, a basal ventricular focus generates anterior forces, yielding mainly upright precordial QRS complexes.

Precordial lead **concordance** describes a pattern when **all** the chest leads (V1-V6) have a similar, **monophasic** morphology. *Positive concordance* is present if all precordial leads exhibit monophasic R waves. This pattern indicates a basal focus within the LV. *Negative concordance* is present when all precordial leads exhibit monophasic QS waves. This pattern is more rare and indicates a focus located either in the apical septum of the LV or the RV free wall.

Clinical Correlation

The most common site of idiopathic ventricular arrhythmias in patients without structural heart disease is the right ventricle,

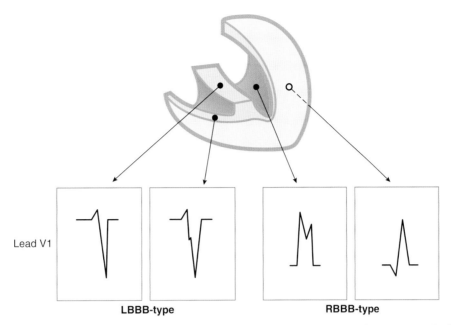

Figure 19-15. LBBB- and RBBB-type morphology in lead V1. The LBBB-type complexes typically reflect a ventricular focus in either the right ventricle or interventricular septum. The slightly narrower complex in the first left box reflects its proximity to the specialized conduction system. The RBBB-type complexes typically indicate a left ventricular focus. Note the qR complex in the box on the far right, suggesting it originates within an infarction related scar.

specifically the RVOT. This is a superiorly located right heart structure; therefore VPCs originating from this location exhibit a LBBB pattern with inferior axis. Less frequently, idiopathic VPCs may arise from the LVOT. Depending on the specific location within the LVOT, either a RBBB or LBBB pattern may be present. But in all cases, outflow tract arrhythmias will have an inferior orientation.

Patients with structural heart disease characteristically have VPCs of left ventricular origin. Post myocardial infarction, the VPC morphology is that of a RBBB if originating from the LV free wall and a LBBB pattern if emerging from a septal location. The frontal plane axis of the complex will vary, depending on the location of the infarction. In general, VPCs derived from an inferior infarction will have a superior

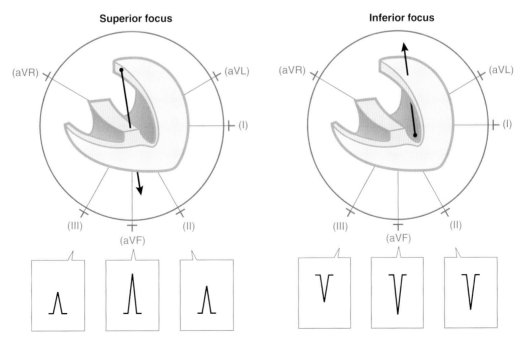

Figure 19-16. Superior versus inferior origin. Ventricular ectopy originating in a superiorly located region (left) have complexes with an inferior mean axis, producing dominant R waves in leads II, III, and aVF. Ectopy derived from an inferior focus (right) will be directed superiorly, with dominant S waves in those leads.

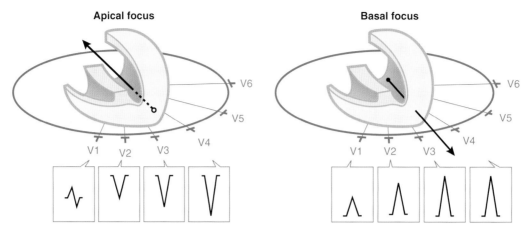

Figure 19-17. Apical versus basal origin. VPCs originating from the LV apex (left) will generally have posteriorly directed forces. Note that lead V1 is an exception in this example due to the RBBB-type morphology. A VPC originating from the base (right) will have forces that direct anteriorly.

axis. VPCs associated with anterior infarctions may demonstrate either a superior or inferior axis, the variability due to the potentially large area of scar, which impacts the exit site of the impulse.

VPCs associated with myocardial infarction may show a qR pattern in contiguous leads, which reflect the area of scar.

Criteria for Ventricular Premature Complex (VPC)
- The complex occurs early relative to the native rhythm and is not preceded by an electrically related P wave.
- QRS duration ≥0.12 seconds.
- Secondary ST segment and T wave abnormalities directed opposite to that of the dominant R wave.
- Supporting criteria:
  - A fully compensatory pause is present.

Ventricular Tachycardia

Ventricular tachycardia (VT) is defined as a series of ≥3 consecutive ventricular complexes at a rate of >100 bpm. VT is not one entity and may be further classified by *duration*, *morphology*, and *mechanism*. Hemodynamic stability and clinical symptoms that occur during VT largely depend on the rate and duration of the arrhythmia, factors that ultimately determine whether cardiac output is preserved.

Duration *Nonsustained* VT terminates spontaneously within 30 seconds (**Figure 19-18**). *Sustained* VT is defined as lasting ≥30 seconds or requiring an intervention such as electrical cardioversion (**Figure 19-19**).

Morphology *Monomorphic* VT has a single QRS morphology from complex to complex, indicating repetitive depolarization from a single focus (or reentry circuit) with the same sequence of activation. *Multiple monomorphic* VT is the term used when multiple separate runs of monomorphic VT are present, each with a unique morphology (**Figure 19-20**). *Polymorphic* VT has a continuously changing QRS configuration, indicating no single site of origin and a changing sequence of activation (**Figure 19-21**). *Torsades de pointes* (twisting of the points) is a unique form of polymorphic VT associated with a long QT interval, characterized by QRS peaks that "twist" around the baseline (**Figure 19-22**). The association with prolongation of the QT interval, whether inherited or acquired (ie, induced by medication or electrolyte abnormalities), distinguishes this arrhythmia from other forms of polymorphic VT. *Pleomorphic* VT has more than one distinct QRS complex within the same episode of VT, but the QRS complex is not changing continuously (**Figure 19-23**). *Bidirectional* VT is characterized by a RBBB pattern accompanied by beat-to-beat alternans in the frontal plane QRS axis (**Figure 19-24**). Typically associated with digitalis toxicity, the mechanism is thought to represent alternating conduction between the two fascicles of the left bundle branch. *Ventricular flutter* describes a very rapid VT (250-350 bpm) with a sine wave appearance that precludes identification of specific QRS morphology (**Figure 19-25**).

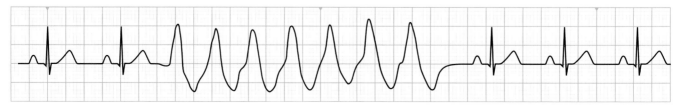

Figure 19-18. Nonsustained monomorphic ventricular tachycardia is defined as a series of ≥3 ventricular complexes at a rate >100 bpm, all with the same QRS morphology, but lasting <30 seconds.

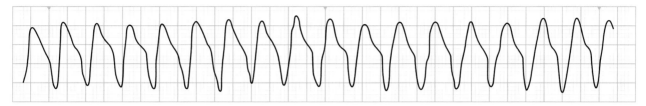

Figure 19-19. Sustained monomorphic ventricular tachycardia. The arrhythmia continues for 30 seconds or more (not shown) with all complexes having the same QRS morphology.

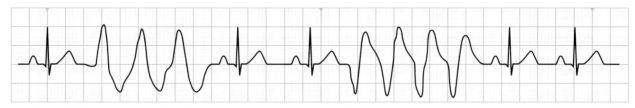

Figure 19-20. Multiple monomorphic ventricular tachycardia. Two separate runs of nonsustained ventricular tachycardia are present, each with a unique morphology.

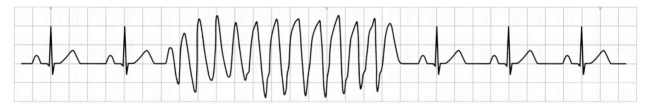

Figure 19-21. Polymorphic ventricular tachycardia has complexes that are changing continuously.

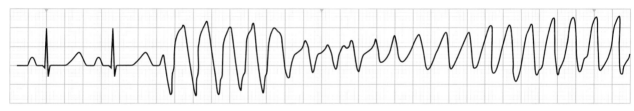

Figure 19-22. Torsades de pointes is a form of polymorphic ventricular tachycardia where the polarity of the complexes appear to spiral. Note the prolonged QT interval of the native complexes.

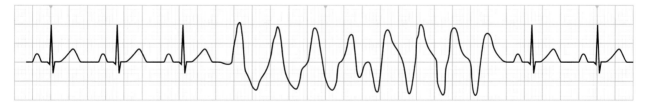

Figure 19-23. Pleomorphic ventricular tachycardia has more than one monomorphic QRS morphology within the same run. Unlike polymorphic VT, the complexes do not change continuously.

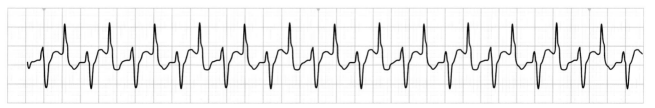

Figure 19-24. Bidirectional tachycardia. The change in morphology and axis is believed due to the focus alternating between the anterior and posterior fascicles of the left bundle branch.

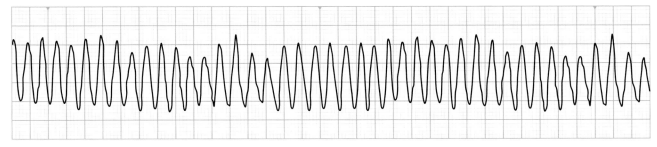

Figure 19-25. Ventricular flutter. This is an extremely rapid form of ventricular tachycardia with no discernible baseline, producing a "sine wave" type appearance.

Mechanism *Focal VT* activates the ventricle from a discrete source, typically due to triggered activity or abnormal automaticity. This is the predominant mechanism of idiopathic VT in patients without structural heart disease. Triggered activity, specifically early afterdepolarizations, is believed responsible for initiating *Torsades de pointes*. VT linked to late afterdepolarizations is associated with conditions that increase intracellular calcium, such as catecholamine excess, hypercalcemia, and digitalis toxicity. *Reentry* is the primary mechanism responsible for monomorphic VT in patients with structural heart disease. This includes patients with coronary artery disease, dilated cardiomyopathy, and other conditions such as arrhythmogenic right ventricular cardiomyopathy, infiltrative and hypertrophic cardiomyopathy. Scars related to myocardial infarction or localized fibrosis from cardiomyopathy cause tissue heterogeneity that set the stage for the reentry circuits we learned about in Chapter 13.

Site of origin With monomorphic VT, all the complexes arise from the same ectopic site, exhibiting the same morphology and axis as the VPC that initiated the arrhythmia. This allows us to apply the concepts we learned in preceding discussion for isolated VPCs to localize the origin of the tachyarrhythmia. Analyzing the ECG morphology and axis provides a roadmap for electrophysiologic mapping and ablation procedures. Akin to the situation with isolated VPCs, ECG localization of VT is most reliable in the absence of structural heart disease, where the arrhythmia arises from a discrete ectopic focus. ECG localization is more challenging in scar-related VT because the vectors reflects the exit site of the impulse as it meanders its way through fibrotic tissue to eventually depolarize normal myocardium.

 FOR BOOKWORMS: Two unusual forms of VT involve reentry that incorporate portions of the His-Purkinje system. *Bundle branch block VT* involves the right and left bundle branches as obligatory limbs of the reentry circuit. Characteristically associated with dilated cardiomyopathy, the morphology of bundle branch block VT is that of a typical LBBB and usually closely resembles the baseline QRS complex. Although uncommon, this form of VT is readily treated by ablation of the right bundle branch.

Verapamil-sensitive, fascicular VT is typically seen in younger patients with structurally normal hearts. Most commonly involving the left posterior fascicle, the mechanism is thought to represent local microreentry. The typical ECG pattern is that of a RBBB with LAFB, reflecting an origin within the left posterior fascicle. And as the name implies, this form of VT responds to verapamil.

Criteria for Ventricular Tachycardia
- A series of ≥3 consecutive ventricular complexes at a rate of >100 bpm.
  - May be defined further according to duration and morphology (see text for details).

Accelerated Idioventricular Rhythm

At times, a sequence of ventricular complexes emerges at a relatively slow rate (45-100 bpm), which is termed *accelerated idioventricular rhythm* (**Figure 19-26**). Unlike ventricular tachycardia, the mechanism of AIVR is thought to result from abnormal automaticity. The ventricular rhythm is considered "accelerated" by virtue of being more rapid than the normal ventricular escape rate (see following discussion). This rhythm is characteristically seen as a "reperfusion arrhythmia"

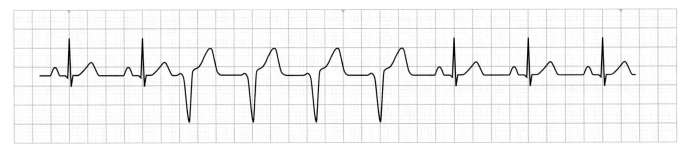

Figure 19-26. Accelerated idioventricular rhythm.

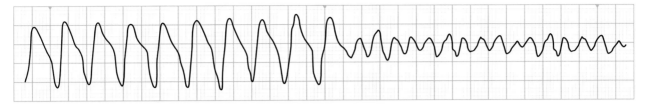

Figure 19-27. Monomorphic ventricular tachycardia degenerating into ventricular fibrillation.

in the setting of acute myocardial infarction. It is usually self-limited and well-tolerated clinically. Different from ventricular tachycardia, AIVR is unlikely to degenerate into ventricular fibrillation.

Criteria for Accelerated Idioventricular Rhythm
- A series of ≥3 consecutive ventricular complexes at a rate ≤100 bpm.

Ventricular Fibrillation

Ventricular fibrillation is a very rapid (>350 bpm), grossly irregular ventricular rhythm with a chaotic, disorganized QRS morphology (**Figure 19-27**). This requires immediate defibrillation, as circulation cannot be maintained in the presence of this lethal arrhythmia.

Ventricular Escape Complexes

Escape complexes are those that emerge from a subsidiary pacemaker following a pause in the native rhythm that is *longer* than the normal cycle length (**Figure 19-28**). Ventricular escape complexes originate below the bundle of His, typically in the Purkinje fibers that intertwine with the cells of the ventricular myocardium. Less frequently, ventricular escape complexes derive from the bundle branches. The actual ventricular myocytes do not normally possess the property of automaticity to generate escape complexes. Like ventricular premature complexes, the morphology of the escape complex is wide (≥0.12 seconds) with secondary ST segment and T wave abnormalities. A pattern of two or more consecutive escape complexes is called a *ventricular escape rhythm*. The escape interval is slow, as the natural automatic rate of the His-Purkinje system is 20 to 40 bpm (**Figure 19-29**).

Criteria for Ventricular Escape Complex
- The complex appears late relative to the cycle of the normal rhythm, emerging due to a failure of a normally faster physiologic pacemaker.
- The complex is wide (≥0.12 seconds) with secondary ST segment and T wave abnormalities.
- There is no electrical relationship to a P wave.
- Two or more consecutive escape complexes define a ventricular escape rhythm.

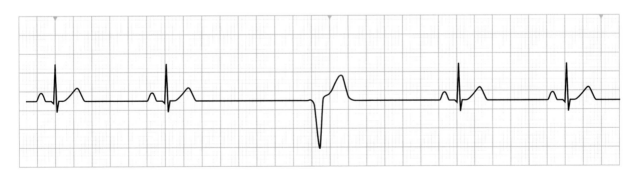

Figure 19-28. A sinus pause followed by a ventricular escape complex.

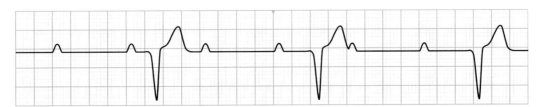

Figure 19-29. Sinus bradycardia with complete AV block and a ventricular escape rhythm.

Chapter 19 • SELF-TEST

1. List the criteria of a ventricular premature complex.

2. Explain the compensatory pause.

3. Under what circumstance will the pause after the VPC be noncompensatory?

4. What is an interpolated VPC?

5. What is a late or end diastolic VPC?

6. A VPC that has a RBBB-type morphology in lead V1 typically originates from what portion of the heart?

7. A VPC that has a LBBB-type morphology in lead V1 typically originates from what portion of the heart?

8. Define the cardiac apex, base, interventricular septum, and free wall.

9. Define idiopathic ventricular arrhythmias.

10. Ventricular arrhythmias that arise from the outflow tracts will have what axis in the frontal plane and why?

11. Define ventricular tachycardia.

12. Torsades de pointes is a form of polymorphic ventricular tachycardia associated with what abnormality of the baseline ECG?

Chapter 19 • SELF TEST

1. • The complex occurs early relative to the native rhythm and is not preceded by an electrically related P wave.
   • QRS duration ≥0.12 seconds.
   • Secondary ST segment and T wave abnormalities directed opposite to that of the dominant R wave.

2. A compensatory pause results because the VPC fails to disturb the normal depolarization of the sinus node. The natural sinus impulse continues and the complex following the VPC arrives "on time."

3. The post-VPC pause will be noncompensatory if there is retrograde depolarization and resetting of the sinus node.

4. An interpolated VPC is one that is interposed between two normal sinus impulses.

5. A late or end diastolic VPC is one that appears late in the cardiac cycle, just after an electrically unrelated P wave.

6. The left ventricle.

7. The right ventricle or the interventricular septum.

8. • The apex is the tip of each cone-like ventricular chamber.
   • The base is defined by a plane that separates the atria from the ventricles.
   • The interventricular septum divides the right and left ventricles.
   • The free wall of each ventricle is that portion of the ventricular myocardium not in contact with the septum or apex.

9. Ventricular arrhythmias that occur in the absence of structural heart disease (eg, an otherwise normal heart).

10. Inferior axis (dominant R waves in leads II, III, and aVF). The reason is the superior location of the ventricular outflow tracts that direct the mean vector inferiorly.

11. A series of ≥3 consecutive ventricular complexes at a rate >100 bpm.

12. Prolongation of the QT interval.

Further Reading

Benito B, Josephson ME. Ventricular tachycardia in coronary artery disease. *Rev Esp Cardiol.* 2012;65:939-955.

Cabrera JA, Sanchez-Quintana D. Cardiac anatomy: what the electrophysiologist needs to know. *Heart.* 2013;99:417-431.

Enriquez A, Baranchuk A, Bricen D, Saenz L, Garcia F. How to use the 12-lead ECG to predict the site of origin of idiopathic ventricular arrhythmias. *Heart Rhythm.* 2019;18:1538-1544.

Gulamhusein S, Yee R, Ko PT, Klein GJ. Electrocardiographic criteria for differentiating aberrancy and ventricular extrasystole in chronic atrial fibrillation: validation by intracardiac recordings. *J Electrocardiography.* 1985;18:41-50.

Hadid C. Sustained ventricular tachycardia in structural heart disease. *Cardiol J.* 2015;22:12-24.

Hai JJ, Lachman N, Syed FF, Desimone CV, Asirvatham SJ. The anatomic basis for ventricular arrhythmia in the normal heart: what the student of anatomy needs to know. *Clin Anat.* 2014;27:885-893.

Haqqani HM, Marchlinski FE. The surface electrocardiograph in ventricular arrhythmias: lessons in localization. *Heart, Lung and Circulation.* 2019;28:39-48.

Haqqani HM, Morton JB, Kalman JM. Using the 12-lead ECG to localize the origin of atrial and ventricular tachycardias: part 2- ventricular tachycardia. *J Cardiovasc Electrophysiol.* 2009;20:825-832.

Hutchinson MD, Garcia FC. An organized approach to the localization, mapping and ablation of outflow tract ventricular arrhythmias. *J Cardiovasc Electrophysiol.* 2013;24:1189-1197.

Josephson ME, Callans DJ. Using the twelve-lead electrocardiogram to localize the site of origin of ventricular tachycardia. *Heart Rhythm.* 2005;2:443-446.

Josephson ME, Horowitz LN, Waxman HL, et al. Sustained ventricular tachycardia: role of the 12-lead electrocardiogram in localizing the site of origin. *Circulation.* 1981;64:257-272.

Kindwall KE, Brown J, Josephson ME. Electrocardiographic criteria for ventricular tachycardia in wide complex left bundle branch morphology tachycardias. *Am J Cardiol.* 1988;61:1279-1283.

Marriott HJL. Differential diagnosis of supraventricular and ventricular tachycardia. *Cardiology.* 1990;77:209-220.

Marriott HJL, Sandler IA. Criteria, old and new, for differentiating between ectopic ventricular beats and aberrant ventricular conduction in the presence of atrial fibrillation. *Prog Cardiovasc Dis.* 1966;9:18-28.

Miller JM, Marchlinski FE, Buxton AE, Josephson ME. Relationship between the 12-lead electrocardiogram during ventricular tachycardia and endocardial site of origin in patients with coronary artery disease. *Circulation.* 1988;77:759-766.

Mond HG, Haqqani HM. The electrocardiographic footprints of ventricular ectopy. *Heart, Lung and Circulation.* 2020;29:988-999.

Park KM, Kim YH, Marchlinski F. Using the surface electrocardiogram to localize the origin of idiopathic ventricular tachycardia. *PACE.* 2012;35:1516-1527.

Pick A, Langedorf R. Parasystole and its variants. *Med Clin North Am.* 1976;60:125-146.

Rosenbaum MB. Classification of ventricular extrasystoles according to form. *J Electrocardiol.* 1969;2:289-297.

Sandler IA, Marriott HJL. The differential morphology of anomalous ventricular complexes of RBBB-type in lead V1. *Circulation* 1963;31:551-556.

Wellens HJJ, Bar FWH, Lie KI. The value of the electrocardiogram in the differential diagnosis of a tachycardia with a widened QRS complex. *Am J Med.* 1978;63:27-33.

Xiong Y, Zhu H. Electrocardiographic characteristics of idiopathic ventricular arrhythmias based on anatomy. *Ann Noninvasive Electrocardiol.* 2020;25:e12782.

Yamada T. Idiopathic ventricular arrhythmias: relevance to the anatomy, diagnosis and treatment. *J Cardiol.* 2016;68:463-471.

20

Wide Complex Tachycardia

▶ INTRODUCTION

Wide complex tachycardia (WCT) is defined as a rhythm with a QRS duration ≥0.12 seconds and a rate >100 bpm. The term is deliberately imprecise, using a general description rather than specific identification of a ventricular or supraventricular origin. WCT poses a unique challenge in electrocardiography, and determining the exact diagnosis often proves difficult and is sometimes impossible. Up until now, we have interpreted the ECG using well-defined criteria. WCT requires a different approach. Here we use ECG clues that help you *predict*, but not *guarantee* the likely diagnosis.

▶ DIFFERENTIAL DIAGNOSIS OF WIDE COMPLEX TACHYCARDIA

A narrow QRS complex requires that both ventricles depolarize in synchrony, concurrently receiving their impulses via the right and left bundle branches. Conduction proceeds uninterrupted through the Purkinje fibers until reaching the ventricular myocardium. Any process that disrupts this continuous passage through the His-Purkinje system will cause **asynchronous activation of the ventricles**, which is the fundamental principle that results in a wide QRS complex. A WCT is a rapid cardiac rhythm that *also* exhibits an alteration of ventricular activation. The causes of WCT include:

- Ventricular tachycardia (VT).
- Supraventricular tachycardia (SVT) with:
  - Aberrant ventricular conduction.
    - Fixed (preexisting anatomical bundle branch block).
    - Functional (physiologic refractoriness during tachycardia).
  - Preexcitation (conduction over an accessory pathway).
  - Other causes of wide QRS (not due to bundle branch block or preexcitation):
    - Ventricular enlargement.
    - Congenital heart disease (eg, Ebstein anomaly).
    - Electrolyte abnormalities (eg, hyperkalemia).
    - Drug effect (eg, flecainide, tricyclic antidepressants).
- Ventricular pacing:
  - Pacemaker-tracked supraventricular arrhythmia.
  - Pacemaker-mediated tachycardia.

In most series, 75 to 80% of WCT is due to ventricular tachycardia. SVT with aberrant conduction (either functional or due to preexisting BBB) is the cause in 15 to 25% of cases. Supraventricular arrhythmias associated with preexcitation and pacemaker-associated rhythms are rare, comprising only 1 to 5% of cases. This means our main task is to differentiate ventricular tachycardia from supraventricular tachycardia with aberrancy, something that greatly impacts clinical decision-making.

▶ THE VT VERSUS ABERRANT SVT TOOLBOX

Electrocardiographers have long sought to find the "Holy Grail" of criteria to distinguish VT from SVT with aberrancy. Although that goal remains elusive, algorithms have been developed in an attempt to predict the likely diagnosis. Before we review the specifics of these approaches, we first need to understand why certain elements are included in the analysis and how to properly perform the measurements. The items in our WCT "toolbox" include examination of the following:

- The atrial-ventricular relationship (AV dissociation).
- Precordial lead QRS morphology (V1-V2 and V6).
- Precordial lead concordance (V1-V6).
- Limb lead morphology (aVR).
- Frontal plane axis.
- QRS duration.
- Ventricular activation velocity.

Each approach to interpretation uses these elements in a variety of combinations and sequences in an attempt to suggest one or the other diagnosis. We introduced many of these concepts in Chapter 16 when we discussed aberrant conduction.

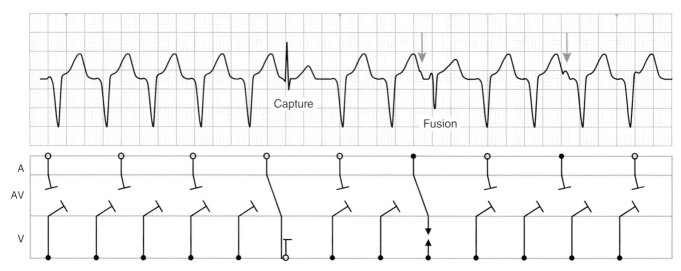

Figure 20-1. Ventricular tachycardia with AV dissociation. P waves are unrelated to QRS complexes except when sporadically conducting to the ventricles with a capture or fusion complex. On occasion, discrete P waves are visible (arrows).

Now we're going to expand the analysis to the unique dilemma posed by a WCT.

Atrial-Ventricular Relationship

In the absence of an AV conduction abnormality, every supraventricular impulse will transmit to the ventricles in a 1:1 ratio. During ventricular tachycardia, the ventricles depolarize more rapidly and independently of the sinus node, typically resulting in **AV dissociation**. This is one of the hallmarks

of VT and provides reliable evidence that a WCT is ventricular in origin. ECG signs of independent atrial and ventricular foci consistent with VT include (1) P waves unrelated to QRS complexes, (2) capture complexes, and (3) fusion complexes (**Figure 20-1**). Unfortunately, these findings are often not appreciable, particularly when the VT rate is rapid. You will have the best chance of seeing evidence of AV dissociation when the VT rate is relatively slow (<150 bpm).

You can optimize your search for hidden P waves by using a "Lewis lead," which amplifies the P wave voltage (**Figure 20-2**).

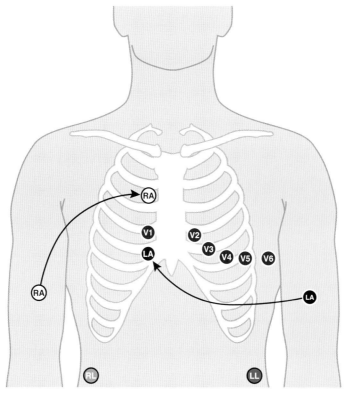

Figure 20-2. Modifying limb lead I into a "Lewis lead" can assist in revealing P waves (see text for details).

To use this technique, move the right arm electrode to the second intercostal space and the left arm electrode to the fourth intercostal space, both at the right sternal border. Then increase the calibration to 1 mV = 20 mm. Analyze this now modified limb lead I to search for evidence of independent atrial and ventricular activity.

BE CAREFUL: Ventricular tachycardia may demonstrate 1:1 retrograde VA conduction, where AV dissociation will be absent. This illustrates that while AV dissociation nearly always confirms that a WCT is ventricular in origin, the absence of this finding does not exclude VT.

CLINICAL TIP: The physical examination may provide clues to AV dissociation, all caused by the independent stimulation of the atria and the ventricles. The jugular pulse may demonstrate "cannon A waves," due to the atria contracting against the closed AV valves. Variable filling of the ventricles may produce beat-to-beat changes in systolic blood pressure. The first heart sound may also vary in intensity.

Precordial Lead QRS Complex Morphology

A supraventricular tachycardia most often results in a wide complex because it encounters either a preexisting or functional bundle branch block. So it is logical that the more the wide complex resembles a typical RBBB or LBBB, the more likely the arrhythmia represents aberrant conduction rather than ventricular tachycardia. Conversely, if the pattern is *incompatible* with a bundle branch block, the diagnosis is ventricular tachycardia. The difficulty arises when a wide complex rhythm closely *resembles*, but is not *identical* to either a right or left bundle branch block. That's when we apply morphologic clues in an attempt to differentiate the two potential diagnoses.

We know that a wide QRS complex results when ventricular depolarization is **asynchronous**, the activation of one ventricle delayed after the other. This occurs when (1) a supraventricular impulse encounters either a fixed or functional bundle branch block, or (2) the impulse originates within the ventricular myocardium. We learned in Chapter 19 that an ectopic complex originating in the left ventricle has features of a RBBB and one arising from the right ventricle or interventricular septum

resembles a LBBB. The reason is that in both left ventricular ectopy and RBBB, the left ventricle is activated first, followed by the right ventricle. Similarly, in both right ventricular ectopy and LBBB, the right ventricle is activated first, followed by the left ventricle. Most septal-based ventricular arrhythmias preferentially exit toward the right ventricle, depolarizing the RV first and the LV free wall afterwards, so again the pattern resembles a LBBB.

So how do we use this knowledge to differentiate SVT with bundle branch block aberrancy from VT? First we inspect lead V1 to determine whether the wide complex resembles a RBBB or LBBB (**Figure 20-3**). If the complex in lead V1 is predominantly positive with a "dominant R wave" (R/S ratio >1), then it has RBBB-type morphology. If a complex in lead V1 is predominantly negative having a "dominant S wave" (R/S ratio <1) with a negative terminal component, then it has LBBB-type morphology. The next step is to examine the QRS complex patterns in leads V1, V2, and V6 and compare them with those of a typical RBBB and LBBB. This analysis forms the basis of the "classical" morphologic criteria that we will discuss later.

Another precordial lead clue for VT is the **absence** of an RS-type complex (RS, rS, Rs) in **any** of the precordial leads. Why should that be? The reason is that the vectors of septal activation and that of the left ventricular free wall are characteristically in different directions, both during normal conduction and in the presence of either a right or left bundle branch block (**Figure 20-4**). This produces a biphasic RS-type complex in one or more precordial lead. In RBBB, a wide, tall terminal R′ wave is found in leads V1 and V2, which will diminish toward leads V3 and V4, with a terminal s wave emerging in leads V5 and V6. In LBBB, a negative QRS (r<S) is present in leads V1 and V2, with increasing R waves toward V5 and V6 (R>s). That explains why SVT with bundle branch block aberrancy nearly always has an RS-type complex in at least *one* precordial lead. This allows us to conclude that if *none* of the precordial leads has an RS-type complex, then VT is the likely diagnosis. To state differently, a precordial lead RS-type complex is consistent with *either* aberrant conduction or VT, but the **absence of a RS-type complex in every precordial lead is nearly always VT**, a result of the complete disruption of normal ventricular depolarization. It is important during this analysis to use a strict definition of a **biphasic RS-type complex** (RS, rS, Rs), which does not include an rsR′, Rsr′, or other QRS combinations that include R or S waves (qR, Qr, qRs, and others).

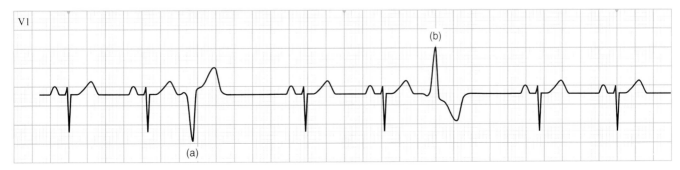

Figure 20-3. In lead V1, VPCs with LBBB-type morphology (a) and RBBB-type morphology (b).

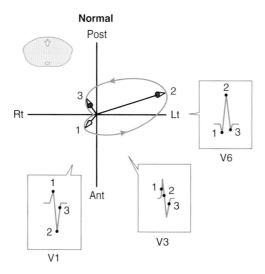

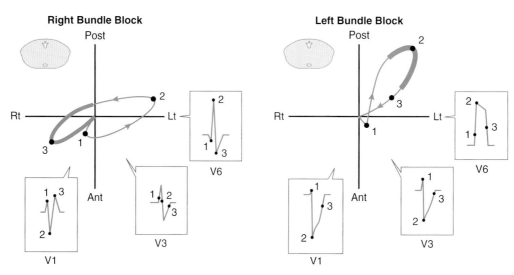

Figure 20-4. The vectors of septal activation (vector 1) and that of the left ventricular free wall (vector 2) are characteristically in different directions, both during normal conduction and in the presence of either a RBBB or LBBB. This results in biphasic, RS complexes in one or more precordial leads.

Precordial Lead Concordance

Concordance is the term used when **all** the QRS complexes in the precordial leads are both **monophasic** and on the **same side of the baseline** (**Figure 20-5**). *Positive concordance* means that all the QRS complexes in leads V1-V6 are monophasic R waves. *Negative concordance* means that every precordial QRS complex demonstrates monophasic QS waves.

 BE CAREFUL: Note that there is no allowance for q or s waves with positive concordance or r waves with negative concordance. The complexes must all be monophasic. Also, don't fall into the trap of describing concordance if most (but not all) of the leads meet the criteria. If you do, you are making a mistake, something you may occasionally find even in some well-regarded scholarly papers and textbooks.

Either positive or negative concordance is a strong indicator that the WCT is of ventricular origin, because it virtually excludes bundle branch type aberrancy. As we just reviewed,

LBBB and RBBB both generate positive and negative deflections in the precordial leads, which is incompatible with the strict definition of concordance.

Positive concordance (all R waves) suggests that the ventricular tachycardia originates from the left-posterior base of the heart, as the impulse is directed toward all of the precordial leads (**Figure 20-6**). An exception is the rare circumstance when a SVT conducts antegrade over a left-sided, posterior, or postero-lateral accessory pathway, which will also show positive concordance.

 BE CAREFUL: Remember the inconsistent and sometimes confusing nomenclature of the cardiac segments and accessory pathways. A left posterior accessory pathway is one that originates in the anatomically true inferior region of the left ventricle. Similarly, a left postero-lateral pathway is more accurately described as infero-posterior. Regardless of the nomenclature, in both circumstances the impulse travels away from the base of the left ventricle, resulting in positive concordance.

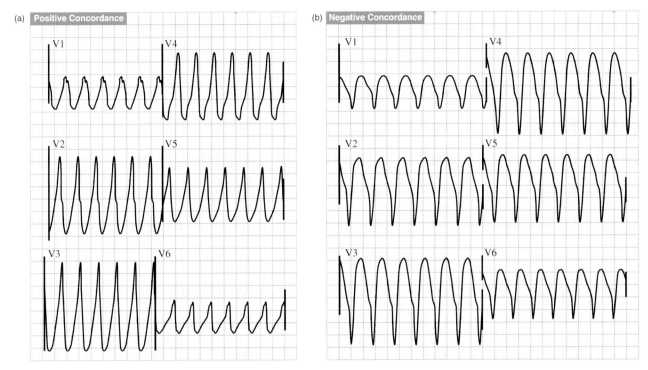

Figure 20-5. WCT showing positive (a) and negative (b) precordial lead concordance.

Negative concordance (all QS waves) strongly indicates the WCT is ventricular tachycardia derived from either the right ventricular free wall or apical-septum of the left ventricle, as the impulse is directed away from all the precordial leads (Figure 20-6). Negative concordance may also be seen in a pacemaker-related tachycardia when ventricular depolarization originates from a lead placed in the right ventricular apex.

Note that the concordance parameters we just discussed are consistent with the precordial lead RS clue we reviewed in the preceding discussion. The "all R waves" seen in positive concordance and the "all QS waves" seen in negative concordance fit within the concept that none of the complexes have an RS morphology, therefore pointing to a diagnosis of VT.

Limb Lead Morphology: The Importance of Lead aVR

Inspection of lead aVR has proven to be a useful tool to differentiate SVT with bundle branch block aberrancy from VT.

The normal septal activation is left-to-right, anterior, and (usually) superior. This is followed by the main ventricular forces, which point leftward, *away* from lead aVR. Accordingly, we expect to see a predominantly negative QRS complex (either a QS or rS) in this lead (**Figure 20-7**). When discussing bundle branch blocks, our focus is usually on the QRS morphology in the precordial leads. But here we draw our attention to the frontal plane. As seen in Figure 20-7, RBBB and LBBB each alter the ventricular activation sequence, but in both circumstances, the main QRS vector in the frontal plane remains leftward, *away* from lead aVR. This means that during normal conduction *and* with bundle branch block, we expect to see a dominant S wave in lead aVR.

Conversely, an **initial dominant R wave** (R, RS, Rs, Rsr´) is not consistent with bundle branch aberration; therefore, its presence in lead aVR suggests that the WCT is ventricular in origin, typically located in the apical or inferior region (**Figure 20-8**).

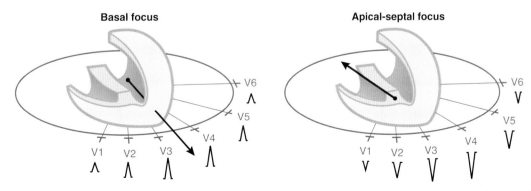

Figure 20-6. Ventricular tachycardia originating from a basal site characteristically generates positive concordance and that from an apical-septal or RV site negative concordance.

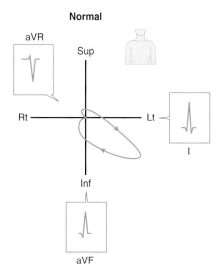

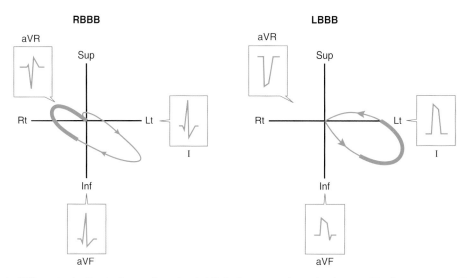

Figure 20-7. The main QRS vector is directed away from lead aVR during normal conduction, and in the presence of RBBB and LBBB. In all cases, a dominant S wave is present in that lead.

BE CAREFUL: A relatively tall initial r (Rs) wave in lead aVR may be seen after inferior wall MI, due to the loss of inferior forces. The net effect is a "reciprocal" enhancement of superior forces. A WCT with a dominant R wave, however, suggests ventricular tachycardia.

Left posterior fascicular block may also produce a relatively tall r wave in lead aVR. But here the positive deflection is a late (qr, qR, Qr) rather than initial wave due to the characteristic configuration of the vector loop (see Chapter 8, Figures 8-15 and 8-16).

VT that arises from locations other than the apex or inferior myocardium will have a main vector that remains directed *away* from lead aVR (**Figure 20-9**). Although this is the same as with normal conduction and with bundle branch blocks, lead aVR still provides clues to help differentiate VT from aberrantly conducted SVT. The common feature of these VT sites is that the *initial deflection*, whether toward or away from aVR, will show slowing, widening, or notching, which is a result of the depolarization originating outside of the specialized conduction system. Accordingly, findings seen in lead aVR that suggest a diagnosis of VT include a broad, initial nondominant r wave, or a notched, dominant Q or QS wave.

At times a WCT may present with a qR complex in lead aVR that resembles RBBB aberrancy. A broad, initial q that is followed by a dominant R wave favors VT. Again this is consistent with slow depolarization initiated within the ventricular myocardium.

Frontal Plane Axis

In most cases of SVT with aberrant conduction, the QRS axis remains either in the normal range or deviates consistent with LAFB (left axis deviation) or LPFB (right axis deviation). Extreme axis deviation (northwest quadrant, between −90 and ±180 degrees) implies a marked deviation from normal ventricular activation that is inconsistent with any combination of complete bundle branch block or fascicular block and therefore is a highly specific indication of VT (**Figure 20-10**). Note that

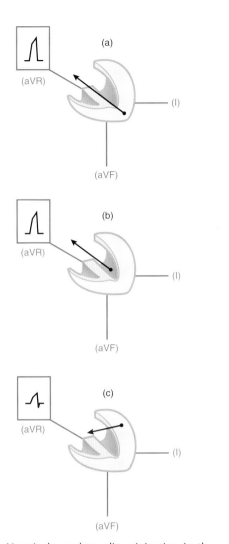

Figure 20-8. Ventricular tachycardia originating in the apex (a), inferior (b), or lateral walls (c) typically produces QRS patterns with an initial, dominant R wave in lead aVR.

a northwest axis suggesting VT is consistent with the *dominant initial R wave in lead aVR* criterion.

Although not as specific as extreme axis deviation, a LBBB-type WCT with right axis deviation favors VT. The reason is that clinical conditions typically associated with LBBB include heart failure, hypertension, and valvular heart disease, all of which are associated with left ventricular enlargement and often left axis deviation. Accordingly, a LBBB-type complex with an unusual right axis likely originates from an ectopic ventricular focus.

 FOR BOOKWORMS: When available, always compare the current ECG with a previous tracing. VT is the likely diagnosis if you find a change in axis and morphology from a previous tracing that shows either a complete LBBB or a RBBB combined with a fascicular block. The rationale is that ventricular aberration cannot occur when only one fascicle is intact at baseline. A supraventricular rhythm that produced impaired conduction in the lone remaining fascicle would produce complete heart block rather than aberration.

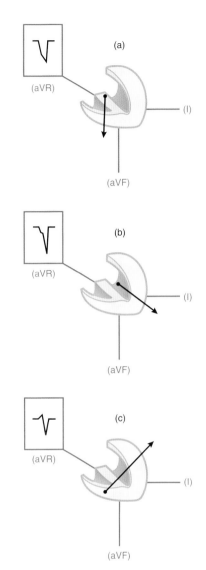

Figure 20-9. The initial deflection is fragmented or delayed when ventricular tachycardia originates in sites with main vectors directed away from lead aVR. Potential QRS patterns are shown for VT originating in the basal septum (a), basal inferior (b), and RV (c). A ventricular origin is suggested by delay of the initial deflection, with a wide or notched S wave or wide nondominant r wave.

QRS Complex Duration

A wider QRS complex duration favors ventricular ectopy over aberrancy, due to the depolarization originating deep within the ventricular myocardium with slow myocyte-to-myocyte conduction. A WCT is more likely ventricular in origin if the QRS complex duration is >0.14 seconds with RBBB-type morphology and >0.16 seconds with LBBB-type morphology.

 BE CAREFUL: A wide complex >0.16 seconds may not be helpful in predicting VT when there is a preexisting bundle branch block, and in the setting of electrolyte disturbance (eg, hyperkalemia) or medication effect (eg, class IA or IC antiarrhythmic drugs and tricyclic antidepressants). In contrast, VT may be associated with a relatively narrow QRS when the focus originates close to the specialized conduction system (eg, septal-based), and in fascicular VT.

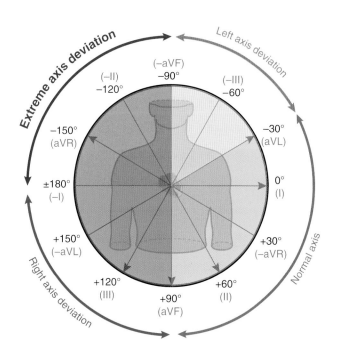

Figure 20-10. Extreme axis deviation (northwest quadrant) is a highly specific predictor of ventricular tachycardia.

 FOR BOOKWORMS: On occasion, a patient with a wide, bundle branch block morphology QRS complex at baseline will develop a WCT that is actually narrower than what is present during sinus rhythm. This favors a diagnosis of VT. The reason is that the ventricular focus originates close to the specialized conduction system, activating the ventricles more in synchrony than at baseline.

Ventricular Activation Velocity

Despite their similar QRS complex appearances, there are important differences between the morphologies of a ventricular ectopic complex and that of a supraventricular impulse conducted with a bundle branch block. A key distinction is the different speed of the initial and terminal portions of ventricular activation.

In the presence of either right or left bundle branch block, the intact bundle branch allows for the normal, rapid activation of the ipsilateral (unblocked) ventricle. Depolarization then proceeds via slow myocyte-to-myocyte conduction to activate the contralateral (blocked) ventricle. Accordingly, we see a relatively narrow initial portion of the QRS complex, followed by a wide mid to terminal portion. In contrast, an impulse that originates in the ventricular myocardium begins with slow myocyte-to-myocyte conduction. The impulse then engages the normal His-Purkinje system to more rapidly depolarize the remaining ventricular myocardium. The net effect is that the initial portion of the QRS is wide and often fragmented, followed by a comparatively narrow terminal portion (**Figure 20-11**).

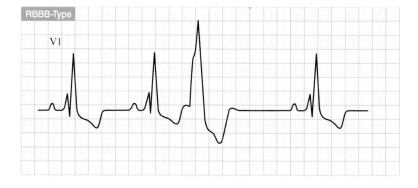

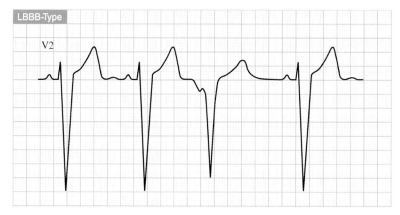

Figure 20-11. (Top) Sinus rhythm with RBBB and a RBBB-type VPC. (Bottom) Sinus rhythm with LBBB and a LBBB-type VPC. With both RBBB and LBBB, the initial deflection is relatively narrow, reflecting normal rapid depolarization via the unblocked portion of the specialized conduction system. With ventricular ectopy of both RBBB- and LBBB-types, the initial depolarization is delayed and fragmented, a result of slow, myocyte-to-myocyte conduction.

Normal (V1)

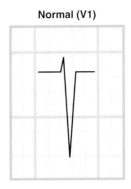

Favors Ventricular Ectopy (V1) or (V2)

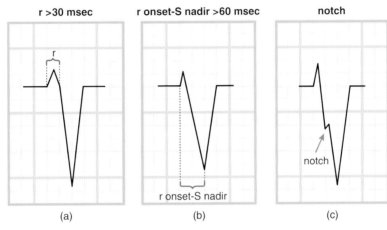

r >30 msec	r onset-S nadir >60 msec	notch
(a)	(b)	(c)

Figure 20-12. LBBB-type complexes in leads V1 or V2. A ventricular origin is favored when (a) the r wave is >30 msec, (b) the rS duration is >60 msec, or (c) the S wave contains a notch. All of the measurements seen here meet those criteria.

Specific measurements of ventricular activation velocity are incorporated into a number of algorithms used for the analysis of WCT. All of the parameters that favor VT are based on the concept of a **slow initial ventricular activation velocity**. Measurements for evaluation include the following:

LBBB-type complex, r wave duration in lead V1 or V2 In a LBBB-type complex, measure the duration of the r wave in leads V1 and V2. A duration >30 msec favors VT (**Figure 20-12a**).

LBBB-type complex, rS duration lead V1 or V2 In a LBBB-type complex, measure the rS duration in leads V1 and V2. The rS duration is measured from the beginning of the r wave to the lowest part of the S wave. A prolonged rS duration >60 msec, favors VT (**Figure 20-12b**).

LBBB-type complex, S wave notch in leads V1 and V2 In a LBBB-type complex, inspect the S wave for a notch or slur, which suggests the slow, fragmented activation typical of a ventricular focus (**Figure 20-12c**).

RS-type complex (RS, Rs, rS) duration in any precordial lead Examine all the precordial leads for a biphasic RS-type complex, regardless of bundle branch type. Measure the

RS duration from the beginning of the R wave to the lowest part of the S wave. An RS duration >100 msec favors VT (**Figure 20-13**).

Favors Ventricular Ectopy
(V1 - V6)
RS duration >100 msec

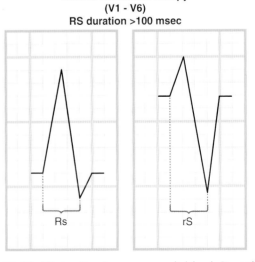

Rs	rS

Figure 20-13. RS duration in any precordial lead. Regardless of morphology, the RS duration is measured in any precordial lead from the beginning of the R wave to the nadir the S wave. An RS duration >100 msec favors VT, as seen in these complexes.

Favors Ventricular Ectopy
(aVR)
r or q >40 msec

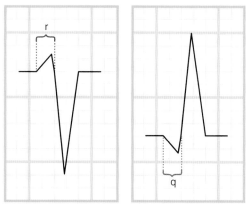

Figure 20-14. Duration of initial nondominant r or q wave in lead aVR. An initial deflection >40 msec favors VT. This is demonstrated here with an rS complex (left) and qR complex (right).

Favors Ventricular Ectopy
(aVR)
Notched QS or Qr

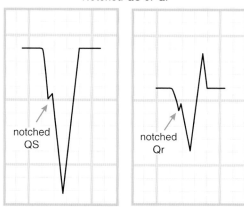

Figure 20-15. In lead aVR, any notch of a dominant QS or Qr wave favors VT.

Initial, nondominant r or q wave duration in lead aVR Examine the QRS complex in lead aVR for an initial r (rS, rSr′) or q (qR, qRs) wave. A wide initial nondominant r or q wave (>40 msec) suggests VT **(Figure 20-14)**.

Notching of initial dominant QS or Qr wave in lead aVR Inspect lead aVR for a predominantly negative QRS complex with an initial negative deflection (QS or Qr). A notched initial QS or Qr wave reflects the fragmented early depolarization typical of a ventricular focus originating outside the specialized conduction system **(Figure 20-15)**.

Lead II initial deflection time In lead II, measure the duration from the onset of the QRS complex until the first reversal of polarity, whether or not the QRS complex is mainly positive

or negative. Depending on the QRS complex morphology, the first change in polarity may be at any of the following: the apex of the initial R or r wave, the nadir of the initial S wave, or any "notch" on the ascending aspect of the initial R wave or descending aspect of the initial S wave. A duration ≥50 msec of these initial deflections supports a diagnosis of VT **(Figure 20-16)**.

Vi/Vt ratio Typically examined in lead aVR, measure the total vertical excursion (in mV) of the initial 40 msec (Vi) and the terminal 40 msec (Vt) of the QRS complex **(Figure 20-17)**. The measurements are made regardless of polarity, encompassing the total excursion of both positive and negative deflections. A Vi/Vt ratio of ≤1 suggests VT, reflecting the slow initial ventricular activation compared with the more rapid late transmission through the specialized conduction system. Conversely,

Favors Ventricular Ectopy
(II)
Initial deflection time ≥50 msec

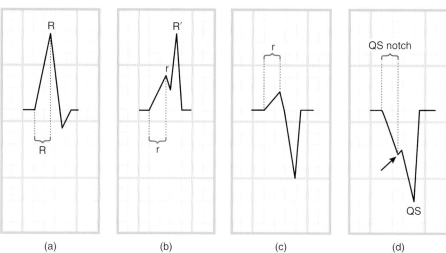

(a)   (b)   (c)   (d)

Figure 20-16. In lead II, an initial deflection time ≥50 msec favors VT. All of the measurements in the complexes seen here meet that criterion (see text for details).

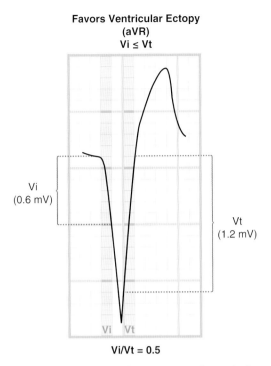

Favors Ventricular Ectopy
(aVR)
Vi ≤ Vt

Vi
(0.6 mV)

Vt
(1.2 mV)

Vi   Vt

Vi/Vt = 0.5

Figure 20-17. Vi/Vt ratio. In lead aVR, measure the vertical excursion of the initial (Vi) and terminal (Vt) 40 msec of the QRS complex. VT is favored if Vi≤Vt. SVT with aberrancy is favored if Vi>Vt. Here the Vi/Vt ratio is 0.5, which favors ventricular ectopy.

a Vi/Vt ratio >1 suggests SVT with aberrancy because of the initial rapid depolarization through the unblocked His-Purkinje system, followed by slow ventricular conduction distal to the blocked fascicle. You can streamline this analysis by simply inspecting the complex, without a mathematical calculation, using your calipers to measure Vi and Vt. If Vi ≤ Vt, then VT is likely. And if Vi > Vt, then SVT with aberrancy is favored.

FOR BOOKWORMS: The original account by Andras Vereckei using the Vi/Vt ratio describes a very specific method of measurement. Vi and Vt are to be measured in the limb or precordial leads that contain a biphasic or multiphasic complex, and in which the onset and end of the QRS complex are clearly visible. The lead selected for determining the Vi/Vt ratio is the one having the fastest initial component. When either the initial or terminal 40 msec of the QRS complex displays both positive and negative deflections, the sum of their absolute values (disregarding polarity) is used as the values for Vi and Vt. This measurement is an integral part of the simplified Vereckei aVR algorithm discussed later. Some authors also find value in measuring the Vi/Vt ratio in lead V2 in subjects with LBBB-type WCT.

BE CAREFUL: There are a number of limitations to using the Vi/Vt ratio. Accurate measurement of Vi and Vt can be difficult without the use of magnification. The morphology of the wide QRS complex may not lend itself to precise identification of the initial and terminal portions. Also, myocardial scar can depress either the initial or terminal activation velocity, which confounds the measurements.

▶ DIAGNOSTIC APPROACH TO THE WIDE COMPLEX TACHYCARDIA

Now that we have identified and learned how to make our measurements, let's start putting them to use. We can consider one approach as "classical," which uses a variety of morphological items in the analysis, but in no specific order. Another type of approach is a step-wise algorithm that applies many of the same concepts but in an ordered pattern. Other methods use a single measurement or point score approach. All have both strengths and weaknesses and frequently do not prove as accurate in "real world" application as described in the original research publication.

Classical Morphologic Approach

The fundamental principle of the classical morphologic method is that the more the WCT resembles a typical right or left bundle branch block, the more likely the complex is supraventricular with aberrant conduction. Conversely, the more "atypical" the wide complex, the more likely it is of ventricular origin. As we discussed, we look at lead V1 to determine the type of bundle branch morphology. Then we examine the morphologies in leads V1, V2, and V6 to see if the patterns are most consistent with either bundle branch block aberrancy or ventricular ectopy.

RBBB-type complexes In lead V1, a triphasic, (eg, rSR′, rsR′, RSR′, rSr′) pattern strongly favors RBBB aberrancy. This is particularly true when there is a small, narrow initial r wave that is followed by an S wave, and accompanied by a tall, wide secondary R′ deflection. Similarly, in lead V6, a triphasic qRs complex with a wide terminal s wave favors aberrancy (**Figure 20-18**).

Ventricular ectopy is suggested by a broad, monophasic R, notched Rr′, or biphasic qR pattern in lead V1. In lead V6, a monophasic QS or biphasic rS complex favors a ventricular origin.

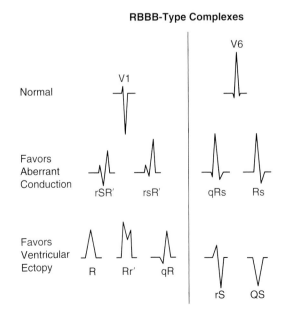

RBBB-Type Complexes

Figure 20-18. Classical morphology approach to RBBB-type complexes.

LBBB-Type Complexes

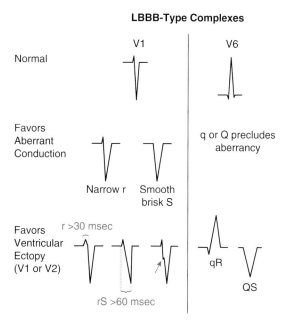

Figure 20-19. Classical morphology approach to LBBB-type complexes.

LBBB-type complexes For this analysis, we inspect *both* leads V1 and V2 (**Figure 20-19**). In these leads, a narrow r wave and smooth, brisk S wave downstroke support LBBB-type aberrant conduction. Unlike RBBB aberrancy, the QRS pattern in lead V6 does not help much to favor aberrant conduction except that any q wave is incompatible with LBBB aberration.

Ventricular tachycardia is suggested in leads V1 or V2 by any of the following (1) a wide initial R wave of >30 msec, (2) a notch or slur on the downstroke of the S wave, and (3) a delayed r wave onset to S wave nadir of >60 msec. Although infrequently seen, the presence of any q wave in lead V6 virtually guarantees a complex of ventricular origin.

Additional items used in the classical diagnostic approach to WCT include our previously reviewed analyses of QRS duration, frontal plane axis, AV dissociation, and comparison with a prior ECG.

BE CAREFUL: A confounding aspect of the classical morphologic criteria is that in approximately 30% of cases, the diagnosis suggested in lead V1-V2 is different from that suggested in lead V6.

Step-wise Algorithms

Multi-step algorithms integrate the concepts we have reviewed in the preceding discussion into an ordered sequence. At each step we are asked to determine whether the evidence favors VT or should proceed to the next step. The most widely accepted of these approaches are the Brugada (**Figure 20-20**) and Vereckei aVR (**Figure 20-21**) algorithms. In contrast to the multi-step algorithms, the Pava lead II algorithm takes a single-step approach (**Figure 20-22**).

Brugada algorithm

- Step one: Inspect the precordial leads. Is there an RS-type complex (RS, Rs, rS) in any precordial lead?
  - Yes—Proceed to the next step.
  - No—VT.
- Step two: In precordial leads with an RS-type complex, measure the duration from the onset of the R wave to the nadir of the S wave (RS duration). Is the RS duration >100 msec in any lead?
  - Yes—VT.
  - No or unable to determine—proceed to the next step.
- Step three: Inspect the entire tracing for evidence of AV dissociation.
  - Yes—VT.
  - No or unable to determine—proceed to the next step.
- Step four: Inspect leads V1, V2, and V6. Apply the classical morphology criteria for LBBB- and RBBB-type complexes. Are criteria for VT met in **both** the right (V1-V2) and left (V6) precordial leads?
  - Yes—VT.
  - No—SVT with aberrancy.

FOR BOOKWORMS: The actual language for the first step of the Brugada algorithm is different than what I described in the preceding discussion. It asks at step one: "absence of an RS complex in all precordial leads?" If yes, the diagnosis is VT. I have chosen what I feel is a more linguistically clear decision point asking you to look for an RS complex in any lead, rather than its absence in all leads.

Vereckei aVR algorithm

- Step one: Is there an initial dominant R (R, RS, Rs, Rsr′) wave?
  - Yes—VT.
  - No—proceed to the next step.
- Step two: Is there an initial nondominant q (qR, qRS, qRs) or r (rS, rSr′) wave with a duration >40 msec?
  - Yes—VT.
  - No or unable to determine—proceed to the next step.
- Step three: Is there a notch present in the initial deflection of a negative onset, predominantly negative QRS complex (QS or Qr)?
  - Yes—VT.
  - No or unable to determine—proceed to the next step.
- Step four: Measure Vi and Vt (Vi/Vt ratio). Is Vi≤Vt?
  - Yes—VT.
  - No—SVT with aberrancy.

Pava lead II single-step method

- Measure the duration of the interval from the onset of the QRS complex until the first reversal of polarity, whether or not the QRS complex is positive or negative. Is the duration ≥50 msec?
  - Yes—VT.
  - No—SVT with aberrancy.

Brugada Algorithm

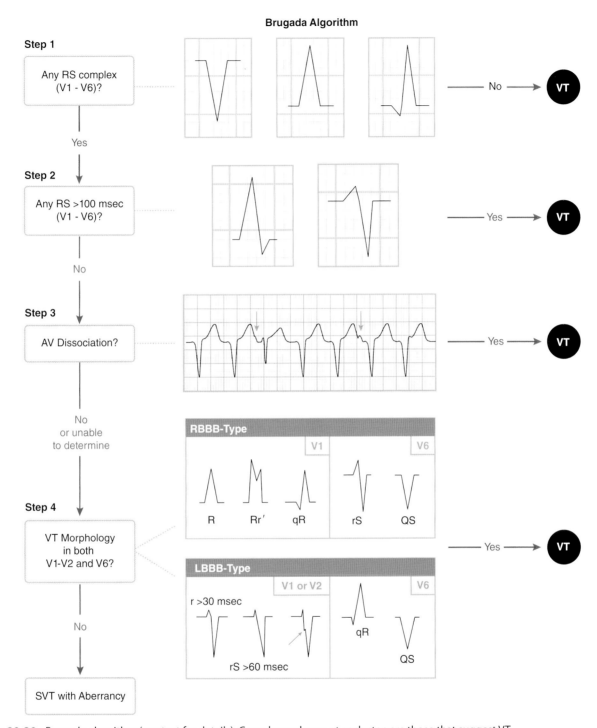

Figure 20-20. Brugada algorithm (see text for details). Complexes shown at each step are those that suggest VT.

BE CAREFUL: The lead II single-step method utilizes a measurement from the beginning of the QRS complex to the first visible reversal of the initial polarity. What is confusing is that the authors of this approach define this measurement as the *R wave peak time*, regardless of whether the deflection is ascending (R wave) or descending (S wave). This is a misnomer because strictly speaking, you cannot legitimately measure the R wave peak time of an S wave. We also learned in Chapter 4 that if the QRS complex is notched, standards call for

the R wave peak time to be measured to the secondary R′ wave, not the first change in polarity that is described in this approach (see Chapter 4, Figure 4-14). To avoid this confusing terminology, I have opted to call this measurement the "initial deflection time."

There are other methodologies that utilize a point score or a Bayesian approach, as well as another multi-step algorithm that combines the QRS complex morphology in lead aVR with analysis of limb lead vectors. For the interested reader, please

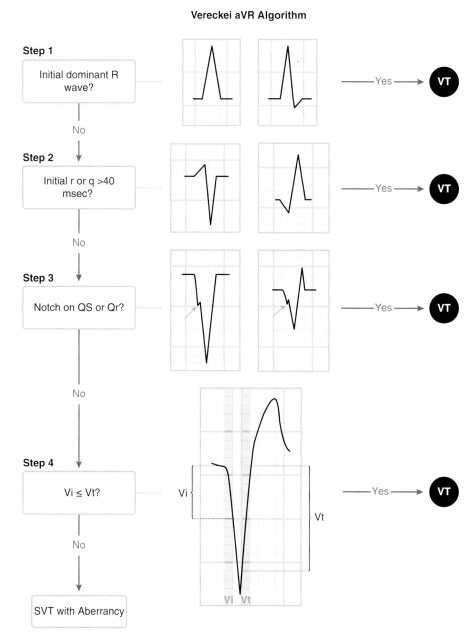

Figure 20-21. Vereckei aVR algorithm (see text for details). Complexes shown at each step are those that suggest VT.

review the suggestions for further study listed at the end of the chapter.

WCT Associated with Preexcitation

This is one of the most difficult problems in electrocardiography. None of the algorithms we discussed earlier can reliably distinguish preexcited SVT from VT because in both cases, ventricular activation begins outside of the specialized conduction system. Fortunately, this circumstance is uncommon. The clinical history and comparison with a prior tracing is key, with preexcitation an appropriate consideration in a young patient without structural heart disease who presents with a WCT. Remember that antegrade conduction over a left posterior (a.k.a. left inferior) or left postero-lateral (a.k.a. left infero-posterior) accessory pathway will show positive concordance

that is indistinguishable from VT originating from a left posterior basal focus.

Pacemaker Related WCT

Ventricular pacing generates a wide QRS complex because the stimulus originates from within the ventricular chamber, outside of the normal His-Purkinje system. For example, a ventricular lead placed within the right ventricle will activate that chamber first followed by the left ventricle, which we have learned will produce a LBBB-type complex. Often the diagnosis is evident because the pacemaker "spike" is seen distinctly. At other times however, the pacemaker stimulus is not readily visible and the diagnosis is unclear. Pacemaker-medicated WCT can occur in two primary circumstances (1) pacemaker-tracked SVT and (2) pacemaker-mediated tachycardia.

Favors VT
(II)
Initial deflection time ≥50 msec

Favors aberrancy
(II)
Initial deflection time <50 msec

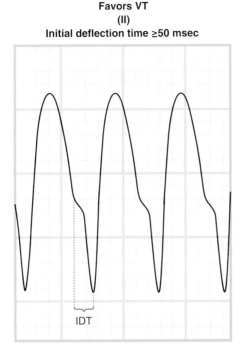

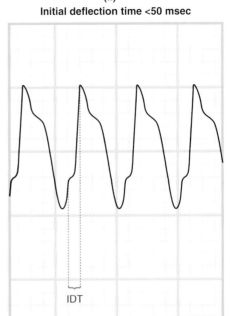

IDT

IDT

Figure 20-22. Pava lead II single-step method. Measure the initial deflection time (IDT), which is the time from the onset of the QRS to the first reversal in polarity. A measurement ≥50 msec suggests VT as seen on the left, whereas the complexes on the right likely represent aberrant conduction.

Pacemaker tracked SVT Dual-chamber pacemakers include a lead that can sense atrial depolarization. Tracking of a supraventricular tachyarrhythmia may induce rapid ventricular pacing, resulting in a WCT. Modern devices are programmed to either cease atrial tracking (mode switch) or limit the upper rate at which the ventricles can be paced in response to an atrial tachyarrhythmia.

Pacemaker-mediated tachycardia Rarely, the two leads of a dual chamber pacemaker may serve as a reentry loop, perpetuating a WCT. This can occur in a patient who has a dual-chamber pacemaker with intact VA conduction. The usual scenario is that a VPC conducts retrograde to the atrium, which is then sensed by the atrial lead. Ventricular pacing follows the tracked atrial depolarization, which sustains the arrhythmia.

 CLINICAL TIP: Pacemaker-mediated tachycardia may be rapidly terminated by placement of a magnet over the pacemaker, which temporarily disables the sensing function of both channels and initiates fixed-rate pacing. We will review pacemaker rhythm interpretation in more detail in an upcoming chapter.

Clinical Correlation

Facing a patient with a WCT is one of the most stressful situations in cardiology. Importantly, you cannot use the patient's clinical status to determine the diagnosis. Some patients may tolerate VT remarkably well, whereas others with SVT will be unstable. In the hemodynamically stable patient, you should quickly acquire a full 12-lead ECG, obtain a clinical and medication history, and perform a pertinent physical examination. Laboratories should be drawn for electrolytes and cardiac biomarkers. When available, always obtain a prior ECG to compare with the current tracing. This may provide evidence of a baseline bundle branch block or preexcitation. There may also be isolated ventricular or aberrantly conducted supraventricular complexes that you can compare with the morphology of the WCT.

 BE CAREFUL: Even under the duress of facing a patient with an apparent WCT, make sure to obtain a high-quality ECG, because artifacts can mimic an arrhythmia.

▶ PUTTING THINGS TOGETHER

We've just discussed the many options for analyzing a WCT. Unfortunately, no single method provides diagnostic certainty. So what approach do I recommend? I advise first applying the clues that are easy to remember, can be identified rapidly, and are highly specific for VT (**Figures 20-23** and **20-24**). Even then, your diagnosis must be considered as probable, rather than definitive.

Scan the tracing for northwest axis, positive or negative precordial lead concordance, and a dominant R wave in lead aVR. Other valuable clues take a little more time or require a specific measurement. Examine lead V1 to determine the bundle branch block type, and then apply the classical morphologic criteria. Look for AV dissociation, and if the patient's condition allows, utilize a Lewis lead in your search for P waves. Inspect lead II and look for an initial deflection time ≥50 msec. If you cannot make a determination after

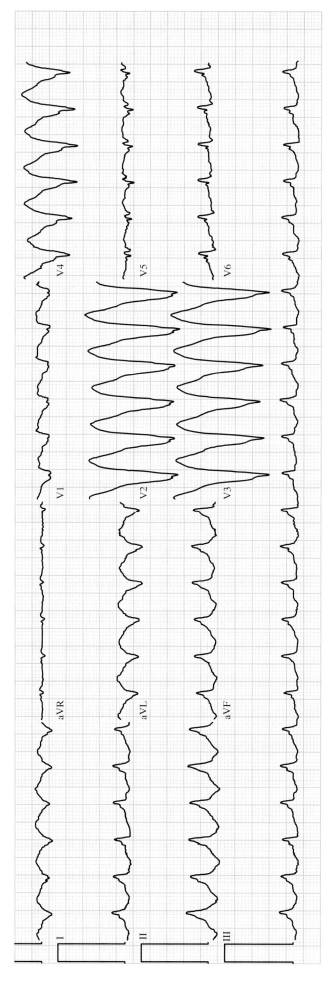

Figure 20-23. Wide complex tachycardia, likely ventricular tachycardia. Findings suggesting this diagnosis include the very wide QRS, an LBBB-type complex with right axis deviation, an S wave notch in lead V1, and by applying the Brugada algorithm. This tracing is recorded at double standardization, which does not affect the analysis.

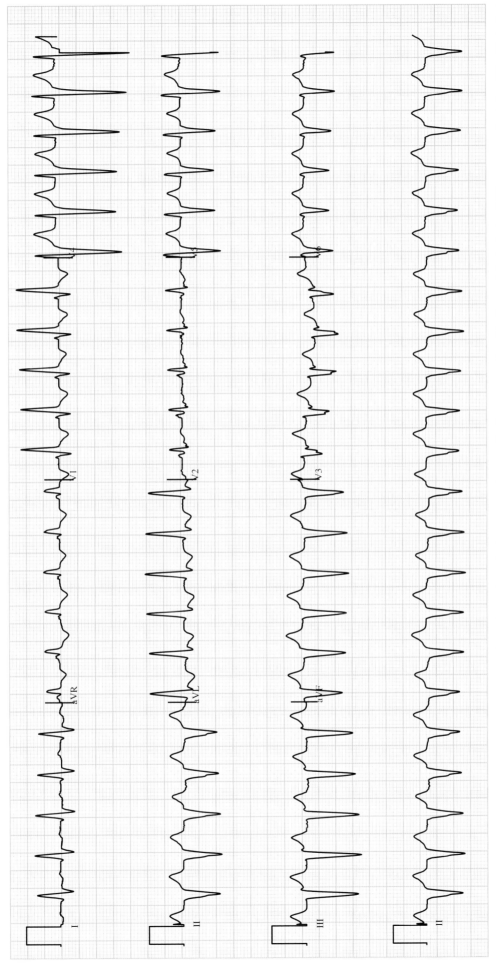

Figure 20-24. Wide complex tachycardia, likely supraventricular tachycardia with aberrant conduction. Findings suggesting this diagnosis include the RBBB-type complex in lead V1 with typical rsR´ morphology and by applying the Brugada algorithm.

a brief inspection, analyze the tracing with the multi-step Vereckei or Brugada algorithms. A frustrating reality is that you will sometimes find that the various methodologies we discussed in this chapter will lead you to different diagnostic conclusions.

Remember that >75% of patients with WCT will prove to have VT, with an even greater percentage found in those with structural heart disease. My best practical advice is to follow the famous British adage (with slight modification) . . .

Keep Calm
Carry On
When Uncertain
Cardiovert-em'!

Chapter 20 • SELF-TEST

1. A wide complex requires what abnormality of ventricular activation?

2. What is the most likely cause of a wide complex tachycardia?

3. In what situations can supraventricular tachycardia result in a wide complex tachycardia?

4. What ECG findings indicate AV dissociation?

5. How do you determine whether a wide complex is of RBBB- or LBBB-type?

6. Define positive and negative concordance.

7. What frontal plane axis is highly suggestive of ventricular tachycardia?

8. In a LBBB-type complex, what QRS findings in lead V1 or V2 suggest ventricular tachycardia?

9. In a RBBB-type complex, what QRS findings in lead V1 suggest aberrant conduction?

10. In lead aVR, what QRS findings suggest ventricular tachycardia?

11. An impulse that originates within the ventricular myocardium begins with slow, myocyte-to-myocyte conduction. True or false?

12. In the presence of either fixed or functional bundle branch block, the initial ventricular activation speed is normal, transmitted through the unblocked fascicle. True or false?

ANSWERS

Chapter 20 • SELF-TEST

1. Asynchronous.

2. Ventricular tachycardia.

3. • Fixed or functional bundle branch block.
   • Preexcitation.
   • Ventricular enlargement.
   • Congenital heart disease.
   • Electrolyte abnormality.
   • Drug effect.
   • Pacemaker related.

4. Capture and fusion complexes.

5. Examine lead V1. A predominantly positive complex (R/S ratio >1) is of RBBB-type. A predominantly negative complex (R/S ratio <1) is of LBBB-type.

6. With positive concordance, all the complexes are monophasic R waves. With negative concordance, all the complexes are monophasic QS waves.

7. Northwest quadrant (between −90 and ±180 degrees).

8. • An r wave duration >30 msec.
   • An rS duration >60 msec.
   • A notched or slurred S wave.

9. A triphasic, (rSR′, rsR′, RSR′, rSr′) pattern strongly favors RBBB aberrancy.

10. • An initial dominant R wave.
    • An initial nondominant r or q wave >40 msec.
    • A QS or Qr complex with a notch on the initial downstroke.

11. True.

12. True.

Further Reading

Alzand BSN, Crijns HJGM. Diagnostic criteria of broad QRS complex tachycardia: decades of evolution. *Europace.* 2011;13:465-472.

Brugada P, Brugada J, Mont L, Smeets J, Andries EW. A new approach to the differential diagnosis of a regular tachycardia with a wide QRS complex. *Circulation.* 1991;83:1649-1659.

DePonti R, Bagliani G, Padeletti L, Natale A. A general approach to a wide QRS complex. *Card Electrophysiol Clin.* 2017;9:461-485.

Garner JB, Miller JM. Wide complex tachycardia – ventricular tachycardia or not ventricular tachycardia. That remains the question. *Arrhythm Electrophysiol Rev.* 2013;2:23-29.

Jastrzebski M, Kukla, P, Czarnecka D, Kawecka-Jaszcz K. Comparison of five electrocardiographic methods for differentiation of wide QRS complex tachycardias. *Europace.* 2012;14:1165-1171.

Jastrzebski M, Sasaki K, Kukla P, Fijorek K, Stec S, Czarnecka D. The ventricular tachycardia score: a novel approach to electrocardiographic diagnosis of ventricular tachycardia. *Europace.* 2016;18:578-584.

Kashou AH, Noseworthy PA, DeSimone CV, Deshmukh AJ, Asirvatham SJ, May AM. Wide complex tachycardia differentiation: a reappraisal of the state of the art. *J Am Heart Assoc.* 2020;9: e016598.

Katritsis DG, Brugada J. Differential diagnosis of wide QRS tachycardias. *Arrhythm Electrophysiol Rev.* 2020;9:155-160.

McGill TD, Kashou AH, Deshmukh AJ, LoCoco S, May AM, DeSimone CV. Wide complex tachycardia differentiation: an examination of traditional and contemporary approaches. *J Electrocardiography.* 2020;60:203-208.

Pava LF, Perafan P, Badiel M, et al. R-wave peak time at DII: a new criterion for differentiating between wide complex QRS tachycardias. *Heart Rhythm.* 2010;7:922-926.

Vereckei A. Current algorithms for the diagnosis of wide QRS complex tachycardias. *Curr Cardiol Rev.* 2014;10:262-276.

Vereckei A, Dura G, Szenasi G, Altemose GT, Miller JM. A new algorithm using only lead aVR for differential diagnosis of wide QRS tachycardia. *Heart Rhythm.* 2008;5:89-98.

Pacemaker Electrocardiography

▶ INTRODUCTION

In 400 BCE, Hippocrates observed that persons who suffered severe attacks of swooning without any manifest cause died suddenly. The artificial electronic pacemaker has been one of the great technological advances in cardiology, able to provide a remedy for many of the conditions that were recognized by Hippocrates more than two millennia ago. Until the development of the pacemaker, there were few options for patients with conduction system failure. Today's sophisticated devices are used to treat not only bradyarrhythmias and heart block, but also have antitachycardia functions and play an increasing role in the treatment of heart failure.

Up until now we have discussed ECG findings that record the heart's native electrical system (**Figure 21-1**). Artificial electronic pacemakers either integrate with, or completely replace natural conduction, requiring an entirely new set of terms and abbreviations. But fear not, because we're going to take this slowly and there's a table of abbreviations with definitions at the end of the chapter to help you.

▶ WHAT IS A PACEMAKER?

There are three basic components of any pacemaker (1) a **generator** (battery or power supply), (2) one or more **electrodes** (wires or leads), and (3) **circuitry** (computer or logic) (**Figure 21-2**). The generator is a battery-based power supply, sealed within a stainless steel or titanium case that is typically placed in a subcutaneous pocket below the clavicle. Also encased is the computer microprocessor, which can be programmed with a variety of functions. The generator is connected to the myocardium via one or more electrodes that are inserted transvenously into the right atrium, right ventricle, or both chambers. A third electrode may be placed through the coronary sinus and extended into an epicardial coronary vein to depolarize the left ventricle. Leadless pacemakers are a recent development where an entire self-contained system is implanted within the myocardial chamber. The electrode input and circuitry of the pacemaker that is devoted to a particular chamber of the heart is called its **channel** (eg, atrial or ventricular channel).

A **single-chamber** pacemaker is one with an electrode in only one chamber, either the right atrium or right ventricle.

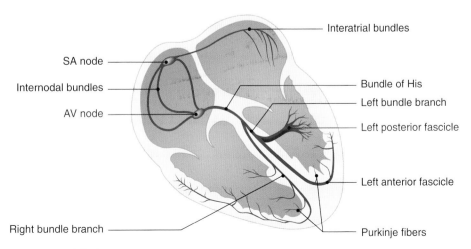

Figure 21-1. Conduction system of the heart.

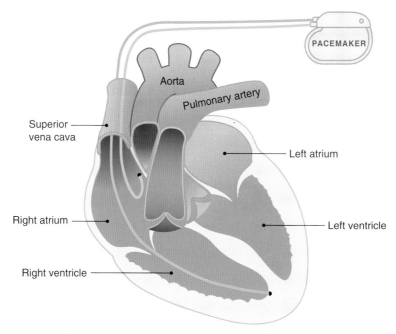

Figure 21-2. Dual-chamber pacemaker. The atrial lead (pink) is typically inserted in the right atrial appendage. The ventricular lead (orange) is typically placed in the right ventricular apex or septum.

A **dual-chamber** pacemaker contains leads in both the right atrium and right ventricle. A **biventricular** pacemaker includes leads to activate both the right and left ventricles. If a dual-chamber pacemaker also has a left ventricular electrode, the device is termed a **dual-chamber biventricular** pacemaker.

The Pacemaker ECG Complex

A pacemaker complex looks different than any other we've seen so far. The pacemaker delivers electrical energy to the myocardium, seen as a **stimulus artifact** or "spike" that appears prior to atrial or ventricular depolarization (**Figure 21-3**). Like all aspects of electrocardiography, the polarity and amplitude of the stimulus artifact relate to its direction of depolarization, which is positive if directed toward, or negative if directed away from a given lead. The amplitude of the artifact also reflects the energy delivered, a programmable function that is determined by the **pacing threshold** at implant and during regular follow-up. Another factor is that the size of the artifact depends on whether the electrodes are **unipolar** or **bipolar** (**Figure 21-4**). A bipolar lead has the negative electrode (cathode) and the positive electrode (anode) in close proximity at the tip of the catheter. The current flows from the generator to the cathode tip, stimulating the myocardium and returning to the anode to complete the circuit. The short distance between the two electrodes produces a small pacemaker artifact. In contrast, a unipolar electrode tip contains only the cathode, the metal housing of the pacemaker generator serving as the anode. Completion of the electrical circuit across the large distance between the cathode and anode produces a large pacemaker artifact.

 CLINICAL TIP: Most modern pacemaker lead systems are bipolar, the small distance between the two terminals minimizing the likelihood of interference from outside electromagnetic forces. Unipolar leads are thinner and simpler in design than bipolar electrodes, but are prone to electrical interference as well as inadvertent stimulation of skeletal muscle.

 BE CAREFUL: The pacemaker artifact of a bipolar lead is small and may be easily overlooked, particularly the atrial spike. You may also need to check the filter settings of the electrocardiograph. If the setting of the low-pass (high-frequency) filter is lowered to help eliminate noise from nearby electrical devices, it may also suppress high-frequency pacemaker signals. A different issue occurs with a unipolar lead, where the large stimulus artifact can give the impression of ventricular capture, where in actuality none has occurred.

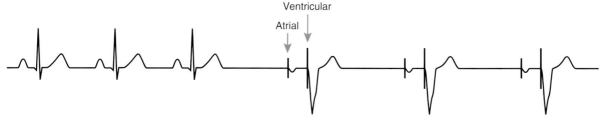

Figure 21-3. Atrial and ventricular pacemaker stimulus deflections.

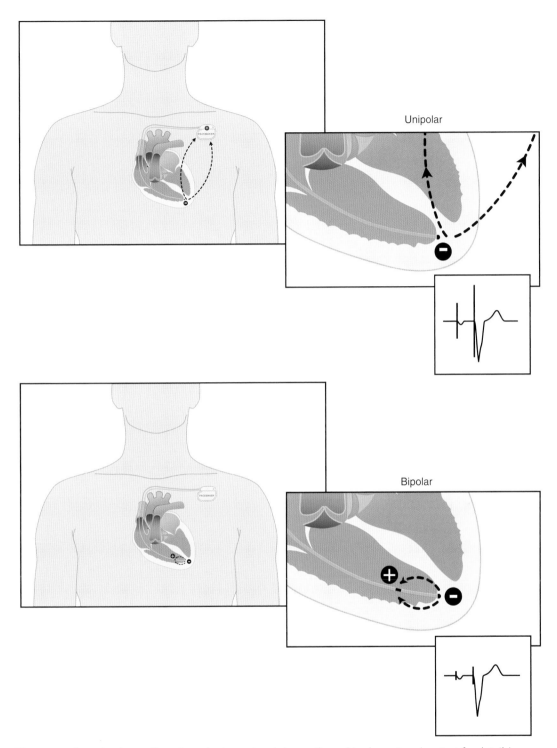

Figure 21-4. The pacemaker stimulus artifact of a unipolar system is larger than a bipolar system (see text for details).

The energy delivered by the generator and electrode stimulates its respective chamber, the right atrium, right ventricle or left ventricle, alone or in concert. Depolarization or "capture" of each chamber generates characteristic ECG findings (**Figure 21-5**).

Atrial pacing The atrial pacing lead is typically positioned in the right atrial appendage. This is close to the sinus node, so we expect that an atrial pacemaker depolarization will be similar in

appearance to a normal P wave. If the atrial lead is placed lower in the atrium, the atrial-paced vector will be directed superiorly, resulting in a negative deflection in the inferior leads.

Ventricular pacing The ventricular electrode is typically placed in the right ventricular apex or septum. The delivered energy depolarizes the right ventricle first; following which the impulse transmits to the left ventricle via myocyte-to-myocyte conduction. This produces a ventricular pacemaker

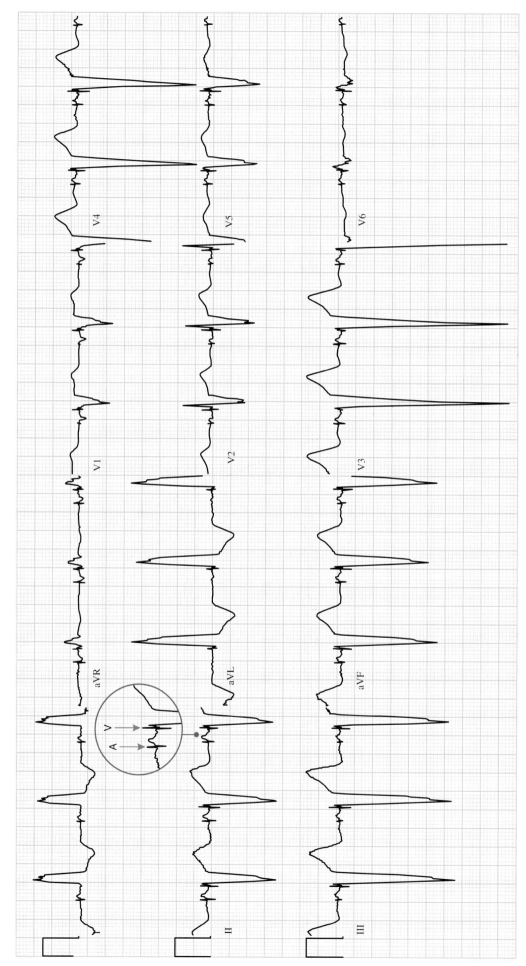

Figure 21-5. 12-lead ECG showing atrial (A) and ventricular (V) pacemaker depolarizations.

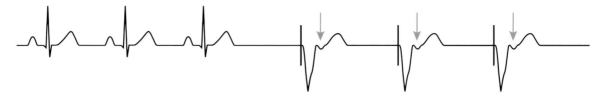

Figure 21-6. Retrograde atrial depolarization (arrow) may occur with ventricular pacing.

depolarization with a LBBB-type configuration, namely a wide, negative QRS complex in lead V1 (dominant S wave) with a discordant T wave. Does this sound familiar? It should because this is the same concept that we discussed in Chapter 19 why a VPC originating in the right ventricle has a LBBB pattern. With LBBB, right ventricular pacing, and a right ventricular VPC, the right ventricle depolarizes first followed by the left ventricle. And with the lead typically placed low in the right ventricular apex, depolarization proceeds from apex-to-base, inferiorly-to-superiorly, resulting in a frontal plane axis with marked left axis deviation. On occasion, the pacing lead is placed in the right ventricular outflow tract (RVOT), which is a more superior structure. If so, the LBBB configuration remains, but depolarization now proceeds inferiorly, which results in a positive deflection in leads II, III, and aVF.

At times, retrograde conduction to the atrium occurs, and an inverted P′ wave may be visualized after the ventricular depolarization (**Figure 21-6**).

BE CAREFUL: In a minority of the time (~10%), uncomplicated RV apical pacing results in a dominant R wave in lead V1, instead of the expected dominant S wave. However, this pattern should at least raise the suspicion that the electrode is not placed properly in the RV and may have been

inadvertently positioned in the LV, entering through a patent foramen ovale, atrial septal defect, or ventricular septal defect. Rarely, the lead has perforated the RV, and either resides within the LV chamber or has entered the pericardial space to migrate along the epicardial surface of the LV.

Dual-chamber pacing As the name implies, dual-chamber pacing stimulates both the right atrium and right ventricle. The device initiates atrial pacing, and after an AV delay, ventricular pacing.

Biventricular pacing As with an intrinsic LBBB, right ventricular pacing produces delayed activation of the left ventricular lateral wall. This results in cardiac *dyssynchrony*, which may induce *de novo* or worsen preexisting left ventricular dysfunction. Adding a left ventricular pacing electrode allows for biventricular pacing and **resynchronization** of right and left ventricular depolarization. The LV electrode is inserted through the ostium of the coronary sinus located within the right atrium and optimally passed into a posterolateral epicardial cardiac vein (**Figure 21-7**). This allows the device to initiate depolarization of the LV via the lateral wall. The depolarization wave spreads anteriorly and to the right, producing a RBBB-type pattern (dominant R wave in lead V1), and typically a negative deflection in lead I (**Figure 21-8**). LV pacing

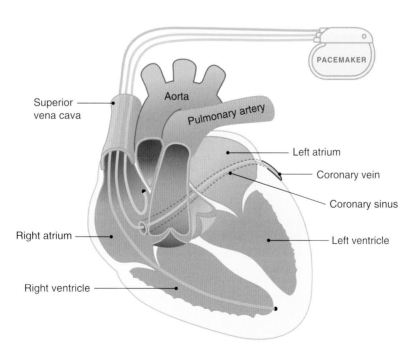

Figure 21-7. Biventricular pacemaker system. For left ventricular pacing, a lead (green) is placed within the coronary sinus and extended into a posterolateral epicardial vein. Combined with a right atrial lead (pink) and right ventricular lead (orange) the system provides dual chamber, biventricular pacing that is used for resynchronization therapy.

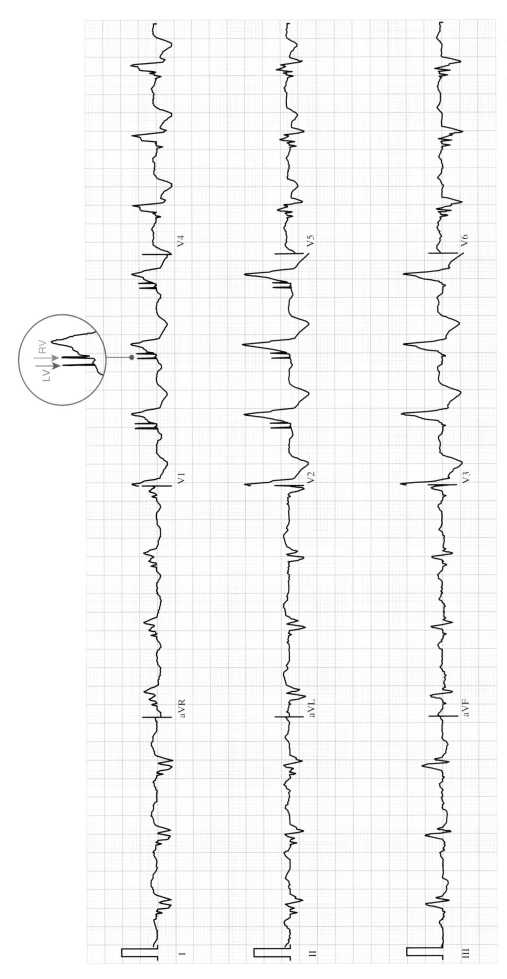

Figure 21-8. 12-lead ECG showing left ventricular (LV) followed by right ventricular (RV) pacing. Note the dominant R wave in lead V1 (RBBB-type) and dominant S wave in lead I, which are characteristic findings of LV pacing. This example clearly shows both the LV and RV pacemaker artifact. More commonly, only the LV pacemaker artifact is evident, with the RV stimulus hidden within the QRS complex. Compare this tracing with Figure 21-5, which is an example of isolated RV pacing with a typical dominant S wave in lead V1 (LBBB-type) and dominant R wave in lead I.

is followed by the RV, the stimulus artifact of the latter often hidden within the QRS complex. The biventricular pacemaker complex is therefore a hybrid, representing the relative activation of each ventricle that varies according to the programming.

 FOR BOOKWORMS: Direct pacing from the His bundle and left bundle branch are evolving techniques intended to maintain physiologic pacing. Both avoid the electrical and mechanical dyssynchrony induced by isolated RV pacing.

Pacemaker Complex Conundrums: Fusion and Pseudofusion

At times, the pacemaker depolarization may fortuitously coincide with intrinsic conduction, resulting in a **fusion** complex. This may occur with isolated ventricular pacing where the native impulse occurs with virtually the same timing as that of the pacemaker. The simultaneous spontaneous and artificial activation results in a ventricular QRS complex that is a cross between the native and paced morphology (**Figure 21-9**). This also occurs with a dual-chamber pacemaker system, where intrinsic atrial conduction to the ventricles happens to be nearly identical to the programmed AV interval. A **pseudofusion** complex is one where a pacemaker spike is present in the vicinity of the QRS complex, but the timing of the stimulus is such that it arrives when the ventricle is naturally refractory, precluding further activation. Both fusion and pseudofusion complexes represent normal pacemaker function that reflects the coincidental timing of intrinsic depolarization and pacemaker stimulation.

 FOR BOOKWORMS: Because the pacemaker leads are inside the heart, one would think the device would detect the intracardiac electrogram before being recorded by the surface ECG. In reality the opposite is true. After each chamber is depolarized, it takes a short period of time before the device can "see" the P wave and QRS complex. This explains the occurrence of fusion and pseudofusion complexes and why they usually represent normal pacemaker function.

To Pace or Not to Pace, That Is the Question

The first pacemakers were rudimentary devices, pacing only one chamber at a time at a preset interval. The disadvantages of these "fixed rate" pacemakers were obvious, producing competition between native and pacing activity and leading to AV dissociation. Advances in pacemaker technology provided multiple leads with sophisticated **sensing** capabilities that allowed for pacing *on-demand*, as well as programming to maintain AV synchrony. In response to a sensed intracardiac event, the pacemaker may **inhibit** or **trigger** an output in the same or a different chamber. The combination of pacing and sensing parameters are called **modes**, which may be programmed for optimal physiologic performance.

 FOR HISTORY BUFFS: In 1958, the first completely internal pacemaker was implanted into Arne Larsson, a 43-year-old man who suffered with complete heart block and recurrent Adams-Stokes attacks. Cardiac surgeon Ake Senning and physician engineer Rune Elmqvist performed the procedure in Stockholm, Sweden. Mr. Larsson went on to receive >20 pacemaker revisions, dying at the age of 86 of noncardiac disease.

The Pacemaker Programming Code

The pacing and sensing modes are categorized according to a three-to-five position code (I-V), which refers to the way the device interacts with the underlying cardiac rhythm (**Table 21-1**). For most clinical settings, three positions are adequate with the fourth used when necessary.

Position I The first position indicates the chamber(s) where pacing occurs. "A" refers to the atrium, "V" indicates the ventricle, and "D" denotes dual or both the atrium and ventricle. The letter "O" is utilized when all pacemaker function has been programmed off.

Position II The second position represents the chamber(s) where sensing occurs, again using "A" for atrium, "V" for ventricle, and "D" for dual. The letter "O" is utilized when there is no sensing function.

Position III The third position identifies how the pacemaker responds to a sensed event. "I" indicates that a sensed event inhibits the next scheduled pacing stimulus and resets the timing cycle (see following discussion). This designation applies

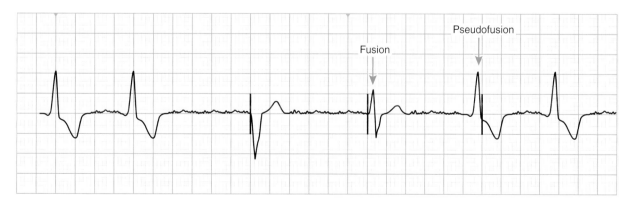

Figure 21-9. Fusion and pseudofusion complexes. A fusion complex is a hybrid of intrinsic and pacemaker depolarization. The pacemaker stimulus of a pseudofusion complex does not depolarize the myocardium. The native rhythm in this example is atrial fibrillation.

TABLE 21-1	Five Position Pacemaker Code				
Position	I	II	III	IV	V
CATEGORY	Chamber(s) Paced	Chamber(s) Sensed	Response to Sensing	Rate Modulation	Multisite Pacing
LETTER	O = None A = Atrium V = Ventricle D = Dual (A + V)	O = None A = Atrium V = Ventricle D = Dual (A + V)	O = None I = Inhibited T = Triggered D = Dual (I + T)	O = None R = Rate modulation	O = None A = Atrium V = Ventricle D = Dual (A + V)

to both single and dual-chamber pacemakers (eg, AAI, VVI, DDI). "T" indicates that a sensed event triggers pacing, either in the same chamber or in another after an AV delay. Although included in the coding system, isolated use of the triggered mode is mainly obsolete. "D" is applicable only to dual-chamber systems and indicates dual functionality that *combines* inhibition and triggering (eg, VDD, DDD). Let's break down what that combination means. If the pacemaker senses spontaneous atrial or ventricular activity, the next scheduled pacing stimulus in that chamber is *inhibited* and the timing cycle resets. That's simple enough and is equivalent to the function of a single-chamber pacemaker. But what about the triggering component? In a dual-chamber pacemaker, this begins with either a sensed or paced atrial event, whereupon the pacemaker now awaits evidence of intrinsic ventricular conduction. If after a programmed AV delay no ventricular activity is detected, then ventricular pacing occurs, *triggered* by the sensed atrial impulse. "O" in position III is used in conjunction with an "O" in the second position (eg, AOO, VOO, DOO) and indicates the absence of both inhibition and triggering function.

Position IV The fourth position of the pacemaker code refers to rate modulation, which is designated with an "R." Pacemakers with this functionality have a sensor that increases the pacing rate in response to physical activity (ie, rate responsiveness). If the function is available but not activated, the letter may be placed in parenthesis (R).

Position V The fifth position is used infrequently and is not needed for routine electrocardiography. It provides a way to designate multisite pacing, defined as stimulation sites in both atria (biatrial), both ventricles (biventricular), more than one stimulation site in a single chamber, or any combination thereof.

 CLINICAL TIP: You can remember the order of the three-position pacemaker code with the acronym PaSeR. That's P for the chamber(s) paced, S for the chamber(s) sensed, and R for the response to sensing.

 FOR BOOKWORMS: You will most often encounter single-chamber pacemakers programmed to VVI mode and dual-chamber devices programmed to DDD mode, with or without rate modulation. There are circumstances where a number of other modes are used, only a few of which we will discuss later. The others are used infrequently and beyond the scope of this discussion. For the interested reader, please review the selections for further study at the end of the chapter.

▶ PACEMAKER TIMING CYCLES

Introduction

Once the mode is set, the pacemaker is programmed with an internal set of timed instructions that govern the sensing and pacing behavior. Pacemaker timing cycles determine the functions associated with an atrial sensed event (P wave), paced atrial output (A), ventricular sensed event (R wave), and paced ventricular output (V). Note that the terminology of pacemaker timing cycles is defined from the perspective of the device (**Figure 21-10**). For example, a native P wave detected by the atrial channel is "atrial sensed (As)" and a native R wave detected by the ventricular channel is "ventricular sensed (Vs)."

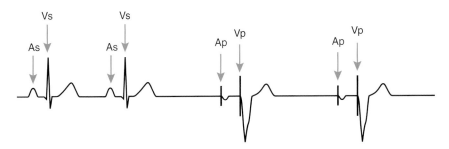

Figure 21-10. Pacemaker timing cycles are defined from the perspective of the device. From the atrial channel, the complexes are termed atrial sensed (As) or atrial paced (Ap). From the ventricular channel, the complexes are termed ventricular sensed (Vs) or ventricular paced (Vp).

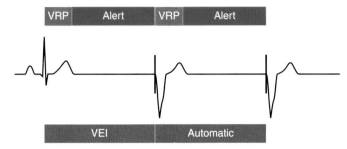

Figure 21-11. The ventricular escape interval (VEI) (blue bar) is the period between a sensed ventricular complex and the next ventricular output. The automatic (pacing) interval is the time between two consecutive ventricular outputs (blue bar). As seen here, the automatic interval is usually programmed to be the same as the VEI. The ventricular refractory period (VRP) (red bar) is the time after a sensed or paced event that the device will note, but not respond to an incoming signal. The alert period (green bar) follows the VRP where the device resumes full ventricular sensing and response functions.

Atrial pacing is "atrial paced (Ap)," and ventricular pacing is "ventricular paced (Vp)."

There are other terms unique to our discussion of pacemaker timing cycles (**Figure 21-11**). One is the **automatic interval**, also called the **pacing, basic** or **demand interval**, which is the period between two consecutive paced events (either Vp-Vp or Ap-Ap). Another is the **escape interval**, which is the period between a sensed cardiac event and the next pacemaker stimulus. In most circumstances, the automatic interval is programmed to be identical to the escape interval, so for practical purposes the terms may be used interchangeably.

Another important term is **refractory period**, which is used differently when discussing pacemakers than is customary in cardiac electrophysiology. We learned in Chapter 3 that the refractory period of a myocyte is that portion of the action potential where the cell is either partially (relative refractory period) or completely (effective refractory period) unable to depolarize the myocardium in response to an outside stimulus. Pacemaker refractory periods are *programmed* parameters that are intended to prevent the device from inappropriately sensing a signal that could result in a detrimental pacemaker response. Any signal "seen" during a channel's refractory period is effectively "ignored," meaning it will not be tracked or reset a timing cycle. This is intended to prevent a potentially deleterious inhibited or triggered response. The conclusion of the refractory period marks the beginning of the **alert period**, where the pacemaker can once again respond to any sensed intrinsic activity.

In a moment we'll discuss more about these and other timing cycles in single and dual-chamber devices. But first, we need to adjust the way we measure the timing of cardiac events.

Time to Talk Timing Cycles

We are accustomed in electrocardiography to measuring heart rate in terms of beats per minute (bpm). The precise programming of pacemaker timing cycles requires that we think in

intervals**, using milliseconds (msec) instead (**Figure 21-12**). We learned in Chapter 5 that you can convert back and forth from HR in bpm to cycle length intervals in msec by using these two versions of the same formula:

$$HR \text{ (bpm)} = 60{,}000/\text{cycle length (msec)}$$
$$\text{Cycle length (msec)} = 60{,}000/HR \text{ (bpm)}$$

Pacemaker timing cycles range from simple to extremely complex. For each chamber there are programmed intervals for pacing, sensing, and a variety of refractory periods. Let's begin our discussion with the essentials, starting first with single-chamber pacemakers. Then we can move on to the more complex dual-chamber devices.

Single-Chamber Timing Cycles

Single-chamber ventricular pacemaker   A single lead ventricular pacemaker is most appropriate when the native rhythm is atrial fibrillation, eliminating the need for an atrial lead. The first timing cycle to discuss is the **lower rate interval** (LRI), which is the longest period the device will wait after one ventricular event before delivering a stimulus. The ventricular LRI is determined by programming the **ventricular escape interval** (VEI), which, in practice, begins after either a sensed or paced ventricular event. If the VEI elapses without intrinsic ventricular activity, the device will deliver a ventricular stimulus.

Figure 21-13 shows an example of a single-chamber ventricular pacemaker, programmed in a VVI mode. After either a paced or sensed ventricular event, the pacemaker starts an internal "stopwatch," awaiting the next intrinsic ventricular depolarization. If none is detected before the elapse of the VEI, the device will deliver a ventricular pacemaker stimulus and reset the timer, starting another VEI. That was easy! You can see that the VEI sets the LRI, which determines the slowest HR allowed (**lower rate limit**). The patient's heart rate may exceed the lower rate limit (LRL), but in no case can it drop below this number. And remember, the "I" in VVI means that if the pacemaker detects an intrinsic ventricular depolarization before it reaches the end of the VEI, the next scheduled pacemaker output is *inhibited*, holding off on ventricular pacing and resetting the internal timing clock to await the next impulse (complexes 3 and 5).

The next timing cycle to discuss in a single-chamber ventricular device is the **ventricular refractory period** (VRP). This is a programmed interval after either a sensed or paced ventricular event where the device "ignores" any detected signal. Why do we need this? One reason is that the VRP is intended to prevent inappropriate sensing of large T waves that the device might mistake as another ventricular depolarization, a phenomenon known as "double counting."

Single-chamber atrial pacemaker   **Figure 21-14** is an example of a single-chamber atrial pacemaker programmed in an AAI mode. This type of device is appropriate when there is sinus node dysfunction with intact AV conduction. Such patients need careful assessment because AV node dysfunction may develop over time in patients who might originally have

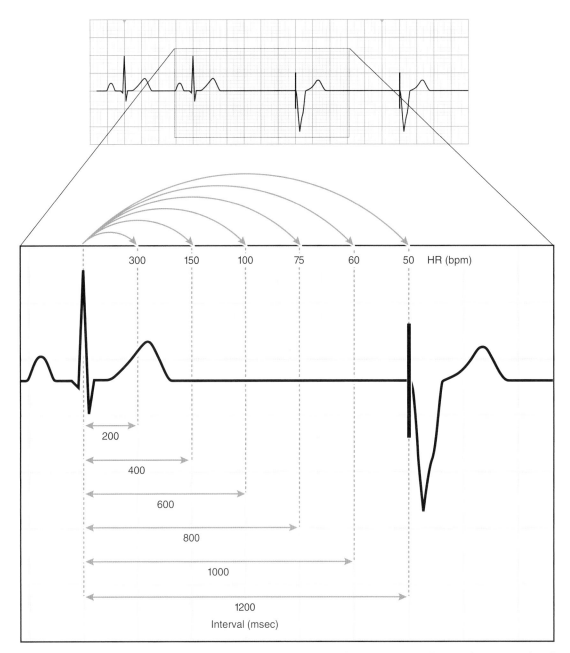

Figure 21-12. Pacemaker timing cycles are analyzed and programmed in intervals measured in milliseconds (msec) rather than heart rate (HR) in beats per minute (bpm).

only sinus node disease. Akin to the situation with ventricular pacing, the **atrial escape interval** (AEI) sets the LRI for atrial pacing in the AAI mode. After either a sensed or paced atrial event, the device awaits the next atrial depolarization. If none is detected by the elapse of the AEI, the device delivers an atrial pacemaker stimulus. Should intrinsic atrial activity be detected, the device will inhibit the next scheduled atrial pacing output and reset the timing cycle (complex 3). Remember that with AAI mode pacing, there is no ventricular channel to detect ventricular events (complex 5) so the atrial pacing cycle remains unaffected (complex 6). However, after each atrial paced or sensed event, an **atrial refractory period** (ARP) is programmed to prevent inappropriate sensing of "far-field" intrinsic ventricular

events by the atrial channel. In other words, the ARP prevents the atrial channel from "being fooled" that something happening in the ventricle is mistaken for an atrial depolarization.

Dual-Chamber Pacemaker Timing Cycles

The advantage of a dual-chamber pacemaker is the ability to emulate normal physiology. The device has an atrial and ventricular channel, each capable of sensing and pacing its respective chamber. The internal computer logic coordinates the output of the two channels to maintain AV synchrony. The most common programming of a dual-chamber pacemaker is in DDD mode, with or without rate modulation. With this programming, four ECG patterns are possible (**Figure 21-15**).

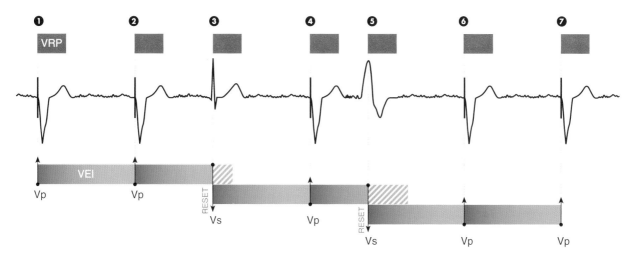

Figure 21-13. VVI mode pacemaker function. The native rhythm is atrial fibrillation. After the first ventricular-paced complex, ventricular pacing occurs on demand as determined by the programmed VEI (complexes 2, 4, 6, 7). If an intrinsic ventricular event is sensed before the VEI times out (hatched), the timing cycle resets and generates a new timing cycle. Here a sensed native QRS (complex 3) and a sensed VPC (complex 5) each inhibit ventricular pacing and reset the timing cycle. The ventricular refractory period (VRP) begins after each paced or sensed ventricular event.

- Atrial pacing and ventricular pacing (AV sequential pacing).
- Atrial pacing and ventricular sensing (atrial pacing).
- Atrial sensing and ventricular pacing (P-synchronous pacing).
- Atrial sensing and ventricular sensing (normal sinus).

As you might imagine, the timing cycles associated with dual-chamber pacemakers are more numerous and complex than for single-chamber devices. Parameters must be set for atrial and ventricular sensing and pacing that include both lower and upper-rate behavior. The timing relationship between the atrial and ventricular channels must be established. A variety of refractory periods are present, intended to mitigate the potential for inappropriate pacemaker function. Wow, that sounds complicated! Well it is, and you may wonder why do you need to know this anyway? The reason is that you are going to encounter puzzling pacemaker ECGs that appear to indicate malfunction, when they really represent normal programming. Yes, it's OK to ask for help from a pacemaker specialist or company representative, but a basic understanding of dual-chamber timing cycles and function will help you better differentiate normal from abnormal pacemaker behavior.

CLINICAL TIP: The *pacemaker syndrome* is a complication of single-chamber ventricular pacing, manifested by reduced cardiac output and hypotension. Patients exhibit retrograde VA conduction or AV dissociation that results in atrial contraction against a closed AV valve. This creates a sensation of "cannon A waves" in the neck and generates a hemodynamic response that produces exercise intolerance and lowers blood pressure. Dual-chamber pacing is intended to emulate normal physiology, maintaining AV synchrony and thereby avoiding the pacemaker syndrome.

Let's review the essentials of timing cycles of a dual-chamber pacemaker programmed in DDD mode. The first item to consider

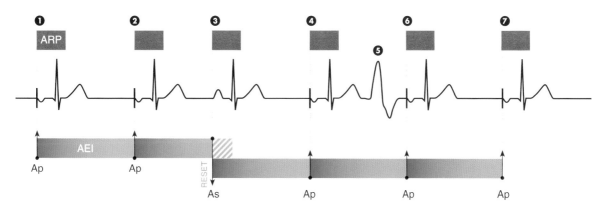

Figure 21-14. AAI mode pacemaker function. After the first atrial-paced complex, atrial pacing occurs on demand as determined by the programmed AEI (complexes 2, 4, 6, 7). If an intrinsic atrial event is sensed before the AEI times out (hatched), the timing cycle is reset and generates a new timing cycle (complex 3). Note that there is no ventricular sensing with AAI mode pacing, so the VPC (complex 5) is unsensed and does not reset the atrial timing cycle. The atrial refractory period (ARP) begins after an atrial-paced or sensed event.

Atrial pacing - Ventricular pacing

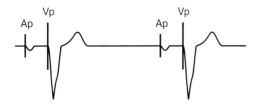

Atrial pacing - Ventricular sensing

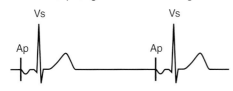

Atrial sensing - Ventricular pacing

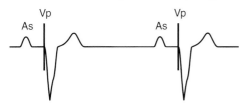

Atrial sensing - Ventricular sensing

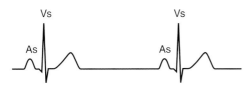

Figure 21-15. The four types of ECG complexes seen with DDD mode programming.

is the **lower rate interval**, which like a single-chamber ventricular pacemaker, is the longest time allowed after one ventricular event before the device will deliver a ventricular pacing output.

But in a dual-chamber device this interval is divided into two portions, the **ventricular-atrial interval** (VAI) and the **AV interval** (AVI) (**Figure 21-16**). The VAI interval, also called the **atrial escape interval** (AEI), is the time between a sensed or paced ventricular event and the next atrial pacemaker stimulus. The AVI is the delay between a sensed or paced atrial event and delivery of a ventricular pacing stimulus, programmed to emulate the normal PR interval.

Figure 21-16 shows an example where both the atrium and ventricle are paced and the device is programmed with a LRI of 1200 msec and an AV interval of 200 msec. Once these two parameters are programmed, the pacemaker automatically calculates a VAI of 1000 msec. You can see here that after the device delivers a ventricular impulse, it waits for 1000 msec to see if there is intrinsic atrial activity. Finding none, it paces the atrium and now awaits native ventricular conduction. Again finding none, it delivers a ventricular stimulus. So you can see that the LRI of a dual-chamber pacemaker is the *combination* of the VAI and the AVI. Like a single-chamber VVI device, the LRI is the longest period allowed between two ventricular events. But with DDD programming, the device must account for atrial activity and AV conduction *in advance* of the next ventricular stimulus.

Figure 21-17 shows what happens if the device detects native conduction. If the device detects intrinsic atrial activity before the elapse of the VAI, atrial pacing is inhibited, the timing cycle is reset, and a new AVI is established (complex 4). Similarly, if the device detects native ventricular depolarization before reaching the end of the VAI, it will inhibit ventricular output, reset the timing cycle, and establish a new VAI (complex 6). Finally, if the device detects native ventricular depolarization after an atrial event, but before elapse of the AVI, ventricular pacing is inhibited and a new VAI begins (complex 8).

Now let's add in the concept of dual-chamber refractory periods (**Figure 21-18**). The **total atrial refractory period** (TARP) modifies the sensing function of the atrial channel such that any detected intrinsic atrial activity will not be tracked. The first portion of the TARP is identical to the AVI, which

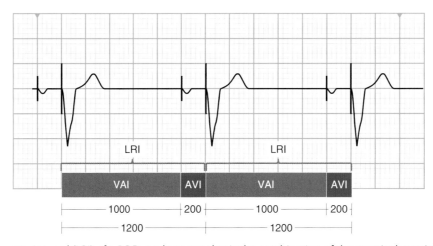

Figure 21-16. The lower rate interval (LRI) of a DDD mode pacemaker is the combination of the ventricular-atrial interval (VAI) (blue bar) and atrial-ventricular interval (AVI) (light blue bar). Here the device is programmed with an LRI of 1200 msec and AVI of 200 msec; therefore, the device will calculate a VAI of 1000 msec.

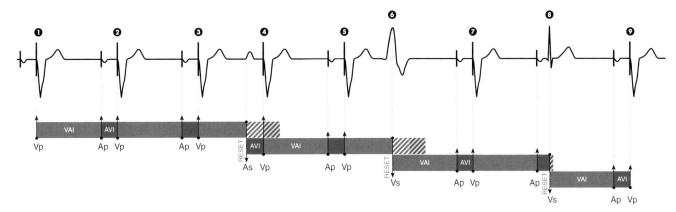

Figure 21-17. DDD mode timing intervals. After the first dual-chamber paced complex, complexes 2, 3, 5, 7, and 9 demonstrate dual chamber, atrial and ventricular pacing on demand as determined by the programming of the LRI (combination of VAI and AVI). Complex 4 is an atrial premature complex that occurs before the VAI elapse (dark blue hatched), resetting a new AVI, LRI, and VAI timing cycle. The new AVI of complex 4 passes without a sensed ventricular event so ventricular pacing follows the atrial sensed event. Complex 6 is a VPC, which occurs before the VAI elapse, resetting a new VAI and LRI. Complex 8 is an atrial paced complex on demand with intrinsic ventricular conduction. The ventricular sensed event of complex 8 occurs prior to the elapse of the AVI (light blue hatched), resetting a new VAI and LRI.

begins after atrial sensing or pacing. Immediately following a ventricular sensed or paced event is the **post-ventricular atrial refractory period** (PVARP). This prohibits tracking of a rapid atrial arrhythmia, as well as any atrial depolarization conducted retrograde from the ventricles, something that might induce a pacemaker-mediated tachycardia (see following discussion). Both the AVI and PVARP are individually programmable, the sum of which determines the duration of the TARP. The elapse of the TARP marks the onset of the **atrial tracking interval** (ATI), where normal atrial sensing resumes.

As with single-chamber ventricular devices, a **ventricular refractory period** begins after either a paced or sensed ventricular event, designed to avoid mistaking a T wave for an R wave.

 FOR BOOKWORMS: A concern for dual-chamber pacemakers is the phenomenon of inappropriate "far-field" sensing and "cross-talk." Far-field sensing is when the channel of one chamber inappropriately detects an *intrinsic* signal from another chamber. Examples are a native P wave detected by the ventricular channel or a native QRS complex detected by the atrial channel. Cross-talk is defined as the inappropriate sensing of a *device stimulus* from one chamber by the channel of another chamber. The most common manifestation is when an atrial pacing stimulus "spills over" and is detected by the ventricular channel, which mistakes the impulse as a ventricular depolarization. Should this occur, the device wrongly inhibits ventricular output, which is a potential catastrophe for a patient who is pacemaker-dependent. In order to combat this, dual-chamber devices are programmed with a **post-atrial ventricular blanking period** (PAVBP), where for a short period after atrial pacing the ventricular sensing channel is completely disabled. Another protection against cross-talk is **ventricular safety pacing** (VSP), which will deliver a ventricular stimulus if a depolarization is detected within a short window after the PAVBP when cross-talk might also occur. The ventricular output is delivered with a shortened AV interval, providing a clue that ventricular safety pacing is active.

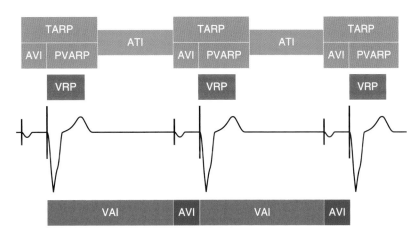

Figure 21-18. The total atrial refractory period (TARP) is comprised of the AVI and the post-ventricular atrial refractory period (PVARP). After elapse of the TARP, the atrial tracking interval (ATI) resumes (green bar). The ventricular refractory period (VRP) (red bar) is programmed separately from the atrial refractory periods (light red bars).

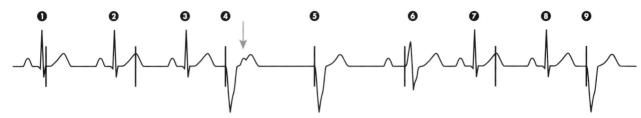

Figure 21-19. VOO mode pacemaker function. Asynchronous, fixed-rate pacing artifacts are noted throughout the tracing. Capture is possible if the stimulus arrives when the ventricle is not naturally refractory (complexes 4, 5, 6, 9). The intrinsic sinus rhythm is unaffected. The small deflection present on the upslope of the T wave of complex 4 (arrow) represents a P wave that cannot conduct because it arrives when the ventricle is refractory after pacemaker capture. Complex 6 is a fusion complex that represents the combined contributions of intrinsic conduction and pacemaker depolarization. Complex 1 represents pseudofusion with a pacemaker artifact that appears in the vicinity of the QRS complex, but without ventricular depolarization.

Miscellaneous Modes and Functions

Asynchronous pacing (VOO, AOO, DOO) There are times when you want to completely disable the sensing function of the pacemaker. A common situation is when you want to avoid inappropriate sensing of electrical interference, such as might occur with the use of electrocautery during surgery. With asynchronous pacing the device functions in a fixed rate mode, stimulating the chambers at a predefined interval without regard to the native rhythm (**Figure 21-19**).

CLINICAL TIP: Placing a magnet over the pacemaker will temporarily disable all sensing functions and convert the device to asynchronous, fixed-rate pacing, the rate of which differs by manufacturer. The underlying programming is unaffected and the device returns to all the original timing cycles on removal of the magnet. The *magnet rate* is also used to determine the status of the pacemaker power source. A change in the original magnet rate from when the device is new is an indicator of battery depletion.

Asynchronous pacing once raised the concern that the pacemaker stimulus would fall on the T wave, considered a "vulnerable period" during repolarization, which might precipitate ventricular tachycardia. Clinical experience indicates this risk is extremely small and limited to situations of acute myocardial ischemia or marked electrolyte imbalance.

Rate modulation Also called *rate-adaptive* or *rate-responsive pacing*, both single and dual-chamber devices may include a function that increases the pacing rate in response to the patient's level of activity. If present, a fourth letter "R" is added to the description of the pacemaker mode (eg, VVIR, DDDR).

Hysteresis This is a special function where after a sensed event, the escape interval is programmed to be *longer* than the automatic interval (**Figure 21-20**). If the intrinsic rate falls below the hysteresis escape rate, the device will pace at the automatic rate until again exceeded by the spontaneous rate. For example, a device programmed to VVI mode with hysteresis might allow for a VEI of 1200 msec (50 bpm) and a pacing interval of 1000 msec (60 bpm). The concept of hysteresis is to improve the opportunity for native conduction, but pace at a sufficient rate on demand.

Upper rate behavior We have discussed that a dual-chamber pacemaker has the ability to track atrial activity. This is desirable in an attempt to maintain normal physiology, but it may be detrimental in the presence of a supraventricular tachyarrhythmia. With simple DDD programming, the TARP provides a "built-in" **upper rate limit** (URL) to rapid heart rates (**Figure 21-21**). We know the atrial channel can only track an intrinsic P wave during its alert period, which begins after the PVARP. As the atrial rate increases, the P wave eventually encounters the period where the impulse is untracked and fails to produce a ventricular output. The next atrial impulse arrives during the atrial alert period and is tracked normally. The net effect is a fixed-ratio, 2:1 atrial sensed-ventricular paced sequence. The problem with this function is that on reaching the TARP the rapid heart rate

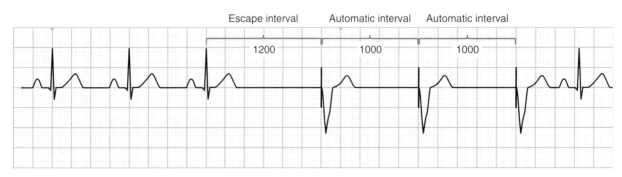

Figure 21-20. Hysteresis (VVI mode). The escape interval (1200 msec) after a sensed event is programmed longer than the pacing/automatic interval (1000 msec).

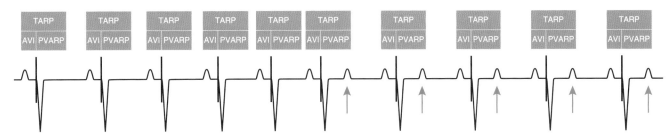

Figure 21-21. Upper rate behavior (2:1 response). The tracing demonstrates atrial sensing and ventricular pacing with an increasing atrial rate. On reaching the TARP, a sensed atrial depolarization will fail to trigger a ventricular-paced response (arrows). This causes an abrupt drop in ventricular rate as now only every other P wave results in a paced ventricular output.

is precipitously cut in half, something that is likely to be clinically symptomatic, particularly for an active patient who might reach the heart rate limit while exercising. Fortunately there is a programming solution that we will now discuss.

Modern pacemakers have a separate programmable timing circuit for the fastest rate at which atrial activity can be tracked in a 1:1 fashion. The **maximum tracking rate** (MTR) is set by programming the **maximum tracking interval** (MTI). If the device detects atrial activity that exceeds the MTR, the pacemaker will begin upper rate "behavior" that modifies the tracking response and limit the effective heart rate (**Figure 21-22**). This typically involves widening the AVI, which extends the time to ventricular depolarization, and hence the TARP, bringing it closer to the next P wave. Eventually the P wave reaches the TARP, preventing the atrial impulse from being tracked, effectively "dropping" a single ventricular stimulus. The cycle then resets creating an ECG pattern that is "Wenckebach-like." The widening of the AVI until an absent ventricular paced complex is analogous to the prolongation of the PR interval and eventual failure of conduction that occurs with Mobitz type I block.

Mode switching   Another means of preventing dual-chamber tracking and pacing of rapid atrial arrhythmias is automatic mode switching. If the device detects a rapid atrial arrhythmia (eg, atrial flutter, atrial tachycardia, or atrial fibrillation), it typically converts the programmed mode from DDD to either DDI or VDI. Both these modes effectively function as VVI-programmed devices, but retain atrial sensing *without* tracking, which avoids triggering a rapid ventricular pacing response.

The original programming mode is automatically restored if the device detects the arrhythmia has reverted back to sinus rhythm.

FOR BOOKWORMS: There are additional programmable functions designed to emulate normal physiology whether at rest, during sleep, or while exercising. Programming also exists to limit potentially deleterious RV pacing by promoting intrinsic conduction. For the interested reader please review the selections for further study.

Pacemaker-Mediated Tachycardia

Dual-chamber pacemakers may participate in a **pacemaker-mediated tachycardia** (PMT). We mentioned earlier that a ventricular depolarization may conduct retrograde through the AV node into the atria (see Figure 21-6). If so, the retrograde atrial impulse from either an intrinsic or paced ventricular depolarization may be detected by the atrial channel, triggering a ventricular response. The cycle can then repeat, initiating a reentrant arrhythmia. Here the pacemaker acts as the antegrade limb of the loop with the AV node serving as the retrograde limb (**Figure 21-23**). This is analogous to what we learned in Chapter 18 when we discussed the mechanism of SVT involving an accessory pathway (AVRT). But instead of a congenital atrioventricular bypass connection, here the dual-chamber pacemaker serves as the accessory AV pathway.

Looking back at our discussion of timing cycles, you can now see the importance of the PVARP in preventing a PMT. Retrograde AV conduction would most likely occur just after

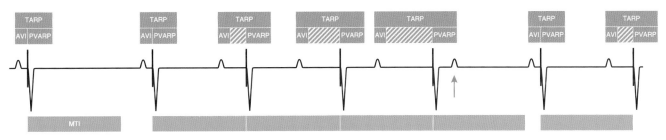

Figure 21-22. Upper rate behavior (Wenckebach-like response). The tracing demonstrates atrial sensing and ventricular pacing with an increasing atrial rate that arrives earlier than allowed by the maximum tracking interval (MTI) (blue bar). The device responds by extending the AVI interval over baseline (hatched), prolonging the time to ventricular pacing and the PVARP that follows. Eventually a P wave encroaches on the TARP and is no longer tracked, "dropping" a ventricular-paced response. Atrial sensing with ventricular pacing resumes afterwards, producing a Wenckebach-type pattern.

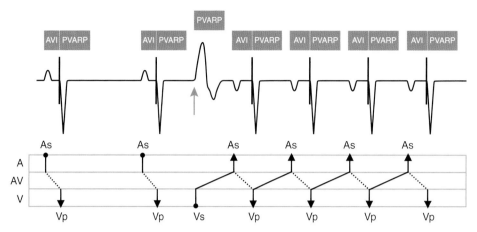

Figure 21-23. Pacemaker-mediated tachycardia (PMT). A VPC (arrow) initiates retrograde atrial conduction that falls outside the PVARP. The atrial depolarization is sensed by the atrial channel, which triggers a ventricular pacing response (dashed line). The cycle repeats, perpetuating a PMT.

ventricular depolarization, which should fall within the PVARP. During this interval, atrial sensing is ignored, thereby preventing the retrograde impulse from initiating a PMT. This arrhythmia can result only if the retrograde conduction reaches the atrial channel beyond the PVARP.

 CLINICAL TIP: If encountering a suspected PMT, place a magnet over the pacemaker. This temporarily inactivates all sensing functions, converting the device to asynchronous, fixed-rate pacing. This will interrupt the PMT so you can attempt to remedy the inciting cause, either with medications or adjustment of the pacemaker programming.

Pacemaker Malfunction and Troubleshooting

Abnormal ECG pacemaker findings can be grouped into two broad categories, **pacing malfunction** (failure to capture or output and pacing at an inappropriate rate) and **sensing malfunction** (undersensing and oversensing). Both do occur, but it is common that what is initially thought to be pacemaker malfunction actually represents one or more of the special programming features we discussed earlier. Let's now review the differential diagnosis of suspected pacemaker malfunction.

Failure to capture refers to the presence of an atrial or ventricular pacemaker stimulus without capture of the respective chamber (**Figure 21-24**). This most commonly occurs early

after implantation with lead dislodgement. In a mature device, the fault more often lies with a defective electrode. This may take the form of an **insulation break**, which causes the current from the generator to leak out into the surrounding chamber, or a **lead fracture** that prevents delivery of the energy to the myocardium. Another cause of capture failure is inadequate pacemaker voltage. A rise in pacing threshold routinely occurs in the first few weeks after implantation. Normally, an adequate safety margin is programmed at implant, but if not, the pacemaker output may be too low to depolarize the myocardium. The pacing threshold may also rise in the setting of tissue fibrosis, myocardial ischemia, metabolic and electrolyte disorders, as well as treatment with some antiarrhythmic medications (eg, flecainide, propafenone). Finally, a nearly depleted pacemaker may not be able to provide adequate voltage for the stimulus to capture the myocardium.

 BE CAREFUL: A ventricular pacemaker spike without capture may be a pseudofusion complex (see Figure 21-9). As we discussed earlier, this results because the pacemaker escape interval is timed coincidentally with that of a native complex. By the same concept, asynchronous pacing initiated by placement of a magnet will likely result in some impulses that arrive when the ventricle is naturally refractory and will fail to capture (see Figure 21-19).

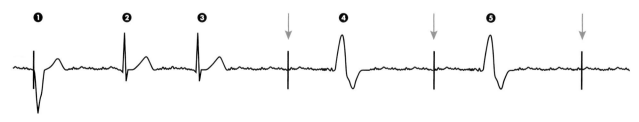

Figure 21-24. Pacemaker malfunction—failure to capture. The native rhythm is atrial fibrillation with a ventricular pacemaker in VVI mode. Complex 1 demonstrates a normal pacemaker depolarization, but there are pacemaker stimuli occurring on demand that fail to capture the ventricles (arrows). Complexes 4 and 5 are ventricular escape complexes.

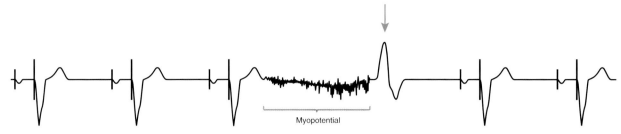

Figure 21-25. Pacemaker malfunction—oversensing. The native rhythm is dual chamber, atrial and ventricular pacing in DDD mode. Myopotentials from skeletal muscle inappropriately suppress both the atrial and ventricular channels of the pacemaker, causing a pause. The wide complex (arrow) is a ventricular escape complex.

Failure to output (failure to pace) refers to the absence of a pacemaker stimulus when expected. The reasons overlap with those causing capture failure including lead fracture and insulation break as well as complete dislodgement of the electrode from the generator. Most causes of failure to output are due to oversensing, where the system is inappropriately inhibited (see following discussion).

BE CAREFUL: As we mentioned earlier, bipolar pacing results in a small, sometimes inapparent stimulus artifact, something particularly common in the atrium. A quick check is to place a magnet over the device, which should alter the heart rate and confirm capture.

Pacing at abnormal rates This is a rare example of pacemaker malfunction, and suspected abnormal findings can nearly always be explained by programming analysis. True dysfunction may be present if there is impending battery depletion, as the device lowers the pacing rate as a means to conserve energy. An extremely rare complication related to generator depletion is a "runaway pacemaker," which results in a markedly elevated pacing rate. High pacing rates also occur with a PMT, but as we discussed, this represents normal function that can be alleviated with a change in programming.

BE CAREFUL: Remember that a pacemaker stimulus that appears at a lower rate than expected may represent hysteresis. Conversely, a stimulus that appears at a greater rate than expected may represent an activity response.

Oversensing Detection of signals not derived from intrinsic cardiac activity is one form of oversensing. Examples include sensing of skeletal myopotentials or electrical interference ("noise") from medical or electromechanical devices. Oversensing may result in pauses (**Figure 21-25**) in either a single or dual-chamber pacemaker. In a dual-chamber device, the atrial channel may track these noncardiac signals, producing either rapid ventricular tracking or a mode switch response. Examples of "functional" oversensing of either intrinsic or device-related cardiac signals are inappropriate T wave sensing (double counting), far-field detection, and cross-talk. These events are unusual with proper programming of refractory periods.

Undersensing Failure to recognize intrinsic cardiac events as programmed is termed undersensing. On the ECG, undersensing demonstrates a pacemaker stimulus where it isn't anticipated (**Figure 21-26**). This may result from either suboptimal lead positioning that prevents detection of an intracardiac electrogram or actual lead dislodgment. Other causes include a change in the intracardiac signal due to fibrosis, ischemia, or metabolic and electrolyte imbalance.

BE CAREFUL: Sensing is absent in devices programmed into asynchronous mode (VOO, DOO). The ECG may have been recorded when the device was temporarily programmed into this mode or when a magnet was applied. Fusion and pseudofusion complexes may also give the appearance of undersensing. Finally, cardiac events that fall within the pacemaker refractory periods will not be sensed by design.

CLINICAL TIP: Oversensing leads to underpacing. Undersensing leads to overpacing.

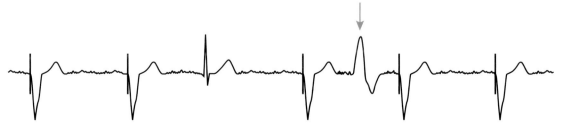

Figure 21-26. Pacemaker malfunction—undersensing. The native rhythm is atrial fibrillation with a ventricular pacemaker in VVI mode. The device fails to sense the VPC (arrow) and reset, delivering an inappropriate ventricular stimulus at the automatic interval.

Pacemaker Potpourri

Post-pacing T wave inversion Ventricular pacing may result in T wave inversion in unpaced complexes that resemble those found in myocardial ischemia. The etiology is believed to be the result of local depolarization changes at the pacing site. The findings may persist for months to years after cessation of pacing, leading to the term "memory T waves."

Diagnosis of myocardial infarction Like the situation with an intrinsic LBBB, the diagnosis of acute myocardial infarction in a patient with ventricular pacing is a particular challenge. Ventricular pacing generates a wide complex with secondary repolarization abnormalities opposite in polarity to the direction of the main QRS complex deflection. For example, leads with a predominantly negative QRS complex will show ST segment elevation and an upright T wave. One of the more specific ECG findings suggesting acute MI in paced complexes is ≥5 mm ST segment elevation in leads with a predominantly negative QRS complex. Reliable criteria however are lacking, and key to the diagnosis remains clinical evaluation. When available, comparison with prior tracings may indicate new findings that assist with the diagnosis.

Implanted cardiac defibrillator (ICD) All cardiac defibrillators also function as pacemakers and may be combined with pacing function that is single chamber, dual chamber, or biventricular. What is different with these devices is the magnet response, which in an ICD temporarily inhibits the antitachycardia function, but does not alter the pacemaker programming. As we learned previously in this chapter, application of a magnet over a standard pacemaker temporarily converts the programming to asynchronous pacing.

Final Thoughts

Modern pacemakers are extraordinarily sophisticated devices with increasingly complex programming. When reading pacemaker ECGs, your first task is always to evaluate the native rhythm, which is a necessary part of determining pacemaker function. Seek out information about the pacemaker manufacturer, which is provided on a card given to every patient at the time of implant. Without knowing the exact programming, it may not be possible to distinguish normal from abnormal pacemaker function from a single ECG. When necessary, it's reasonable to make statements in your reporting such as "suspected" or "possible" pacemaker malfunction. Often an exact diagnosis requires using the manufacturer's programmer to examine the device's internal marker channels, which allows you to evaluate what the device is "thinking." Above all, don't be discouraged if you find this topic daunting, because most pacemaker ECGs are straightforward and device malfunction is rare. **Table 21-2** should help you with the multitude of new terms and abbreviations we introduced in this chapter.

TABLE 21-2	Pacemaker Timing Cycle Glossary	
Term (Abbreviation)	**Definition**	**Comment**
Alert period	The timing cycle following a refractory period where the device can sense and respond to intrinsic activity.	Dual-chamber devices have separate alert periods for each chamber.
Atrial escape interval (*single chamber atrial device*) (**AEI**)	The period after an atrial sensed event until the next atrial pacemaker output.	In the absence of hysteresis, the atrial escape interval equals the automatic (pacing) interval.
Atrial escape interval (*dual-chamber device*) (**AEI**) or (**VAI**)	See ventricular-atrial interval.	In dual-chamber pacing, ventricular-atrial interval preferred.
Asynchronous (*fixed rate*) pacing	The pacing output is delivered at a preset rate with the sensing function completely disabled.	Placing a magnet over the device will initiate asynchronous pacing.
Atrial refractory period (*single-chamber atrial device*) (**ARP**)	The period after an atrial event (paced or sensed) where any further atrial sensed event is ignored.	Be careful not to confuse this with the total atrial refractory period (TARP) in dual-chamber devices.
Atrial tracking interval (**ATI**)	The period after the TARP where atrial sensing and tracking function resumes.	Also known as atrial alert interval.
Automatic interval (pacing, basic or demand interval)	The period between two consecutive paced events (Vp-Vp or Ap-Ap).	In the absence of hysteresis, the automatic interval equals the escape interval.
AV interval (**AVI**)	In dual-chamber pacing, the period between an atrial event (paced or sensed) and the delivery of a ventricular output.	
Cross-talk	Inappropriate sensing of device output originating in one chamber by another.	Example: An atrial pacemaker stimulus detected by the ventricular channel.

(Continued)

TABLE 21-2	Pacemaker Timing Cycle Glossary (Continued)	
Term (Abbreviation)	**Definition**	**Comment**
Escape interval	The period between a sensed cardiac event and the next pacemaker output.	In the absence of hysteresis, the escape interval equals the automatic interval.
Far-field sensing	An intrinsic signal originating in one chamber inappropriately detected by another.	Examples are a P wave detected by the ventricular channel or a QRS complex detected by the atrial channel.
Hysteresis	A programmable function where the escape interval after a sensed event is greater than the automatic interval.	Allows more opportunity for intrinsic depolarization before the next pacemaker output.
Lower rate interval/ Lower rate limit (**LRI/LRL**)	The interval that sets the heart rate below which pacing will occur.	In dual-chamber pacing, comprised of the VA and AV intervals.
Maximum tracking interval/ Maximum tracking rate (**MTI/MTR**)	In dual-chamber pacing, the interval that sets the maximum rate the device will track an atrial sensed event in a 1:1 relationship.	Also called upper rate interval (URI) or upper rate limit (URL).
Pacemaker-mediated tachycardia (**PMT**)	A perpetuated arrhythmia where the pacemaker acts as the antegrade limb and the AV node as the retrograde limb of the circuit.	Typically, a VPC induced retrograde atrial impulse falls outside of the PVARP, triggering ventricular pacing and initiating a repetitive cycle.
Post-atrial ventricular blanking period (**PAVBP**)	A short interval after delivery of an atrial output where the ventricular sensing is completely disabled.	Intended to prevent cross-talk.
Post-ventricular atrial refractory period (**PVARP**)	In dual-chamber pacing, the period after a ventricular event (paced or sensed) when the atrial channel will not track a sensed event.	Intended to prevent a premature or retrograde atrial depolarization from initiating a pacemaker-mediated tachycardia.
Refractory period	In pacing, a period following a sensed or paced event where any sensed event will not track or reset a timing cycle.	Dual-chamber devices have separate refractory periods for each chamber.
Total atrial refractory period (**TARP**)	Combination of the AVI and PVARP.	In a dual-chamber device, determines the upper rate behavior 2:1 response.
Upper rate interval/ Upper rate limit (**URI/URL**)	See Maximum tracking interval/rate.	
Ventricular-atrial interval (**VAI**)	In dual-chamber pacing, initiated by a ventricular event (paced or sensed) and ending with the next atrial paced event.	Also called the atrial escape interval, don't confuse with the identical term used with a single-chamber atrial pacemaker.
Ventricular escape interval (**VEI**)	The interval after a ventricular sensed event and the next pacemaker output.	In the absence of hysteresis, the ventricular escape interval equals the automatic (pacing) interval.
Ventricular refractory period (**VRP**)	The period after a ventricular event (paced or sensed) where any further ventricular sensed event is ignored.	

Chapter 21 • SELF-TEST

1. A ventricular pacemaker placed in the right ventricular apex typically shows what type of QRS complex morphology in lead V1?

2. What is the difference between a ventricular fusion and pseudofusion complex?

3. What is the purpose of adding a left ventricular lead to right ventricular pacing?

4. Define the first four letters of the pacemaker programming modes.

5. Pacemaker timing cycles are converted from heart rate in beats per minute into what unit of measurement?

6. In a single-chamber ventricular pacemaker, define the automatic and escape intervals.

7. Define hysteresis in a ventricular pacemaker programmed to VVI mode.

8. What are the four possible ECG patterns associated with a dual-chamber pacemaker programmed to DDD mode?

9. In a dual-chamber pacemaker programmed to DDD mode, what comprises the lower rate interval?

10. In a dual-chamber pacemaker programmed to DDD mode, what comprises the total atrial refractory period (TARP)?

11. Explain a typical mechanism of a pacemaker-mediated tachycardia in a dual-chamber pacemaker programmed to DDD mode.

12. How can you quickly interrupt a pacemaker-mediated tachycardia?

13. Myopotential inhibition of pacemaker output is an example of what type of pacemaker malfunction?

14. "Double counting" of a large T wave as a QRS is an example of what type of pacemaker malfunction?

15. Failure to recognize a VPC is an example of what type of pacemaker malfunction?

QUESTIONS

Chapter 21 • SELF-TEST

1. LBBB-type configuration.

2. A fusion complex is a hybrid that represents both intrinsic ventricular depolarization and that from the pacemaker stimulus. A pseudofusion complex is one where a pacemaker artifact appears in the vicinity of the QRS complex without any evidence of pacemaker capture.

3. A left ventricular lead allows for pacing of both ventricles (biventricular) and alleviation of cardiac dyssynchrony.

4. • Position I: Chamber(s) paced (O = none, A = atrium, V = Ventricle, D = Dual, A + V).
   • Position II: Chamber(s) sensed (O = none, A = atrium, V = Ventricle, D = Dual, A + V).
   • Position III: Response to sensing (O = none, I = inhibited, T = triggered, D = dual, I + T).
   • Position IV: Rate modulation (O = none, R = rate modulation).

5. Milliseconds.

6. In a single-chamber ventricular device, the automatic interval (also known as the pacing, basic, or demand interval) is the programmed period between two consecutive paced outputs. The ventricular escape interval is the period between a ventricular sensed event and the next ventricular output. In the absence of hysteresis, the automatic interval is identical to the escape interval.

7. After a sensed event, the programmed ventricular escape interval is longer than the automatic (pacing) interval. This is utilized to allow added time for intrinsic conduction while pacing at an effective rate on demand.

8. • Atrial pacing-ventricular pacing.
   • Atrial pacing-ventricular sensing.
   • Atrial sensing-ventricular pacing.
   • Atrial sensing-ventricular sensing.

9. The combination of the ventricular-atrial interval (VAI) and AV interval (AVI). This represents the time interval between two ventricular outputs.

10. The combination of the AV interval (AVI) and post-ventricular atrial refractory period (PVARP).

11. A VPC results in retrograde atrial depolarization that arrives beyond the PVARP. The atrial depolarization is sensed by the atrial channel, which then generates a triggered ventricular response. The cycle repeats, perpetuating a PMT.

12. Place a magnet over the device, which temporarily inhibits sensing function and converts the device to asynchronous pacing.

13. Oversensing.

14. Oversensing.

15. Undersensing.

Further Reading

Alasti M, Machado C, Rangasamy K, et al. Pacemaker-mediated arrhythmias. *J Arrhythm*. 2018;34:485-492.

Aqualina O. A brief history of cardiac pacing. *Images Paedeatr Cardiol*. 2006;8:17-81.

Atlee JL, Bernstein AD. Cardiac rhythm management devices (Part I): indications device selection and function. *Anesthesiology*. 2001;95:1265-1280.

Atlee JL, Bernstein AD. Cardiac rhythm management devices (Part II): perioperative management. *Anesthesiology*. 2001;95:1492-1506.

Bernstein AD, Daubert JC, Fletcher RS, et al. The revised NASPE/BPEG generic code for antibradycardia, adaptive-rate, and multisite pacing. *PACE*. 2002;25:260-264.

Harper RJ, Brady WJ, Perron Ad, Mangrum M. The paced electrocardiogram: issues for the emergency physician. *Am J Emerg Med*. 2001;19:551-560.

Hayes DL, Vlietstra RE. Pacemaker malfunction. *Ann Intern Med*. 1993;119:828-835.

Jacob S, Panaich SS, Maheshwari R, Haddad JW, Padaniliam BJ, John SK. Clinical applications of magnets on cardiac rhythm management devices. *Europace*. 2011;13:1222-1230.

Jastrezebski M, Kukla P, Fijorek K, Czarnecka D. Universal algorithm for diagnosis of biventricular capture in patients with cardiac resynchronization therapy. *PACE*. 2014;37:986-993.

Locati ET, Bagliani G, Testoni A, Lunati M, Padeletti L. Role of surface electrocardiograms in patients with cardiac implantable electronic devices. *Card Electrophysiol Clin.* 2018;10:233-255.

Mond HG. Interpreting the normal pacemaker electrocardiograph. *Heart Lung Circ.* 2019;28:233-236.

Mond HG. The footprints of pacing lead position using the 12-lead electrocardiograph. *Heart Lung Circ.* 2020; https://doi.org/10.1016/j.hlc.2020.08.029.

Mulpuru SK, Madhavan M, McLeod CJ, Cha YM, Friedman PA. Cardiac pacemakers: function, troubleshooting and management. *J Am Coll Cardiol.* 2017;67:189-210.

Sgarbossa EB, Pinski SL, Gates KB, Wagner GS. Early electrocardiographic diagnosis of acute myocardial infarction in the presence of ventricular paced rhythm. *Am J Cardiol.* 1996;77:423-424.

Sharma PS, Ellenbogen KA, Trohman RG. Permanent His bundle pacing: the past, present and future. *J Cardiovasc Electrophysiol.* 2017;28:458-465.

Venkatachalam KL. Common pitfalls in interpreting pacemaker electrocardiograms in the emergency department. *J Electrocardiol.* 2011;4:616-621.

Zhang S, Zhou X, Gold MR. Left bundle branch pacing. *J Am Coll Cardiol.* 2019;74:3039-3049.

SECTION V
Medications, Metabolic, and More

Medication Effects and QT Syndromes

▶ INTRODUCTION

In this chapter we will review how the ECG is affected by medications, both cardiac and noncardiac. We'll pay special attention to medications that prolong the QTc interval, which may predispose to life-threatening arrhythmias. Afterwards, we'll discuss hereditary QT syndromes and other channelopathies that may pose a similar risk.

▶ MEDICATIONS

Action Potential Review

Before we go into detail about the effect of medications on the ECG, let's review our old friend the action potential (**Figure 22-1**). Antiarrhythmic medications exert their effect by altering ion channels, the opening and closing of which determine the phases of the action potential. Here is a summary of what we reviewed in detail in Chapter 3.

Nonpacemaker cell **Figure 22-1a** displays the typical action potential of a nonpacemaker cell of the ventricular myocardium. Remember that there are five distinct phases (phases 0-4).

Phase 0 (rapid depolarization) is the rapid upstroke of the action potential that represents depolarization. A stimulus from adjacent cells opens gated sodium (Na^+) channels, causing the membrane potential to become less negative. When the voltage reaches the threshold potential, typically in the range of -60 mV to -70 mV, even more Na^+ channels open to permit a rapid, self-sustaining entry of Na^+ ions into the cell, coining the term "fast response."

Phase 1 (early rapid repolarization) is the initial repolarization of the cell. It reflects the final closing of the gated Na^+ channels and opening of outward K^+ channels. There is a net loss of positive ions from the cell, which lowers the transiently positive membrane potential to approximately 0 mV.

Phase 2 (plateau) represents a delay in repolarization. Slow Ca^{2+} channels open that allow a weak, inward flow of Ca^{2+} into the cell. K^+ continues to exit the cell as Ca^{2+} slowly enters. There is a near balance of inward-flowing Ca^{2+} ions and outward-flowing K^+ ions, which produces the plateau.

Phase 3 (terminal rapid repolarization) restores the negative membrane potential. K^+ ions continue to exit the cell as the slow Ca^{2+} channels are inactivated. The membrane potential becomes progressively more negative until repolarization is complete.

Phase 4 (resting) represents the time between action potentials. This is when a nonpacemaker cell establishes a stable resting membrane potential of -90 mV using the three-step process we reviewed in Chapter 3 that includes (1) the Na^+/K^+–ATPase pump, (2) K^+ diffusion out of the cell via open channels, and (3) the balancing of electrostatic and chemical forces.

Pacemaker cell **Figure 22-1b** displays the typical action potential of a pacemaker cell of the SA node. The action potential of pacemaker cells of the AV junction has a similar configuration. Remember there are key differences between the action potential of a pacemaker cell compared with that of a nonpacemaker cell.

Phase 0 (slow depolarization) in pacemaker cells has a slower upstroke and lower amplitude than nonpacemaker cells, hence the term, "slow response." Depolarization in pacemaker cells is dependent on the slow influx of Ca^{2+}. The fast Na^+ channels responsible for the rapid phase 0 response in nonpacemaker cells are inactivated in pacemaker cells.

Phase 3 (repolarization) represents inactivation of the Ca^{2+} channel and the opening of K^+ channels, which result

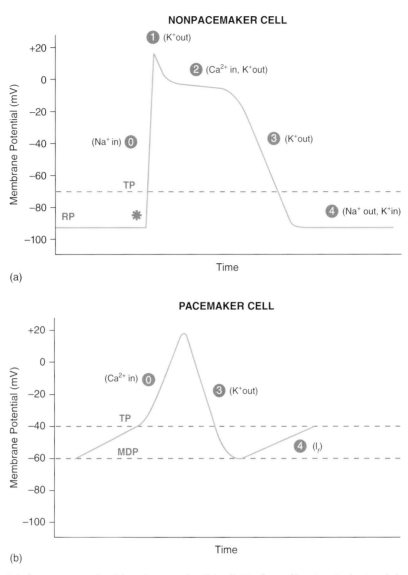

Figure 22-1. Action potential of a nonpacemaker (a) and pacemaker (b) cell. The flow of key ions is depicted during each phase (see text for details). Abbreviations: resting potential (RP), threshold potential (TP), maximum diastolic potential (MDP), funny current (I_f), depolarizing stimulus (*).

in repolarization of the cell, typically to a level of −60 mV. The action potential of pacemaker cells does not have a true phase 1 or phase 2.

Phase 4 (diastolic depolarization) in pacemaker cells demonstrates the property of automaticity, characterized by a gradually upward slope and absence of a true resting potential. This means that these cells can reach their threshold potential, typically −30 to −40 mV, and initiate depolarization on their own without an outside stimulus. Because of a number of unique characteristics, this primary pacemaker current is termed the "funny current" (I_f). Another current contributing to pacemaker function is mediated by the oscillatory exchange of Na^+ and Ca^{2+} ions and is termed the "calcium clock."

Proarrhythmia

An important concern with antiarrhythmic agents and many noncardiac medications is the potential for *proarrhythmia*.

This is the term used to describe either provoking *de novo* or increasing the frequency of cardiac arrhythmias. This is particularly true for agents that **prolong the QTc interval**, which may lead to *torsades de pointes* (TdP). We learned in Chapter 19 that TdP is a polymorphic ventricular tachycardia characterized by QRS peaks that "twist" around the baseline (**Figure 22-2**). Medications that prolong the QTc interval characteristically do so by blocking one or more repolarizing K^+ currents in nonpacemaker cells, thereby prolonging phase 3 of the action potential. The presence of QTc interval prolongation due to medications and other contributing factors such as electrolyte disturbances (eg, hypokalemia and hypomagnesemia) and myocardial ischemia, defines an *acquired* or *secondary* QTc prolongation syndrome. This distinguishes this entity from a *hereditary* or *primary* prolonged QTc syndrome that is associated with a genetic mutation of cardiac ion channels (discussed later under inherited channelopathies).

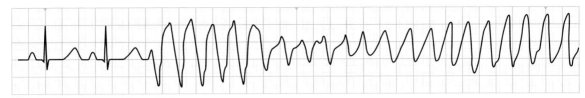

Figure 22-2. *Torsades de pointes.* The peaks of the QRS complexes twist around the baseline. Note the prolonged QT interval of the native complex.

 FOR BOOKWORMS: Prolongation of phase 3 of the action potential in nonpacemaker cells increases the potential for early afterdepolarizations (see Chapter 13). These oscillations are a form of triggered activity that generates additional action potentials. Propagation of these depolarizations may induce repetitive ventricular premature depolarizations and TdP. Note that QTc interval prolongation is not the sole determinant of the potential for drug-induced TdP. Additional factors play a role, including whether the drug promotes dispersion of refractoriness in the ventricular myocardium, resulting in heterogeneity of tissue repolarization that sets the stage for reentry. The underlying electrophysiologic mechanisms for the development of TdP are complex and subject to continuing debate.

QT or Not QT: That Is the Question

Let's pause a moment to review the significance of the QT interval and how to measure it properly. The QT interval represents the sum of ventricular depolarization and repolarization. The QT interval includes the QRS complex, which records ventricular activation and early repolarization. The remainder of the QT interval represents the completion of ventricular repolarization, which begins at the J point and concludes with the end of the T wave. As we discussed in Chapter 4, accurate measurement of the QT interval can be vexing because of a variety of issues. These include (1) difficulty in the proper identification of the end of the T wave, (2) accounting for differences in the QT interval in various leads, (3) variability of the QT interval with heart rate and gender, and (4) factoring in the effect of the QRS duration.

Measure the QT interval in the lead with the longest QT duration. Inspect leads II and V5 initially, but remember that the most accurately determined QT interval may be in another lead. Note that the QT interval may normally vary in different leads by as much as 40 msec, a term called *QT dispersion*. Be sure to identify the true end of the T wave and not mistakenly measure a superimposed U wave or P wave. It is often helpful to use the tangent method of measurement, drawing a line from the maximum downslope of the T wave until it intersects the baseline (**Figure 22-3**).

The normal QT interval varies with the heart rate. As the heart rate slows, the QT interval lengthens; and as the heart rate rises, the QT interval shortens. Therefore, the measured QT interval requires a mathematical correction for heart rate called the **QTc**. A variety of methods exist for calculating the QTc. The most common method is the Bazett formula, which is the QTc = QT interval (measured in seconds) divided by the

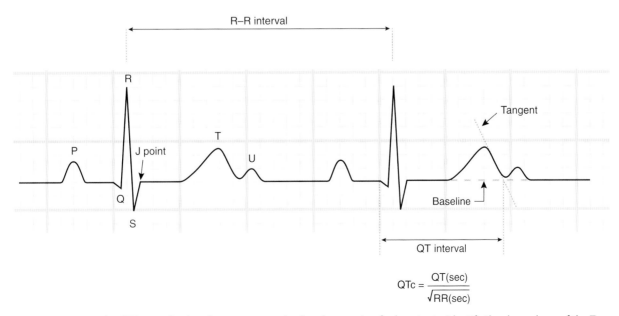

$$QTc = \frac{QT(sec)}{\sqrt{RR(sec)}}$$

Figure 22-3. Measuring the QT interval using the tangent method and correcting for heart rate. Identify the downslope of the T wave and draw a line until intersecting a baseline derived from the TP segment. The QT interval is the distance from the onset of the Q wave to this point. Dividing the QT interval in seconds by the square root of the R-R interval in seconds derives a corrected QT interval (QTc).

square root of the R-R interval (measured in seconds). The formula assumes a stable R-R interval and is most valid between the heart rates of 60 and 100 beats per minute (bpm).

Tables exist that calculate the normal range of QTc, but these are not always available at the bedside. A quick way to evaluate for QT prolongation, valid between a heart rate of 60 to 100 bpm, is to assess whether the QT interval is less than half of the R-R interval. It's easy to use this method by counting the number of small boxes for each interval and doing a simple calculation, checking whether the number of boxes you count for the QT interval is less than half those of the R-R interval. A QT interval more than half of the R-R interval is potentially abnormal and a more formal mathematical calculation is warranted.

The QTc is also affected by gender. Women normally have a longer QTc than men.

Although there remains considerable debate, it's reasonable to use the following guidelines for the upper and lower limits of the corrected QT interval (QTc). Values that are outside these require further evaluation for QTc interval prolongation or shortening, either of which may predispose a patient to life-threatening arrhythmias.

Men: >390 msec to <450 msec

Women: >390 msec to <460 msec

 BE CAREFUL: Manual measurements of the QT interval are more accurate than the values derived on automated digital ECG machines. They often use a multiple-lead algorithm that measures the QT interval from the earliest Q wave in *any* lead to the latest T wave in *any* lead. Consequently, the values for the automated QT and QTc intervals are frequently longer than one found in any individual lead.

Antiarrhythmic Agents

Agents used to treat cardiac arrhythmias exert their effects by altering the Na⁺, K⁺, and Ca²⁺ ion channels we discussed earlier as well as by modifying beta-adrenergic mechanisms. The medications alter the phases of the action potential, impacting conduction and refractoriness, which ultimately translate into findings recorded on the ECG (**Figure 22-4**). Antiarrhythmic drugs have been traditionally classified into four major groups (I-IV) that are based on their predominant mechanism of action. This is a gross oversimplification because many of the agents have actions that target multiple ion channels. In addition, there are antiarrhythmic drugs that do not fall into one of the classical four categories. Despite these limitations, the original grouping as introduced in 1970 by Miles Vaughan Williams is useful to predict both the potential therapeutic and adverse effects of these agents as well as the expected electrocardiographic findings. Let's go over the basics of the major drug categories and how they impact the ECG.

Class I—Na⁺-channel blockers
All class I drugs act by modulating or blocking voltage-gated Na⁺ channels at phase 0 of the action potential. The class is divided into three subgroups (IA, IB, IC) depending on whether the degree of Na⁺-channel

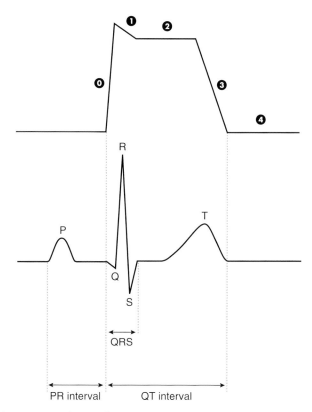

Figure 22-4. Phases of a ventricular myocardial cell action potential as related to the surface ECG.

blockade is moderate (IA), weak (IB), or strong (IC). Some agents also have K⁺-channel modulating properties that affect repolarization. The differing Na⁺ and K⁺ blocking properties predict their varying effects on the ECG (**Figure 22-5**).

Class IA agents include quinidine, procainamide, and disopyramide. They moderately block and decrease the rate of rise of phase 0 of the action potential, which can result in a mild widening of the QRS complex. Agents in this class also block K⁺ channels, prolonging repolarization. This can produce a significant and clinically important prolongation of the QTc interval.

Class IB agents are lidocaine and mexiletine, as well as the antiepileptic medication phenytoin. These agents exhibit weak Na⁺-channel blockade and may slightly shorten the QTc interval. Overall, there is minimal effect on the ECG.

Class IC agents include flecainide and propafenone. They have the most profound Na⁺-channel blockade, thereby slowing phase 0 depolarization and producing the greatest QRS complex prolongation. Repolarization is unaffected; therefore the overall action potential duration is unchanged.

Class II—Beta-adrenergic blockers
Class II drugs act by inhibiting sympathetic activity via the blockade of beta-adrenergic receptors. Among many others, medications in this class include atenolol, metoprolol, carvedilol, and propranolol. These medications reduce SA node automaticity, which may produce sinus bradycardia. They also slow AV node conduction, which prolongs the PR interval in sinus rhythm and reduces the ventricular rate in the setting of some atrial arrhythmias.

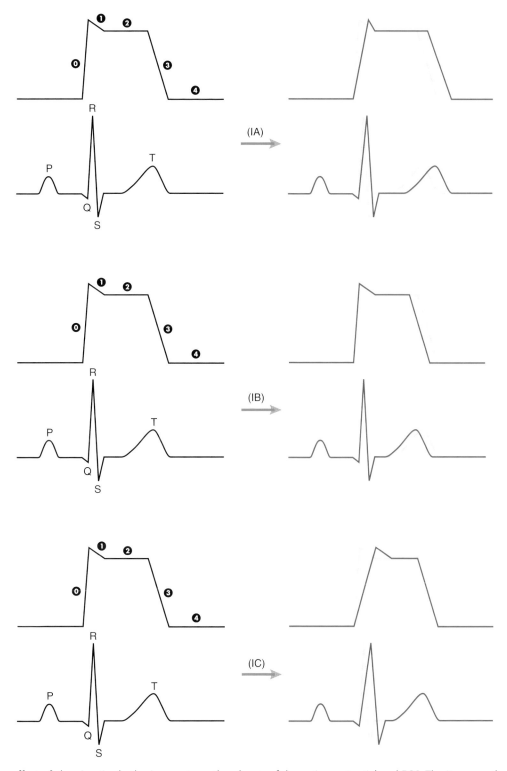

Figure 22-5. The effect of class I antiarrhythmic agents on the phases of the action potential and ECG. The items on the right side of the figure illustrate the drug effect (red) versus the baseline findings (gray). Class IA drugs (top) mildly increase the QRS complex and prolong the QTc interval. Class IB drugs (middle) minimally alter the ECG with slight QTc interval shortening. Class IC drugs (bottom) prolong the QRS complex with minimal effect on the QTc interval.

Class III—K⁺-channel blockers Class III agents include sotolol, amiodarone, dronedarone, and ibutilide. These complex agents have a predominant action of blocking K⁺ channels. This prolongs repolarization and widens the QTc interval

(**Figure 22-6**). Medications in this class have varying properties that overlap into other classes. Amiodarone, despite increasing the QTc interval, has a low propensity for inducing TdP. It prolongs repolarization in a more homogenous manner, avoiding

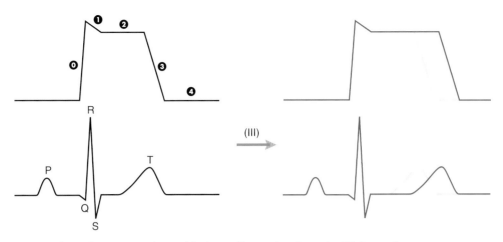

Figure 22-6. Class III agents have the greatest phase 3 blocking effect and prolong the QTc interval.

the tissue dispersion and heterogeneity that promotes reentry. Other agents in this class have a higher risk of TdP.

Class IV—Ca²⁺ channel blockers Agents in class IV include nondihydropyridine medications such as diltiazem and verapamil. Their predominant action is to block the slow calcium channels in both the SA and AV nodes. This decreases automaticity and reduces AV conduction, which can slow the sinus rate, prolong the PR interval, and reduce the ventricular response in the presence of atrial arrhythmias.

FOR BOOKWORMS: An updated classification system of antiarrhythmic agents has been developed. The Modernized Oxford Classification introduces additional categories for agents that have targets outside of the original Vaughan Williams classification. In addition to the original classes I-IV, the new categories are: Class 0—blockers of ion channels involved in automaticity, Class V—mechanically sensitive channel blockers, Class VI—gap junction channel blockers, and Class VII—upstream target modulators affecting structural remodeling. Also introduced in this new scheme are subclasses within each category.

Another concept influencing the effect of an antiarrhythmic drug is that of *use dependence*. This refers to the relationship between the pharmacologic effects of an agent relative to heart rate. Ion channel blockers that show use dependence have a greater effect at higher heart rates. In contrast, agents with *reverse-use dependence* exert a greater effect at slower heart rates.

Digitalis

Digitalis glycosides (eg, digoxin) do not fall into any of the Vaughan Williams drug categories. They have a complex therapeutic action that includes inotropic effects that increase the force of cardiac contraction in ventricular myocardial cells and vagotonic actions that slow conduction through the AV node. The electrophysiologic properties and ECG findings associated with digitalis depend on the specific tissues involved (eg, atrial and ventricular myocardium versus the specialized conduction

system) and whether the drug is acting within a therapeutic or toxic range.

The positive inotropic effect of digitalis in ventricular myocardial cells works by inhibiting the activity of Na⁺/K⁺–ATPase. When this pump is inhibited, less Na⁺ is removed from the cell thereby increasing the concentration of intracellular Na⁺ and decreasing the concentration of intracellular K⁺. Ultimately, the Na⁺ ions are exchanged for Ca²⁺ ions, which increase the force of cardiac muscle contraction. The speed of repolarization is enhanced, shortening the refractory period. This is believed to explain the ECG findings of **digitalis effect**, which is a characteristic "scoop" of the ST segment, depression of T wave amplitude (without changing direction), and shortening of the QTc interval (**Figure 22-7**).

Digitalis slows conduction by enhancing vagal tone, prolonging the effective refractory period of the AV node. This increases the PR interval in sinus rhythm and decreases the ventricular response in the setting of atrial arrhythmias.

Digitalis toxicity is associated with a multitude of cardiac arrhythmias, which are due to more than one electrophysiologic mechanism. At high concentration, digitalis reduces the resting potential of phase 4, augmenting the rate of diastolic depolarization. This leads to hyper-automaticity, which may produce ectopic and accelerated rhythms throughout the atrium, AV junction, and the ventricles. High levels of intracellular Ca²⁺ during phase 4 may induce triggered activity with delayed afterdepolarizations. AV conduction abnormalities may produce varying degrees of AV block. The following list includes the multitude of cardiac arrhythmias associated with digitalis toxicity.

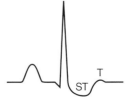

Figure 22-7. Digitalis effect characteristically shows a ST segment "scoop" and shortening of the QTc interval.

- Sinus and AV conduction abnormalities.
  - Sinus bradycardia.
  - SA block.
  - First-degree AV block (may not represent clinical toxicity).
  - Second-degree AV block.
  - High grade and third-degree AV block.
- Atrial arrhythmias.
  - Atrial premature complexes.
  - Atrial tachycardia (characteristically with AV block).
  - Accelerated AV junctional rhythm and tachycardia.
  - AV junctional rhythm associated with atrial fibrillation and complete AV block.
- Ventricular arrhythmias.
  - Ventricular premature complexes (often multiform).
  - Ventricular bigeminy.
  - Ventricular tachycardia (including bidirectional).
  - Ventricular fibrillation.

 CLINICAL TIP: Do not rely on measurement of the serum digoxin level to exclude a toxic medication effect. A value within the "therapeutic range" listed by the laboratory may still be clinically toxic. For example, consider an elderly patient with atrial fibrillation treated with digoxin presenting with complete AV block and an accelerated junctional rhythm. You don't need a digoxin level in order to recognize the medication is demonstrating a toxic pharmacologic effect and that you need to discontinue the drug and consider administering digoxin-binding antibodies as an antidote. Also pay attention to interactions of digoxin with other medications, as well as electrolyte abnormalities (particularly hypokalemia), which may potentiate digoxin toxicity.

Psychotropic Medications

Psychoactive medications are recognized to have significant electrophysiologic effects that can lead to cardiac arrhythmias. They have properties that modify cardiac ion channels that affect the action potential as well as anticholinergic effects that impact heart rate.

Antidepressants Tricyclic antidepressant medications (eg, amitriptyline, imipramine, nortriptyline) have properties of class IA type Na^+-channel blockers. At therapeutic levels, the effects on the ECG are usually minimal, but can include mild prolongation of the PR interval, QRS complex, and QTc interval. Increased drug levels may result in significant QTc prolongation (**Figure 22-8**). Toxic levels of tricyclic agents produce characteristic ECG findings. In addition to QRS complex and QTc interval prolongation, tricyclic drug toxicity results in an abnormal QRS complex morphology consisting of deep, slurred S waves in leads I and aVL along with an increase in R wave amplitude and the R/S ratio in lead aVR, findings that reflect a rightward shift of the terminal 40 msec of the frontal plane QRS vector. In contrast, selective serotonin uptake inhibitors (SSRIs) appear to have a low risk of drug-induced QTc interval prolongation and TdP. The exception is citalopram, which in higher doses (>40 mg/day) is reported to increase the QTc interval and is associated with cardiac arrhythmias.

Antipsychotics Phenothiazines and related medications have anticholinergic properties that can increase the heart rate. Thioridazine, and to a lesser extent chlorpromazine is associated with QTc prolongation. Haloperidol, particularly when administered intravenously in higher doses, has been associated with QTc prolongation, TdP, and sudden death. The higher risk attributed to the intravenous versus oral administration is a subject of debate and confounded by additional risk factors for QTc interval prolongation. Some second-generation antipsychotic agents have been associated with QTc interval prolongation, but a relationship with TdP is unconfirmed. Of medications in this class, ziprasidone is reported to have the greatest QTc interval prolonging effect.

Opiates Methadone is a synthetic opioid agonist that is associated with QTc prolongation and TdP. The risk appears to be dose-related and higher in individuals undergoing long-term treatment.

Other Medications

Many other medications are associated with QTc prolongation. These include macrolide antibiotics (eg, erythromycin, azithromycin, clarithromycin), fluoroquinolone antibiotics (eg, ciprofloxacin, levofloxacin, gatifloxacin), antifungals (eg, fluconazole, itraconazole, ketoconazole), and antimalarial agents (eg, chloroquine, hydroxychloroquine).

 CLINICAL TIP: The list of potential QTc interval-prolonging medications discussed in this chapter is but a representative sample of an exhaustive list. As noted, not every drug that increases the QTc interval is associated with TdP. However, use caution when prescribing multiple agents that might increase the risk when used in combination. Also be aware of coexistent risk factors that include female gender, electrolyte abnormalities, and baseline bradycardia. Concern is greatest when the QTc is >500 msec and/or there is a drug-induced increase of the QTc >60 msec.

► INHERITED CHANNELOPATHIES

Hereditary (congenital) long QT syndrome (LQTS) results from one of a number of genetic mutations that alters the function of cardiac ion channels responsible for repolarization. LQTS is not one disorder and the list of identifiable genetic defects responsible for the various forms continues to expand. In most cases, QTc interval prolongation results from interference with K^+ channels responsible for phase 3 repolarization. At least one known form interferes with a late repolarizing Na^+ current. All forms of LQTS present a risk of TdP, which is higher when accompanied by bradycardia and electrolyte disturbances. Different from the acquired form of LQTS is the role of sympathetic activity, where a sudden surge in tone can be a trigger for TdP. Inherited LQTS may be "uncovered" when QTc interval prolongation becomes evident after treatment with a potentiating medication.

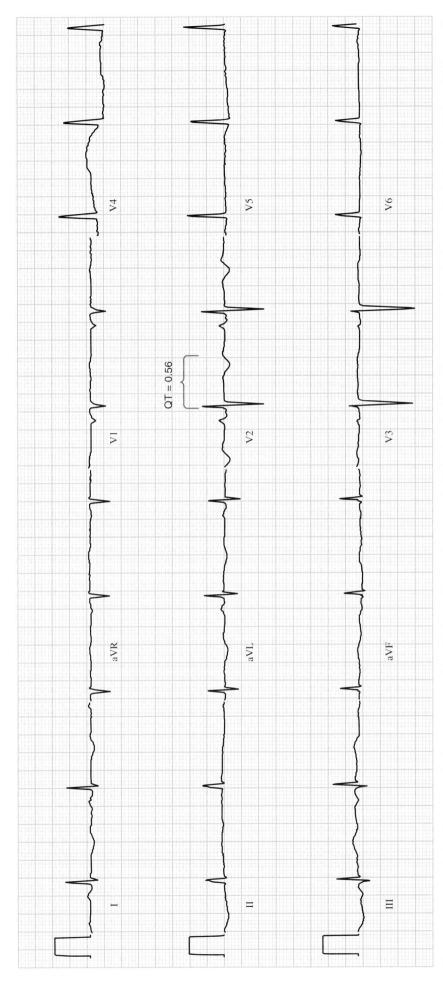

QT = 0.56

Figure 22-8. 12-lead ECG showing marked prolongation of the QTc interval in a patient treated with both a tricyclic antidepressant and a quinolone antibiotic. Here, the QT (and QTc) interval is 0.56 sec.

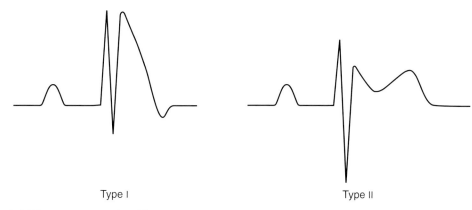

Type I   Type II

Figure 22-9. Brugada ECG patterns, types I and II.

Short QT syndrome (SQTS) is a rare, genetically heterogeneous syndrome associated with marked shortening of the QTc interval and sudden cardiac arrest. Paroxysmal atrial fibrillation is also common in this disorder. The syndrome should be suspected when a patient has unexplained cardiac arrest or syncope, a family history of same, and an unusually short QTc interval. Universally accepted diagnostic criteria for the lower limit of the QTc interval are lacking, but it is reasonable to consider a short QTc interval in men as <360 msec and <370 msec in women. Most patients with SQTS have a QTc interval of ≤340 msec. In diagnosing SQTS, other causes of a short QTc interval (eg, digitalis, hypercalcemia) must be absent. Additional ECG findings of SQTS include tall, peaked T waves in the precordial leads with either an absent or very short ST segment. Importantly, the mere presence of a short QTc interval is insufficient to make a diagnosis of SQTS and does not alone impart an increased risk of sudden cardiac death. Diagnosis of SQTS requires a short QTc *and* further investigation into clinical symptoms, family history, and genetic testing.

The Brugada syndrome is a genetic Na^+ ion channelopathy characterized by an increased risk of sudden arrhythmic death in patients with structurally normal hearts and who have specific ECG findings of the *Brugada pattern*. The Brugada pattern ECG refers to a QRS complex that resembles a right bundle branch block with an unusual form of ST segment elevation in the right precordial leads (V1 and V2). Two distinct electrocardiographic Brugada patterns are recognized (**Figure 22-9**). Type 1 is characterized by coved ST segment elevation of ≥2 mm followed by a negative T wave. This is the pattern diagnostically associated with the Brugada syndrome. Type 2 has ST segment elevation of ≥2 mm shaped like a "saddleback" followed by a positive or biphasic T wave. This pattern is considered "suggestive," but not diagnostic of the Brugada syndrome. Confounding the diagnosis is that the Brugada pattern ECG can fluctuate over time and may be evident only in the presence of fever, bradycardia with autonomic imbalance, or after administration of Na^+-channel blocking drugs (eg, flecainide, procainamide, ajmaline).

All hereditary channelopathies share a common theme of a mutation in one or more genes that affect cardiac ion channels. These ultimately impact phases of the action potential involving depolarization and repolarization, which may predispose the patient to life-threatening arrhythmias and sudden cardiac death. Despite their rarity, it is important to recognize these patterns, particularly in patients surviving cardiac arrest so treatment can be appropriately directed and family members screened.

QUESTIONS

Chapter 22 • SELF-TEST

1. Briefly identify the five phases of the action potential of a nonpacemaker cardiac myocyte.

2. Define proarrhythmia.

3. What is the name of the polymorphic ventricular tachycardia associated with prolongation of the QTc interval?

4. Describe the predominant ECG findings of agents in the following subclasses of class I antiarrhythmic drugs:
   • Class IA.
   • Class IB.
   • Class IC.

5. Describe the predominant ECG findings of class III antiarrhythmic drugs.

6. Describe the characteristic ECG findings of digitalis effect.

7. Agents that block depolarizing Na^+ channels and prolong phase 0 of the action potential will result in what ECG finding?

8. Agents that block repolarizing K^+-channel and prolong phase 3 of the action potential will result in what ECG finding?

9. In patients with a prolonged QTc interval, name three risk factors that increase the potential for *torsades de pointes*.

10. Describe the typical Brugada pattern ECG findings that are associated with the Brugada syndrome.

ANSWERS

Chapter 22 • SELF-TEST

1. The five phases of the action potential of a nonpacemaker cardiac myocyte are:
   • Phase 0—rapid depolarization.
   • Phase 1—early rapid repolarization.
   • Phase 2—plateau.
   • Phase 3—terminal rapid repolarization.
   • Phase 4—resting.

2. Proarrhythmia is either the provocation *de novo* or increase in the frequency of cardiac arrhythmias.

3. *Torsades de pointes.*

4. The predominant ECG findings of agents in the following subclasses of class I antiarrhythmic drugs are:
   • Class IA—mild prolongation of the QRS complex and greater prolongation of the QTc interval.
   • Class IB—minimal shortening of the QTc interval with minimal ECG change overall.
   • Class IC—QRS complex prolongation with no significant effect on the QTc interval.

5. The predominant ECG finding of class III antiarrhythmic drugs is the prolongation of the QTc interval.

6. Digitalis effect is a "scoop" of the ST segment, depression of T wave amplitude (without changing direction), and shortening of the QTc interval.

7. QRS complex prolongation.

8. QTc interval prolongation.

9. In patients with a prolonged QTc interval, risk factors that increase the potential for *torsades de pointes* include (1) bradycardia, (2) female gender, and (3) hypokalemia.

10. A complex resembling a RBBB in leads V1-V2 that includes a coved ST segment elevation of ≥2 mm followed by a negative T wave (type I Brugada pattern).

Further Reading

Bayes de Luna A, Brugada J, Baranchuk A, et al. Current electrocardiographic criteria for diagnosis of Brugada pattern: a consensus report. *J Electrocardiol*. 2012;45:433-442.

Beach SR, Celano CM, Noseworthy PA, Januzzi JL, Huffman JC. QTc prolongation, torsades de pointes, and psychotropic medications. *Psychosomatics*. 2013;54:1-13.

Beach SR, Celano CM, Sugrue AM, et al. QT prolongation, torsades de pointes, and psychotropic medications: a 5-year update. *Psychosomatics*. 2018;59:105-122.

Belardinelli L, Antzelevith C, Vos MA. Assessing predictors of drug-induced torsades de pointes. *Trends Pharmacol Sci*. 2003;24:619-625.

Bjerregaard P, Hallapaneni H, Gussak I. Short QT interval in clinical practice. *J Electrocardiol*. 2010;42:390-395.

Brouillette J, Nattel S. A practical approach to avoiding cardiovascular adverse effects of psychoactive medications. *Can J Cardiol*. 2017;33:1577-1586.

Brugada J, Campuzano O, Arbelo E, Sarquella-brugada G, Brugada R. Present status of Brugada syndrome. *J Am Coll Cardiol*. 2018;72:1046-1059.

Dewi IP, Dharmadjati BB. Short QT syndrome: the current evidences of diagnosis and management. *J Arrhythm*. 2020;36:962-966.

Drew BJ, Ackerman MJ, Funk M, et al. Prevention of torsades de pointes in hospital settings. *J Am Coll Cardiol*. 2010;55:934-947.

Fisch C, Knoebel SB. Digitalis cardiotoxicity. *J Am Coll Cardiol*. 1985;5:91A-98A.

Groleau G, Jotte R, Barish R. The electrocardiographic manifestation of cyclic antidepressant therapy and overdose: a review. *J Emerg Med*. 1990;8:597-605.

Kramer DB, Zimetbaum PJ. Long-QT syndrome. *Cardiol Rev*. 2011;19:217-225.

Locati E, Bagliani G, Padeletti L. Normal ventricular repolarization and QT interval. *Card Electrophysiol Clin*. 2017;9:487-513.

Lei M, Wu L, Terrar DA, Luang CLH. Modernized classification of cardiac antiarrhythmic drugs. *Circulation*. 2018;138:1879-1896.

Marriott HJL, Conover MB. Digitalis dysrhythmias. In: *Advanced Concepts in Arrhythmias*. 3rd ed. St. Louis, Mo: Mosby; 1998:179-201.

Morita H, Wu J, Zipes DP. The QT syndromes: long and short. *Lancet*. 2008;372:750-763.

Roden DM. Drug-induced prolongation of the QT interval. *N Engl J Med*. 2004;350:1013-1022.

Shu J, Zhou J, Patel C, Yan G-X. Pharmacology of cardiac arrhythmias—basic science for clinicians. *PACE*. 2009;32:1454-1465.

Tan HL, You CJY, Laurer MR, Sung RJ. Electrophysiologic mechanisms of the long QT interval syndromes and torsades de pointes. *Ann Intern Med*. 1995;122:701-714.

Whalley DW, Wendt DJ, Grant AO. Basic concepts in cellular cardiac electrophysiology: part II: block of ion channels by antiarrhythmic drugs. *PACE*. 1995;18:1686-1704.

Xiong GL, Pinkhasov A, Mangal JP, et al. QTc monitoring in adults with medical and psychiatric comorbidities: expert consensus from the Association of Medicine and Psychiatry. *J Psychosom Res*. 2020;135:110138.

Yap YG, Camm AJ. Drug induced QT prolongation and torsades de pointes. *Heart*. 2003;89:1363-1372.

ECG Miscellany: Electrolytes, Metabolic, and Other Topics

▶ INTRODUCTION

In this chapter we will review a variety of topics including ECG findings associated with electrolyte, metabolic, environmental, and cerebrovascular disorders. We'll finish up with a few miscellaneous ECG items associated with a number of clinical disorders.

Electrolyte Abnormalities

Hyperkalemia Elevations of serum potassium (K^+) produce changes in the ECG that become more profound with the degree of hyperkalemia (**Figure 23-1**). The normal serum K^+ level is 3.5 to 5.3 milliequivalents per liter (mEq/L). ECG findings of mild hyperkalemia (<6.0 mEq/L) typically manifest as peaked, tall, and symmetrical "tent-shaped" T waves. The QT (QTc) interval is either normal or slightly shortened over baseline. Moderate hyperkalemia (6.0-7.0 mEq/L) produces a further increase in T wave amplitude and a widened QRS complex. In addition, P wave amplitude is diminished and the PR interval is prolonged. In severe hyperkalemia (>7.0 mEq/L), P wave amplitude diminishes further and may become unrecognizable despite the presence of sinus rhythm, a finding called *sinoventricular rhythm*. The QRS complex widens and may merge with the peaked T wave. ST segment elevation in leads V1 and V2 may resemble acute myocardial infarction. With further increases in serum K^+ the QRS complex resembles a sine wave. Cardiac arrest may follow from ventricular tachycardia, ventricular fibrillation, or asystole.

Hypokalemia The earliest ECG finding associated with hypokalemia is a decrease in T wave amplitude. Unlike the situation with hyperkalemia, the ECG findings of hypokalemia do not correlate as well with the serum level. With progressive hypokalemia (<2.7 mEq/L), characteristic findings include slight ST segment depression, a flat or inverted T wave and most significantly, a prominent U wave (**Figure 23-2**). The U wave may be so large as to superimpose on the T wave, making accurate measurement of the QT interval difficult and leading to an erroneous diagnosis of QT prolongation.

Hypercalcemia The normal level of serum calcium (Ca^{2+}) is 8.5 to 10.5 mg/dL. The primary ECG manifestation of hypercalcemia (usually >12.0 mg/dL) is shortening of the QT interval. The duration of the ST segment within the QT interval is decreased, a result of shortening of phase 2 of the action potential. ST segment elevation may also be present, mimicking findings of acute myocardial infarction (**Figure 23-3**).

Hypocalcemia QT prolongation is the characteristic finding of hypocalcemia. Here the action potential is prolonged, increasing the duration of the ST segment within the QT interval (**Figure 23-4**).

Metabolic and Environmental Disorders

Thyroid disorders ECG findings associated with hyperthyroidism include sinus tachycardia and nonspecific ST segment and T wave abnormalities. AV conduction delay may be present including prolongation of the PR interval, and rarely, higher degrees of AV block. Thyrotoxicosis may present clinically as atrial fibrillation with a rapid ventricular response. Hypothyroidism is often associated with sinus bradycardia. Severe hypothyroidism (myxedema) may lead to a large pericardial effusion that produces low-voltage complexes. Additional findings include diffusely inverted T waves, intraventricular conduction delay, and AV conduction abnormalities.

Hypothermia A characteristic ECG feature of profound hypothermia is the *Osborn wave*. Described by Joseph Osborn in

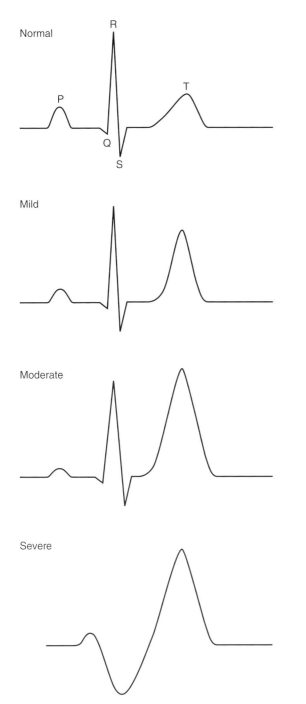

Figure 23-1. Hyperkalemia. Mild hyperkalemia typically produces tall "tent-shaped" T waves. With moderate hyperkalemia, the QRS complex widens, the T wave amplitude increases further, and P waves diminish in size. In severe hyperkalemia the complex may resemble a sine wave.

1953, this J wave deflection is seen in approximately 80% of patients with a core temperature of 30°C or less. It is described as a "dome" or "hump" at the end of the QRS complex and may resemble the ST segment elevation of acute MI (**Figure 23-5**). Additional ECG manifestations of hypothermia include shivering artifacts, PR interval prolongation, QT interval prolongation, and marked bradycardia.

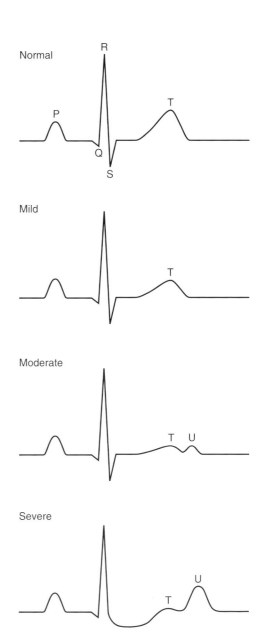

Figure 23-2. Hypokalemia. Mild hypokalemia diminishes the amplitude of the T wave. A U wave is typically seen with moderate hypokalemia, which becomes more prominent with severe lowering of serum potassium.

Cerebrovascular Disease

Cerebrovascular disease may produce a variety of ECG findings. Subarachnoid hemorrhage, in particular, is commonly associated with diffuse T wave inversion, QT interval prolongation, and prominent U waves (**Figure 23-6**). The mechanism is believed to reflect alterations in the autonomic nervous system. The ECG findings are unpredictable and may resemble a pattern of subendocardial ischemia with diffuse ST segment depression and T wave inversion that usually resolve over time.

Miscellaneous ECG Findings

Low voltage Low limb lead voltage is defined when the amplitude of the entire QRS complex (R wave + S wave) in each of

Normal

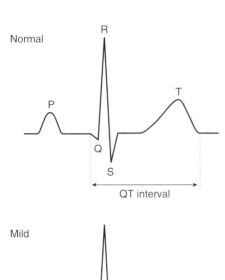

Mild

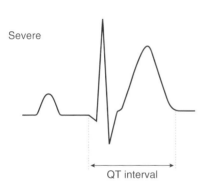

Severe

Figure 23-3. Hypercalcemia. Hypercalcemia shortens the QT interval. ST segment elevation may be seen with severely elevated calcium.

Normal

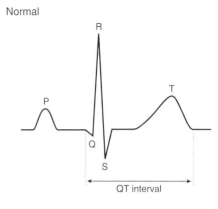

Hypocalcemia

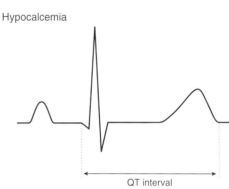

Figure 23-4. Hypocalcemia prolongs the QT interval.

the limb leads is <5 mm. Low precordial lead voltage is when the sum of the R wave and S wave in each of the precordial leads is <10 mm. The causes can be divided into those that interfere with the transmission of electrical voltage to the recording electrodes and those that impair myocardial voltage generation. Fluids, adipose tissue, and air all act as an electrical insulator, attenuating the conduction of cardiac depolarization to the electrocardiograph machine. Examples include large pericardial and pleural effusions (**Figure 23-7**), obesity (**Figure 23-8**), anasarca, and chronic obstructive pulmonary disease with lung hyperinflation (**Figure 23-9**). Primary cardiac causes of low voltage include multiple myocardial infarctions (**Figure 23-10**) and infiltrative cardiomyopathies. The combination of electrocardiographic low voltage that accompanies markedly increased left ventricular wall thickness on echocardiography is a marker for cardiac amyloidosis (**Figure 23-11**).

Low voltage may be seen in the limb leads alone (most common), the precordial leads alone, or in both the limb and precordial leads.

Poor R wave progression Poor R wave progression (PRWP) is the term used to describe the presence of small R waves that increase in voltage from leads V1-V3, but the R wave amplitude in V3 is ≤3 mm. Reverse R wave progression is as above, except that R wave voltage decreases from leads V1-V3. PRWP may be due to a number of clinically important conditions including anteroseptal MI, left ventricular enlargement/hypertrophy (LVH/LVE), and chronic pulmonary disease. PRWP may also be a reflection of cardiac rotation, or represent a normal variant.

One diagnostic "nuance" to note when identifying PRWP is that the presence of low precordial lead voltage makes the additional finding of PRWP moot, and need not be added to the interpretation. Also, do not diagnose PRWP in the setting of LBBB or WPW.

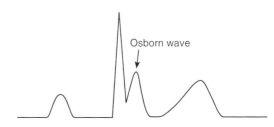

Figure 23-5. Osborn wave of hypothermia.

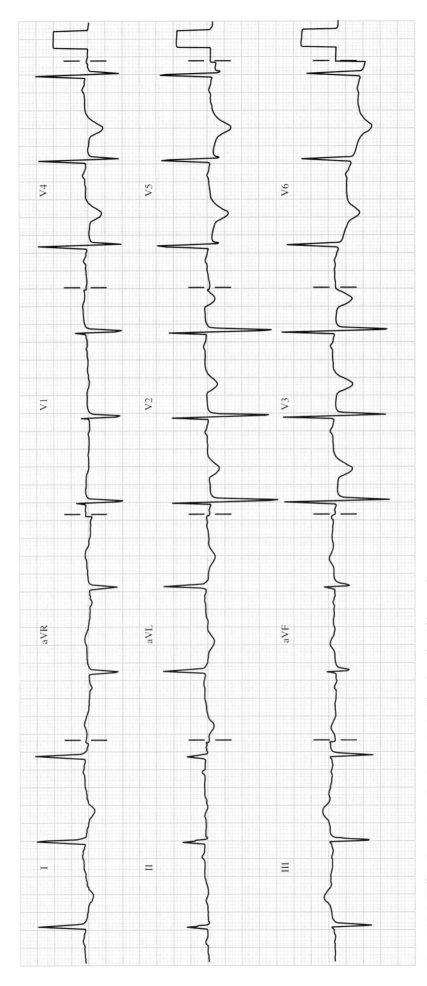

Figure 23-6. Diffuse T wave inversion in a patient with subarachnoid hemorrhage.

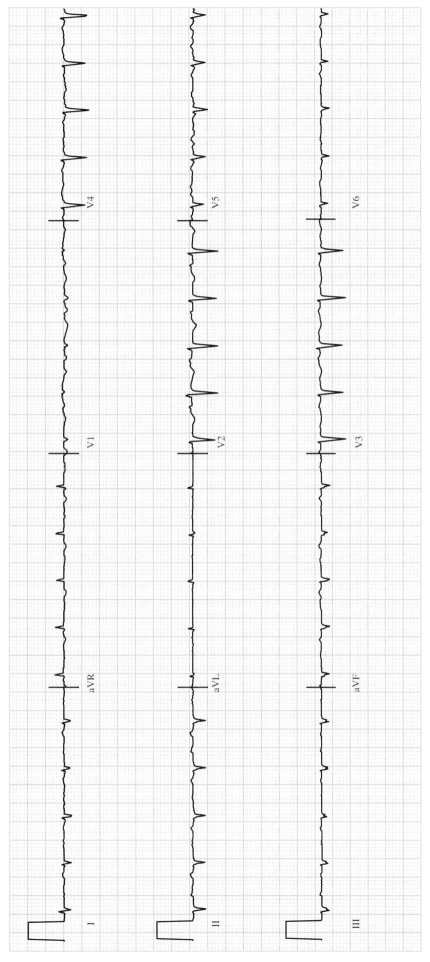

Figure 23-7. Low voltage in the limb and precordial leads seen in a patient with large, malignant pericardial and pleural effusions.

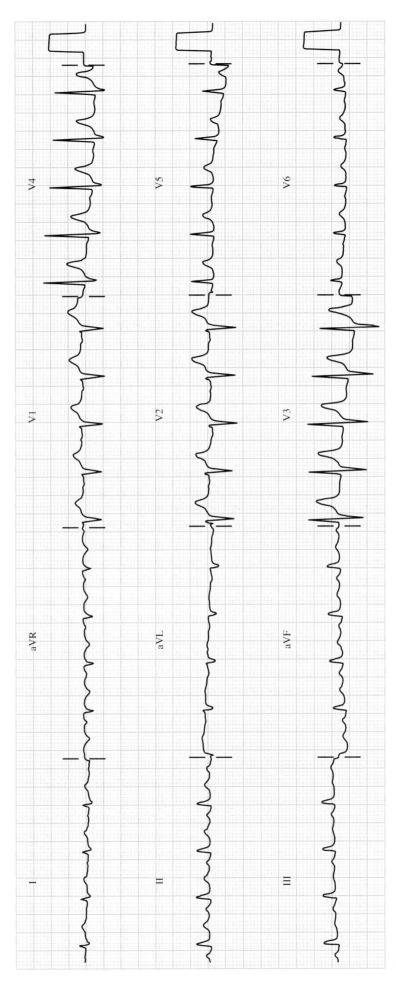

Figure 23-8. Low limb lead voltage in a patient with obesity.

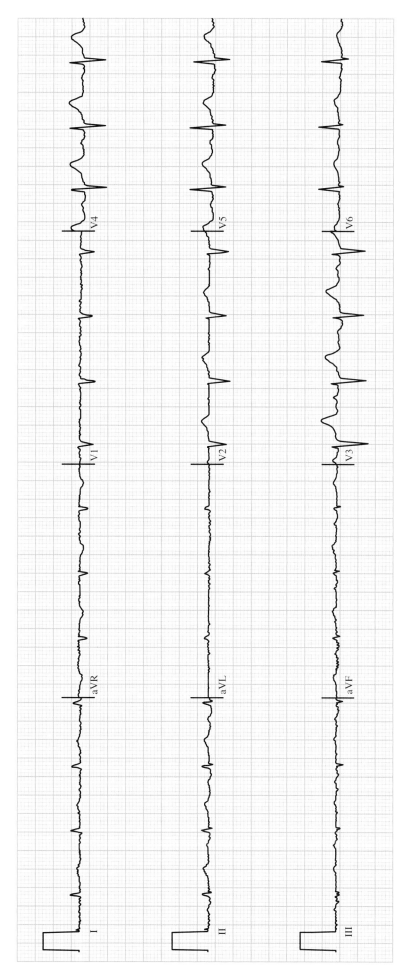

Figure 23-9. Low limb lead voltage in a patient with emphysema.

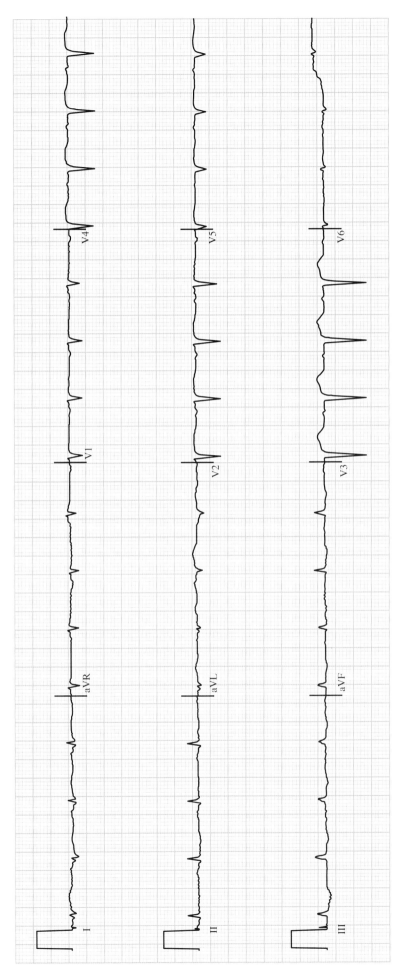

Figure 23-10. Low limb lead voltage in a patient with multiple myocardial infarctions.

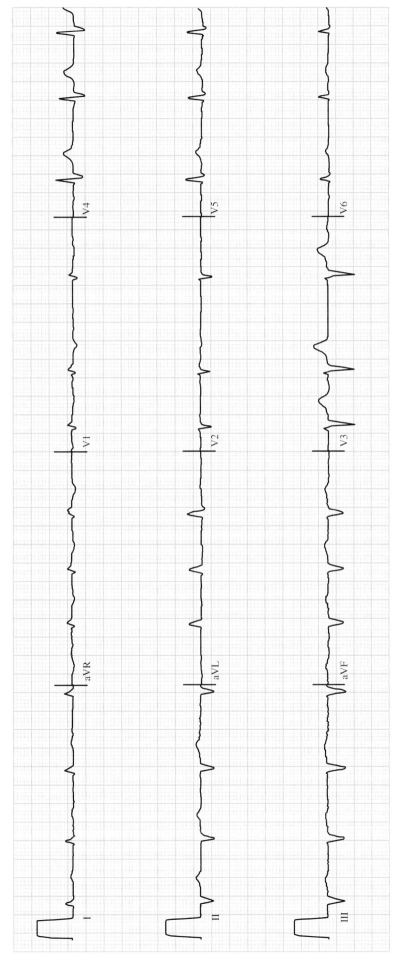

Figure 23-11. Low precordial lead voltage (and borderline in the limb leads) in a patient with cardiac amyloidosis. Echocardiography demonstrated concentric left ventricular hypertrophy. The rhythm is atrial fibrillation.

Anteroseptal wall MI may result in PRWP if some anterior forces in the frontal plane are preserved, producing smaller than normal R waves rather than Q waves in leads V1-V3 (**Figure 23-12**).

Left anterior fascicular block (LAFB) produces PRWP by shifting the initial forces inferiorly and posteriorly (toward the left posterior-inferior fascicle), and away from the anterior recording leads (**Figure 23-13**).

LVE/LVH results in PRWP, as the increased mass of the left ventricle pulls the vector loop posteriorly, reducing anterior forces recorded in the right precordial leads (**Figure 23-14**).

Chronic pulmonary disease, particularly emphysema with hyperinflation, alters the position of the diaphragm within the chest. The lower R wave voltage reflects the relatively low position of the heart in relation to leads V1-V3. Cor pulmonale and type C RVH turns the vector loop posteriorly, away from the anteriorly looking leads (**Figure 23-15**).

Clockwise rotation turns the right ventricle more anterior and to the left, producing smaller R waves in leads V3-V4, moving the dominant R waves out of the recording field beyond V6 (**Figure 23-16**).

Electrical alternans Beat-to-beat voltage changes in the P wave, QRS complex, and T wave, alone or in combination, are termed electrical alternans. This may occur in the setting of a large pericardial effusion as the heart swings within the pericardial space (**Figure 23-17**). The presence of electrical alternans in the setting of a supraventricular tachycardia suggests that the rhythm is an atrioventricular reentrant tachycardia (AVRT) and utilizes an atrioventricular bypass connection as one limb of the circuit. The mechanism of this phenomenon is subject to debate.

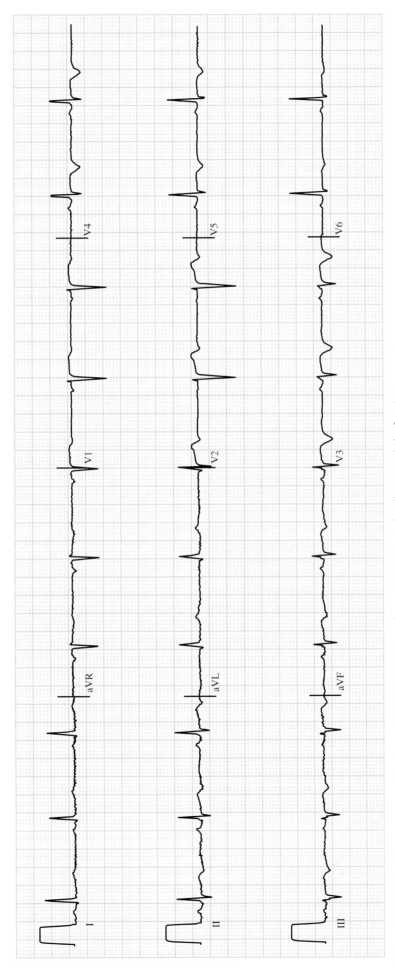

Figure 23-12. Poor R wave progression in a patient with a history of recent anteroseptal wall myocardial infarction.

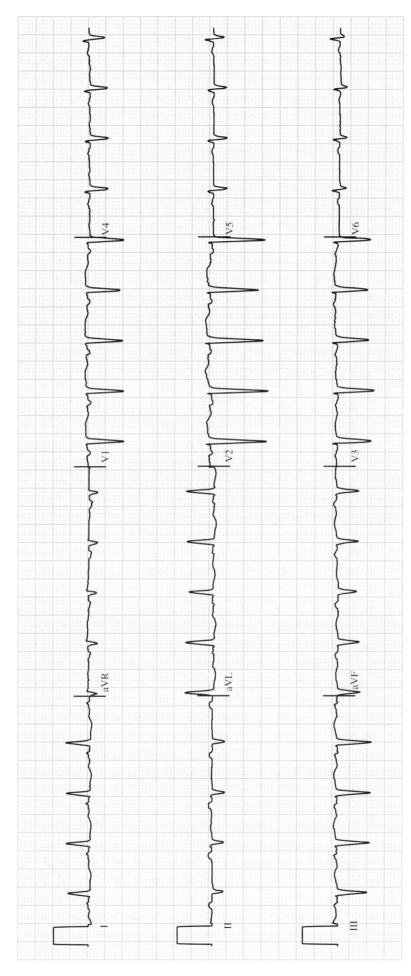

Figure 23-13. Poor R wave progression in a patient with left anterior fascicular block.

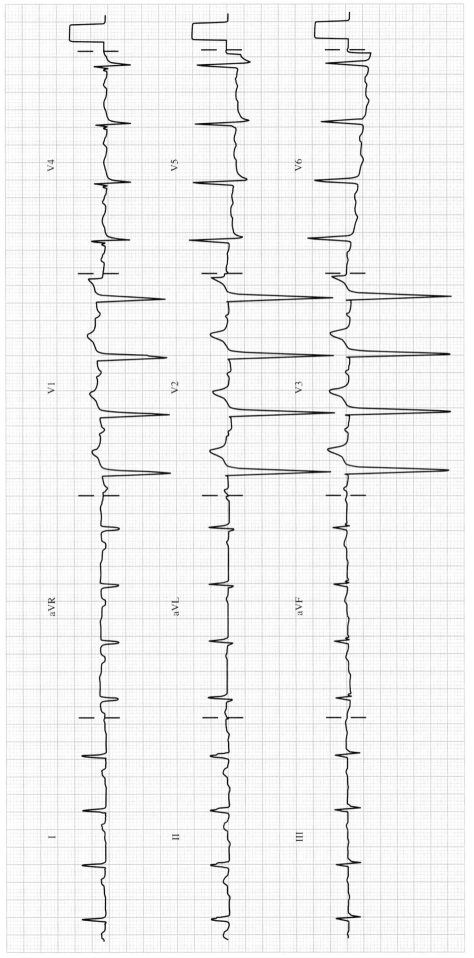

Figure 23-14. Poor R wave progression in a patient with left ventricular enlargement/hypertrophy (Cornell criteria).

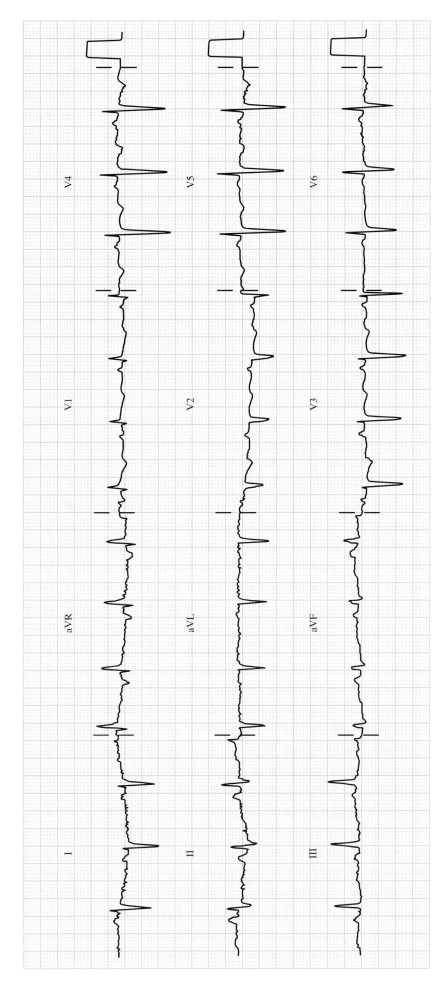

Figure 23-15. Reverse R wave progression in a patient with right ventricular enlargement/hypertrophy.

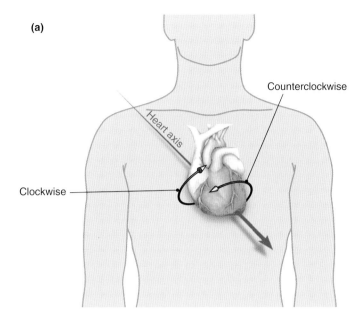

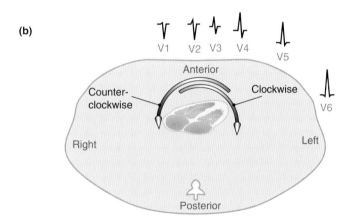

Figure 23-16. The heart can rotate along its long axis, either clockwise or counterclockwise (a). Clockwise rotation brings the transition zone rightward, producing poor R wave progression (b). The direction of rotation is from the perspective of one viewing from below the diaphragm with the patient lying face up.

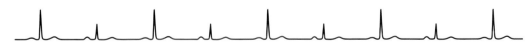

Figure 23-17. Electrical alternans. Note the alternating amplitude of the QRS complexes.

Chapter 23 • SELF-TEST

1. Increased T wave amplitude is a characteristic finding of what electrolyte abnormality?

2. A prominent U wave is a characteristic finding of what electrolyte abnormality?

3. What ECG finding is typical of hypercalcemia?

4. What ECG finding is typical of hypocalcemia?

5. What is the unique ECG finding seen in marked hypothermia?

6. Define low voltage in:
   - The limb leads.
   - The precordial leads.

7. List at least four causes of low voltage.

8. Define poor R wave progression.

9. List at least four causes of poor R wave progression.

10. Define electrical alternans.

Chapter 23 • SELF-TEST

1. Hyperkalemia.

2. Hypokalemia.

3. Shortening of the QT interval.

4. QT interval prolongation.

5. The Osborn wave.

6. Low voltage is defined as:
   - Limb lead voltage <5 mm.
   - Precordial lead voltage <10 mm.

7.
   - Large pericardial or pleural effusion.
   - Anasarca.
   - Obesity.
   - Chronic pulmonary disease, especially with lung hyperinflation.
   - Others include multiple myocardial infarction and infiltrative cardiomyopathies.

8. The presence of small R waves that increase in voltage from leads V1-V3, but the R wave amplitude in V3 is ≤3 mm.

9.
   - Anteroseptal wall myocardial infarction.
   - Left anterior fascicular block.
   - Left ventricular enlargement/hypertrophy.
   - Chronic pulmonary disease.

10. Beat-to-beat voltage changes in the P wave, QRS complex, and T wave, alone or in combination.

Further Reading

Chinitz JS, Cooper JM, Verdino RJ. Electrocardiogram voltage discordance: interpretation of low QRS voltage only in the limb leads. *J Electrocardiol.* 2008;41:281-286.

Diercks DB, Shumaik GM, Harrigan RA, Brady WJ, Chan TC. Electrocardiographic manifestations: electrolyte abnormalities. *J Em Med.* 2004;27:153-160.

Fisch C. Relation of electrolyte disturbances to cardiac arrhythmias. *Circulation.* 1973;47:408-419.

Gupta P, Jain H, Bharaj G, et al. Electrocardiographic changes in emphysema. *World J Cardiol.* 2021;13:533-545.

Kim DH, Verdino RJ. Electrocardiogram voltage discordance: interpretation of low QRS voltage only in the precordial leads. *J Electrocardiol.* 2017;50:551-554.

Llg KJ, Lehmann M. Importance of recognizing pseudo-septal infarction due to electrocardiographic lead misplacement. *Am J Med.* 2012;125:23-27.

Madias JE. Low QRS voltage and its causes. *J Electrocardiol.* 2008;41:498-500.

Surawicz B, Fisch C. Cardiac alternans: diverse mechanisms and clinical manifestations. *J Am Coll Cardiol.* 1992;20:483-489.

Zema MJ, Kligfield P. ECG Poor R-wave progression: review and synthesis. *Arch Intern Med.* 1982;142;1145-1148.

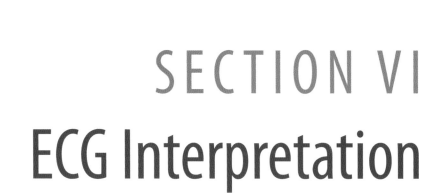

SECTION VI
ECG Interpretation

24

A Step-by-Step Method of Interpretation

We've come a long way on our journey and are now ready to perform comprehensive 12-lead ECG interpretations. There's more than one way to approach an ECG and some of you will find that one method works better for you than others. This chapter presents a method I believe you will find easy to understand and organize. When analyzing each item, return to the relevant chapters to review the diagnostic considerations in detail. You do have flexibility in what order you choose to address each element. But whatever method you use in practice, it's vital that you follow a routine of **structured reporting**. This guarantees that all the key elements are reported consistently in every tracing. One of my teaching "mantras" is: *You can have different styles, but not different standards.*

The following lists the essential elements that should be part of every ECG interpretation, something I like to call "The Diagnostic Dozen."

▶ THE DIAGNOSTIC DOZEN

1. Technical aspects
2. Analyze the rhythm and rate
3. Make your measurements (PR, QRS, QT)
4. Determine the mean frontal plane QRS axis
5. P wave analysis
6. QRS complex analysis
7. Q wave inspection
8. Examine precordial R wave progression
9. ST segment analysis
10. T wave analysis (and U wave if present)
11. Synthesis
12. Comparison and clinical correlation

▶ STEP 1: TECHNICAL ASPECTS

The first step in ECG interpretation is to assess the technical aspects of the tracing. Identify the name, gender, and age of the patient, items that will impact your interpretation. For example, interpreting the ECG of a pediatric patient is very different from that of an adult, a topic best left to textbooks devoted to that subject. And as we reviewed in Chapter 7, the criteria for left ventricular enlargement are different depending on age and gender. Inspect the tracing for overall quality, making sure it is satisfactory and devoid of excessive baseline artifact. If necessary, don't hesitate to request a repeat tracing stating in your report that, "technical artifacts preclude accurate interpretation." Check that the tracing is performed at normal paper speed (25 mm/sec), information that is routinely printed on each ECG. Also check the standardization, which can be confirmed as normal (10 mm/mV) by inspecting the calibration mark that appears either at the beginning or end of each tracing. At times the calibration is performed at half-standard, the machine making the adjustment to fit large complexes on one page. Note that half-standardization can be utilized for only the precordial leads with the limb leads recorded at normal calibration, which will be indicated by a two-tiered calibration mark. Finally, examine the tracing for an obvious lead reversal. As we reviewed in Chapter 4, clues to this include a highly unusual P wave and QRS complex in leads I and aVR, as well as an isolated "flat line" in any of leads I, II, or III.

▶ STEP 2: ANALYZE THE RHYTHM AND RATE

Rhythm and rate are analyzed together in a step-wise fashion. The rhythm is modified by the rate, a simple example being normal sinus rhythm, which is adjusted to sinus *tachycardia* if the heart rate is increased (>100 bpm) or sinus *bradycardia* if decreased (<60 bpm). Oh, if every cardiac rhythm analysis were that simple! In addition to heart rate, evaluation of the cardiac rhythm involves determination of its origin, analysis of atrial and ventricular activity, the AV relationship, assessment of any early or late ectopic complexes, as well as analysis of any pacemaker complexes and rhythms. Wow, that seems pretty complicated. Well it can be, and indeed there are times when the cardiac rhythm cannot be determined. That's not often the case, but if so, it's reasonable to report the tracing with an "undetermined rhythm." Let's now review the essentials of rhythm analysis, for now deferring any modification due to heart rate.

Origin of the Rhythm

Our first task is to determine whether the dominant rhythm is derived from the sinus node, within the atrium, the AV junction, the ventricles, or results from an artificial device. As we proceed, it helps to mentally create a ladder diagram. You may even wish to draw a simple three-tiered laddergram on a copy of the tracing itself, filling in the items below the rhythm strip. As we have done throughout this book, this involves identifying supraventricular activity, ventricular events, and the relationship between the two.

Identify supraventricular activity by searching for (1) P waves of normal morphology and axis, (2) P′ waves with abnormal morphology and axis, (3) the absence of P or P′ waves, and (4) P waves replaced by flutter or fibrillatory waves. Normal P waves indicate a sinus mechanism. Abnormal P′ waves indicate either an ectopic atrial or an AV junctional focus. The differential diagnosis of absent P waves includes sinus arrest, as well as rhythms of AV junctional origin where the retrograde P′ wave is hidden within the QRS complex. Flutter or fibrillatory waves are seen in atrial flutter and atrial fibrillation, respectively.

Ventricular events are analyzed by examination of the QRS complex. Determine whether the QRS complex is narrow or wide. A narrow QRS complex indicates normal ventricular activation resulting from a supraventricular focus. A wide QRS complex may result from an impulse of ventricular origin, as well as supraventricular impulses with aberrant conduction, underlying bundle branch block, or transmission over an accessory pathway. Ventricular paced complexes are also wide.

The AV Relationship

With normal AV conduction, supraventricular events are followed by ventricular depolarization in a 1:1 relationship. Accordingly, there is a P wave before every QRS complex and a QRS complex after every P wave. Examine the tracing and confirm this is the case. If any exceptions are found, consider diagnoses that include various forms of AV block, ventricular-based rhythms, as well as ectopic complexes.

Calculate the Atrial and Ventricular Heart Rates

Once you identify the origin of the rhythm, calculate *both* the atrial and ventricular heart rates. With a 1:1 AV relationship, the atrial and ventricular rates are the same. However, there are many circumstances where this is not the case, including AV conduction abnormalities and a variety of atrial tachyarrhythmias (eg, some atrial tachycardias, atrial flutter). As mentioned in the preceding discussion, the heart rate modifies the rhythm origin,

both for tachyarrhythmias and bradyarrhythmias. For example, a rhythm of atrial origin with a HR >100 bpm is characterized as atrial tachycardia. In addition, it is appropriate to combine the impulse origin, heart rate, and AV relationship together to further define the rhythm. For example, an atrial tachycardia with an atrial rate of 220 bpm and a ventricular rate of 110 bpm, is defined as an atrial tachycardia with 2:1 AV conduction.

Ectopic Complexes

After defining the dominant rhythm, inspect the tracing for ectopic complexes. The origin of these complexes may be atrial, AV junctional, or ventricular. The timing may be early (premature) or late (escape). Supraventricular complexes may conduct normally, demonstrate aberrant conduction, or fail to conduct (blocked). Remember that we have employed a convention that identifies an ectopic complex first by its origin followed by the timing (eg, ventricular premature complex or junctional escape complex).

Pacemaker Complexes and Rhythms

If present, describe any rhythms or complexes associated with a cardiac pacemaker. When evident, it is important to integrate the native rhythm into the interpretation. For example, a patient with sinus rhythm in which every P wave is followed by a tracked ventricular pacemaker stimulus is interpreted as "sinus rhythm with atrial sensing-ventricular pacing." Similarly, the rhythm of a patient with underlying atrial fibrillation that demonstrates a ventricular paced complex after a pause is interpreted as "atrial fibrillation with ventricular pacing on demand."

▶ STEP 3: MAKE YOUR MEASUREMENTS

Measure the PR Interval

This is measured from the beginning of the P wave until the first deflection of the QRS complex, regardless of whether this is a Q wave or an R wave. The PR interval should be measured in the lead that exhibits the longest interval. The normal PR interval is 0.12 to 0.20 seconds.

Measure the QRS Complex Duration

The QRS complex duration is measured in the limb or precordial lead with the longest duration from the beginning of the first deflection (either Q or R wave) to the end of the last deflection. The normal QRS duration is 0.06 to 0.10 seconds.

Measure the QT Interval

Measure the QT interval in the lead with the longest QT duration from the onset of the QRS complex to the end of the T wave. Be sure to identify the true end of the T wave and not mistakenly measure a superimposed U wave or P wave. You may find it helpful to use the tangent method of measurement, drawing a line from the maximum downslope of the T wave until it intersects the baseline (see Figure 4-15). Remember that the normal QT interval varies by heart rate and gender, called the corrected QT interval (QTc).

The normal QTc for men is >390 msec and <450 msec. The normal QTc for women is >390 msec and <460 msec.

STEP 4: DETERMINE THE MEAN FRONTAL PLANE QRS AXIS

Use any of the methods described in Chapter 6 to determine the mean frontal plane axis. The normal mean QRS axis is between −30 and +90 degrees. Computer-based analysis can determine the frontal plane axis with great precision. When determined manually, it is reasonable to report an estimated axis in increments of 15 degrees.

STEP 5: ANALYZE THE P WAVE

Analyze the P wave in terms of duration, amplitude, axis, and morphology. This is best performed by first inspecting lead II in the frontal plane and lead V1 in the horizontal plane. The width of the P wave is measured from where the forward and hind limbs join the baseline. The amplitude of an upright P wave is measured from the upper edge of the baseline to the summit, and should not include the thickness of the line.

In the frontal plane, the contour of the normal P wave is smooth, with an amplitude ≤2.5 mm, a duration of ≤0.11 seconds, and an axis between 0 and +75 degrees. In the horizontal plane, the normal P wave may be upright, inverted, or biphasic (upright followed by inverted) in lead V1. The inverted terminal portion of a normal biphasic P wave is <0.1 seconds in duration and <1 mm in depth.

Abnormalities of P wave morphology and axis may be related to chamber enlargement or an ectopic focus.

STEP 6: ANALYZE THE QRS COMPLEX

Analyze the QRS complex in terms of duration, amplitude, and morphology. A prolonged QRS duration typically represents an interventricular conduction delay associated with a bundle branch block, aberrant conduction, or transmission via an accessory pathway, which are diagnoses that also alter QRS complex morphology. Nonspecific QRS complex widening may also be associated with ventricular enlargement/hypertrophy.

The amplitude of the QRS complex in an individual lead is the sum of the single tallest positive and single deepest negative waveforms of the complex as measured from the baseline. There is wide variation of the maximum normal QRS complex amplitude in individual leads. The normal total QRS complex amplitude should be ≥5 mm in at least one limb lead and ≥10 mm in at least one precordial lead. The differential diagnosis of low voltage is reviewed in Chapter 23. Inspect the tracing for increased voltage in the limb and precordial leads that indicate ventricular enlargement/hypertrophy, the criterion for which we reviewed in Chapter 7.

The normal QRS complex contains waves that are sharp in configuration with a morphology that varies in different leads.

Even though this group of deflections is termed the QRS complex, not every one will contain an individual Q wave, R wave, and S wave. Accordingly, a QRS complex may be described as a QR, QS, or RS wave. Capital and lowercase letters can be used to describe the relative sizes of waves comprising the QRS complex (see Figure 4-12). As noted in the preceding discussion, bundle branch block, aberrancy, and preexcitation all markedly alter the normal QRS complex morphology.

STEP 7: Q WAVE INSPECTION

Inspect each lead for abnormal Q waves indicative of myocardial infarction. Small, narrow Q waves ≤0.03 seconds related to septal depolarization may be normally found in leads I, II, III, aVL, aVF, and V4-V6. A wider Q wave ≥0.04 seconds may be a normal finding in lead III, as is a QS complex in leads aVR and V1.

There are a number of definitions for pathological Q waves. A classic criterion is a Q wave ≥0.04 seconds wide with an amplitude ≥1 mm deep. Specificity is increased when the Q wave has an amplitude that exceeds 25% of the corresponding R wave. These characteristics help to distinguish the pathological Q wave of myocardial infarction from one resulting from normal septal depolarization or other normal variants. As reviewed in Chapter 10, the diagnosis of myocardial infarction requires evidence of pathological Q waves in at least two contiguous leads of a regional group.

STEP 8: EXAMINE PRECORDIAL R WAVE PROGRESSION

Examine the R wave progression, which is the term used to describe the normal increase in R waves across the precordial leads. Poor R wave progression (PRWP) is the term used to describe the presence of small R waves that increase in voltage from leads V1-V3, but the R wave amplitude in V3 is ≤3 mm. As we reviewed in Chapter 23, PRWP may be a normal variant, a reflection of cardiac rotation, or associated with a number of clinically important conditions.

Reverse R wave progression is as above, except that R wave voltage decreases from leads V1-V3.

STEP 9: ANALYZE THE ST SEGMENT

Analyze the ST segment for contour and abnormal deviation from the baseline. Measure the ST segment at the J point compared to a baseline of either the PR segment or TP segment, using whichever appears the most stable and accurate (see Figure 4-11). The normal ST segment is isoelectric, but may be slightly elevated or depressed by <1 mm relative to the baseline. Somewhat greater ST elevation may be a normal finding in leads V2 and V3 (<1.5 mm in women and <2 mm in men younger than age 40 years).

Abnormal ST segment displacement is defined as elevation or depression of ≥1 mm from the baseline in at least two contiguous leads. In leads V2 and V3 the criteria for abnormal ST segment elevation is ≥1.5 mm in women and ≥2 mm in men. Displacement of the ST segment may take different morphologies that may be described as horizontal, upsloping, downsloping, or with more complex patterns (see Chapters 10 and 11).

▶ STEP 10: ANALYZE THE T WAVE (AND U WAVE)

Evaluate the T wave in terms of direction, amplitude, and morphology. The direction of the T wave usually parallels that of a normal QRS complex in that lead. Accordingly, leads that contain a tall R wave will also have an upright T wave. Similarly, leads with a deep S wave will normally have an inverted T wave. The amplitude of an upright T wave is measured from the upper level of the baseline to the peak of the wave. Inverted T waves are measured from the lower level of the baseline to the nadir of the wave. The amplitude of the T wave should not exceed 6 mm in the limb leads, or 10 mm in the precordial leads. The normal T wave configuration is rounded, smooth, and slightly asymmetric, with the terminal portion exhibiting a steeper downslope.

T wave abnormalities may be characterized by abnormal direction, amplitude, and morphology. Their shape may be described as peaked, symmetrical, biphasic, flat, or inverted. Ischemic T waves are characteristically deep, symmetrical, and opposite in direction (>45 degrees) to the main axis of the QRS complex.

If present, inspect the U wave. This is a low amplitude deflection of controversial origin that may be seen following or partially superimposing the T wave. It is more often present at lower heart rates and may be seen best in leads V2 and V3. The amplitude of the U wave should be <25% of the T wave in that lead and normally follows in the same direction.

▶ STEP 11: SYNTHESIS

Once you identify and measure the normal and abnormal findings of the items discussed earlier, you need to synthesize the information into an integrated interpretation. For example, measurement of a prolonged QRS complex of 0.14 seconds with identification of an rSR′ associated with T wave inversion in lead V1 is synthesized as a diagnosis of RBBB. Similarly, the

identification of pathological Q waves in leads II, III, and aVF with a normal ST segment and T wave is synthesized as a diagnosis of inferior wall myocardial infarction, old or of indeterminate age. The key concept of structured reporting is first you *measure* and *identify*, and then you *synthesize* the findings into a diagnosis.

▶ STEP 12: COMPARISON AND CLINICAL CORRELATION

If available, compare every ECG you interpret with a previous tracing. Include a statement in your interpretation such as "compared with ECG of (date/time) there are (new findings) or (no significant change)." And if no prior tracing is available for comparison, state so in your report.

Every ECG interpretation represents an important aspect of clinical patient care. There is a school of thought that every ECG should be interpreted without any consideration of the clinical history, so as not to influence the reader. I disagree. A subtle change found in the ECG of a patient in the emergency department with chest discomfort might prompt a call to suggest a repeat tracing or other clinical recommendation. The same tracing performed in an asymptomatic individual as part of a routine yearly insurance physical would likely not be of the same concern. Yes, the findings and interpretation in each situation are identical, but the clinical history has value. Similarly, a suspicious new conduction abnormality in a hospitalized patient admitted for syncope should prompt a phone call to the treating physician. And even a "routine" ECG may have serious unexpected abnormalities that warrant evaluation. So when in doubt as to the significance of the interpretation, err on the side of caution and contact the treating provider.

A Word About Computer Interpretation

Modern ECG machines are routinely programmed with interpretation software. Beware of relying solely on a computer interpretation. Research demonstrates the limitations of the software, so always interpret the tracing personally. I consider computer-based interpretation as an important preliminary, but not definitive report.

Further Reading

Bagliani G, DePonti R, Leonelli FM. Precision electrocardiography: a rational approach for simple and complex arrhythmias. *Card Electrophysiol Clin.* 2019;11:175-187.

Guglin ME, Thatai D. Common errors in computer electrocardiogram interpretation. *Int J Cardiol.* 2006;106:232-237.

Hurst JW. Electrocardiographic interpretation (1995): can we do better? Part I. *Clin Cardiol.* 1995;18:433-439.

Hurst JW. Electrocardiographic interpretation (1995): can we do better? Part II. *Clin Cardiol.* 1995;18:493-495.

Hurst JW. Current status of clinical electrocardiography with suggestions for the improvement of the interpretive process. *Am J Cardiol.* 2003;92:1072-1079.

Leonelli FM, DePonti R, Bagliani G. Electrocardiographic approach to complex arrhythmias: P, QRS, and their relationships. *Card Electrophysiol Clin.* 2019;11:239-260.

Padeletti L, Bagliani G. General introduction, classification, and electrocardiographic diagnosis of cardiac arrhythmias. *Card Electrophysiol Clin.* 2017;9:345-363.

Schlapfer J, Wellens HJ. Computer-interpreted electrocardiograms: benefits and limitations. *J Am Coll Cardiol.* 2017;70:1183-92.

Smulyan H. The computerized ECG: friend and foe. *Am J Med.* 2018;132:153-160.

25

Diagnostic Criteria

▶ INTRODUCTION

In this chapter you will find the criteria for most of the electrocardiographic diagnoses that you are likely to encounter in clinical practice and on board exams. Minor variations of these criteria have been published.

OUTLINE

ELECTROCARDIOGRAPHIC DIAGNOSES

▶ I. RHYTHM ABNORMALITIES

A. Supraventricular Rhythms and Complexes

Sinus rhythm
- P wave of sinus origin.
  - Normal P wave configuration (upright in leads I, II, and aVF, and inverted in aVR).
  - Normal mean axis (between 0 and +75 degrees).
- Normal PR interval (0.12-0.20 seconds).
- Consistent P wave configuration and PR interval in each lead.
- Constant P-P cycles with only minor variation.
  - Any variation between the longest and shortest cycles is ≤0.12 seconds or ≤10%.
- HR of 60 to 100 bpm.

Sinus bradycardia
- Normal sinus rhythm except for heart rate.
- HR <60 bpm.
  - Comment: Some authors define it as <50 bpm.

Sinus tachycardia
- Normal sinus rhythm except for heart rate.
- HR >100 bpm.

Sinus arrhythmia
- P wave of sinus origin with normal P wave morphology and axis.
- Normal HR.
- Phasic variability of P-P intervals.
- P-P intervals vary from the shortest to longest cycle by either:
  - >0.12 seconds.
  - >10%.
    - Determine this percentage by dividing the difference between the two numbers by the average of the two numbers, then multiplying by 100 to convert to percent.
      - Difference between the two numbers: (Maximum P-P interval − Minimum P-P interval).
      - Average of the two numbers: (Maximum P-P interval + Minimum P-P interval) ÷2.
    - Comment: The cycles used in the above calculation do not need to be consecutive.
- Sinus arrhythmia may be further characterized as respiratory, nonrespiratory, ventriculophasic, and combined with bradycardia (sinus bradyarrhythmia).

Sinus arrest or pause

- Sinus rhythm with sudden absence of P waves at the expected time/cycle.
- P waves and QRS complexes are absent during the pause (except for the emergence of a subsidiary pacemaker).
- The resulting pause is not an exact multiple of the normal cycle length.

Sinoatrial exit block

An abnormality of transmission of the sinus impulse that results in a delay or failure to produce a P wave. Only second-degree SA block can be identified on the surface ECG. Second-degree SA block may manifest in two forms, type I and type II.

Type I second-degree SA block

- Sinus rhythm with normal P wave morphology and axis.
- Normal PR interval.
- Progressive shortening of the P-P interval that is followed by a pause.
- The pause is less than the sum of any two consecutive short cycles.
- Supporting criteria:
  - Group beating is common.

Type II second-degree SA block

- Sinus rhythm with normal P wave morphology and axis.
- Normal PR interval.
- Constant P-P interval with sudden absence of the P wave.
- The pause is an exact multiple (two or more) of the normal cycle length.

Wandering atrial pacemaker within the sinus node

- P wave of sinus origin with normal P wave axis.
- Varying P wave configuration, but remaining upright in leads I, II, and aVF and inverted in lead aVR.
- Constant P-P intervals with minor, normal variation.
- PR interval may have slight variation, but remains within the normal range (0.12-0.20 seconds).

Wandering atrial pacemaker

- Normal sinus rhythm that exhibits gradual, cyclic alteration in P (P′) wave configuration and PR (P′R) interval until two or more sequential atrial complexes appear.
- The P′ wave is nearly normal relative to the native P wave, but may be biphasic or inverted.
- The PR (P′R) interval may have slight variation, but usually remains within the normal range (0.12-0.20 seconds).
- The heart rate is typically either slow (<60 bpm) or at the lower limits of normal.

Wandering pacemaker to the AV junction

- Normal sinus rhythm that exhibits gradual, cyclic alteration in P (P′) wave configuration and PR (P′R) interval until two or more sequential AV junctional complexes appear.
- The junctional complexes display an inverted, retrograde P′ wave that may appear before, within, or after the QRS complex.

- When present before the QRS complex, the P′R interval of the junctional complex is short (<0.12 seconds).
- The heart rate of the junctional rhythm is typically 40 to 60 bpm.

Ectopic atrial rhythm

- A rhythm whose origin is an atrial pacemaker other than the sinus node.
- The P′ wave may be nearly normal, biphasic, or inverted.
  - When inverted P′ waves are present, the rhythm may be termed a "low" atrial rhythm (reflecting the proximity to the AV node).
- The P′R interval may have slight variation, but usually remains within the normal range (0.12-0.20 seconds).
- The heart rate is typically within the normal range.
  - If the HR is <60 bpm, the rhythm is described as a "slow" ectopic atrial rhythm (or ectopic atrial bradycardia).

Atrial premature complex (APC)

- The complex appears early relative to the native rhythm.
- A nearly normal P′ wave is present, but may be biphasic or inverted.
- The P′R interval is typically within the normal range (0.12-0.20 seconds), but may be shorter or longer than that of the baseline sinus complex.
- The P′ wave is followed by a QRS complex identical to the native rhythm.
- Supporting criteria:
  - The complex is followed by a noncompensatory pause.
- Exceptions and modifiers (see text for details).
  - Nonconducted (blocked) APC.
  - APC with aberrant conduction.

Atrial escape complex

- The complex appears late relative to the cycle of the normal rhythm, emerging due to a failure of a normally faster physiologic pacemaker.
- The P′ wave is nearly normal relative to the native P wave, but may be inverted.
- The P′R interval remains within the normal range (0.12-0.20 seconds).
- The QRS complex is identical to the native rhythm.

Sinus node reentrant tachycardia

- P (P′) wave of sinus origin.
  - Normal P (P′) wave configuration (upright in leads I, II, and aVF, and inverted in aVR).
  - Normal mean axis (between 0 and +75 degrees).
- Normal PR (P′R) interval (0.12-0.20 seconds).
- HR >100 bpm.
- Typically paroxysmal onset.
- Usually initiated by and terminated with an APC.

Atrial tachycardia (classical criteria)

- Series of ≥3 monomorphic atrial complexes (P′ waves).
- P′ wave of atrial origin.
  - Morphology and axis are variable, depending on atrial origin.

- Atrial rate >100 bpm (usually 150-240 bpm).
- Regular, 1:1 AV conduction.
  - Physiologic AV conduction delay is common at higher atrial rates.
- Normal P´R interval (0.12-0.20 seconds).
- P´ waves separated by an isoelectric line.
- Comment: There are forms of atrial tachycardia that overlap with atypical forms of atrial flutter (see text for details).

Atrial tachycardia with block
- Repetitive monomorphic atrial complexes (P´ waves).
- Atrial rate >100 to 240 bpm (usually <200 bpm).
- 2:1 or higher degree of AV conduction block.
- P´ waves separated by an isoelectric line.
- Comment: This arrhythmia often historically carries the mechanistically inaccurate name of *paroxysmal* atrial tachycardia (PAT) with block.

Multifocal atrial tachycardia
- Rapid atrial rhythm with ≥3 consecutive P´ waves of different morphologies.
- Atrial rate >100 bpm.
- Absence of a single, dominant atrial pacemaker.
- Variable P´-P´, P´R, and R-R intervals.
- P´ waves separated by an isoelectric line.

Multifocal atrial rhythm
- Atrial rhythm with ≥3 consecutive P´ waves of different morphologies.
- Atrial rate ≤100 bpm.
- Absence of a single, dominant atrial pacemaker.
- Variable P´-P´, P´R, and R-R intervals.
- P´ waves separated by an isoelectric line.

Supraventricular tachycardia (unspecified)
- A series of ≥3 consecutive ectopic supraventricular complexes at a heart rate >100 bpm.
- Narrow complex (unless aberrant conduction or underlying bundle branch block).
- Retrograde P´ waves may be present.
- May be sustained or appear in short paroxysms.
- Comment: Unspecified SVT reflects that the exact underlying mechanism cannot be determined from the surface ECG.

Atrial flutter (typical)
- An atrial rhythm with an atrial rate between 240 and 350 bpm.
- Flutter waves with a continuously undulating "sawtooth" morphology.
  - The polarity of the flutter waves in leads II, III, aVF, V1 depends on the direction of rotation, but is usually negative in the inferior leads and positive in lead V1.
- Conduction ratio is typically 2:1.
- Comment: There are atypical forms of atrial flutter that overlap with forms of atrial tachycardia (see text for details).

Atrial fibrillation
- P waves are replaced by fibrillatory waves with an atrial rate of 350 to 600 bpm.
- The ventricular response is normally irregularly irregular.

B. AV Junctional Rhythms and Complexes

AV junctional premature complex (JPC)
- The complex appears early relative to the native rhythm.
- An inverted, retrograde P´ wave is present that may appear before, within, or after the QRS complex.
- When present before the QRS complex, the P´R interval is short (<0.12 seconds).
- The P´ wave is followed by a QRS complex identical to the native rhythm (unless aberrant conduction).
- Exceptions and modifiers.
  - Abnormalities of both antegrade and retrograde conduction may be present (see text for details).

AV junctional rhythm
- A rhythm whose origin is the AV junction.
- An inverted, retrograde P´ wave is present that may appear before, within, or after the QRS complex.
- When present before QRS complex, the P´R interval is short (<0.12 seconds).
- The heart rate is typically 40 to 60 bpm.

Accelerated AV junctional rhythm
- An AV junctional rhythm with a rate higher than the normal intrinsic rate of the AV junction (>60 bpm).
- Typically has gradual onset and termination.
- Comment: Also called *nonparoxysmal junctional tachycardia*. When the HR is >100 bpm, it may be termed *accelerated AV junctional tachycardia*.

Focal junctional tachycardia
- A rapid rhythm whose origin is the AV junction.
- Junctional rate >100 bpm (typically 110-250 bpm).
- Inverted, retrograde P´ waves that may be present before, within, or after the QRS complex.
- When present before the QRS complex, the P´R interval is short (<0.12 seconds).
- Typically has a paroxysmal onset.
- Comment: This is a rare clinical entity that is also known as *automatic junctional tachycardia* or *paroxysmal* (*ectopic*) *junctional tachycardia*.

AV junctional escape complex
- The complex appears late relative to the cycle of the normal rhythm, emerging due to a failure of a normally faster physiologic pacemaker.
- P´ waves are commonly absent.
- If present, an inverted, retrograde P´ wave may appear before, within, or after the QRS complex.
- When present before the QRS complex, the P´R interval of the junctional complex is short (<0.12 seconds).
- The QRS complex is identical to the native rhythm.

AV junctional escape rhythm
- A pattern of two or more AV junctional escape complexes.

C. Ventricular Rhythms and Complexes

Ventricular premature complex (VPC)
- The complex occurs early relative to the native rhythm and is not preceded by an electrically related P wave.
- QRS duration ≥0.12 seconds.
- Secondary ST segment and T wave abnormalities directed opposite to that of the dominant R wave.
- May have uniform or multiform morphology.
- Supporting criteria:
  - A fully compensatory pause is present.
- Exceptions and modifications (see text for details).
  - Interpolated VPC.
  - Late (end) diastolic VPC.

Ventricular tachycardia (VT)
- A series of ≥3 consecutive ventricular complexes at a rate of >100 bpm.
  - May be defined further according to duration and morphology:
    – Sustained: lasting ≥30 sec.
    – Nonsustained: lasting <30 sec.
    – Monomorphic: single QRS complex morphology.
    – Multiple monomorphic: >1 monomorphic VT is present.
    – Polymorphic: continuously changing QRS complex morphology.
    – Pleomorphic: more than one distinct QRS complex within the same VT episode.
    – Bidirectional: VT typically with a RBBB pattern accompanied by beat-to-beat alternans in the frontal plane (usually associated with digitalis toxicity).
    – Ventricular flutter: A very rapid form of VT (250-350 bpm) with a sine wave appearance.

Torsades de pointes
- A unique form of polymorphic ventricular tachycardia characterized by QRS peaks that "twist" around the baseline.
- Associated with prolongation of the QT interval, whether inherited or acquired.

Accelerated idioventricular rhythm
- A series of ≥3 consecutive ventricular complexes at a rate ≤100 bpm.

Ventricular fibrillation
- A disorganized, rapid (>350 bpm) ventricular rhythm.
- Chaotic, fibrillatory waves of variable rate and amplitude.

Ventricular parasystole
- Ventricular premature complexes in a pattern independent of the intrinsic rhythm.
- VPCs appear with varying coupling intervals, along with interpolated and fusion complexes.
- The interectopic intervals are constant or are multiples of a common denominator.

Ventricular escape complex
- A ventricular complex that appears late relative to the cycle of the normal rhythm, emerging due to a failure of a normally faster physiologic pacemaker.
- There is no electrical relationship to a P wave.

Ventricular escape rhythm
- A series of two or more consecutive ventricular escape complexes.

D. Pacemaker Function, Rhythm, and Complexes

Single-chamber atrial pacing
- A pacemaker stimulus captures the atrium.
- In the absence of conduction abnormality, a native QRS complex follows.
- Comment: The presence of a ventricular lead cannot be excluded.

Single-chamber pacemaker, ventricular pacing on demand
- A pacemaker stimulus captures the ventricles after a pause in the native rhythm.

Single-chamber pacemaker, ventricular pacing with complete control
- A ventricular pacemaker captures the ventricles without evidence of intrinsic ventricular depolarization.

Dual-chamber pacemaker, atrial sensing with ventricular pacing
- A ventricular pacemaker captures the ventricles following a normally sensed P wave.

Dual-chamber pacemaker, atrial and ventricular sensing, and pacing
- A pacemaker rhythm with evidence of both atrial and ventricular sensing and pacing.

Biventricular pacemaker (with or without atrial pacemaker)
The paced complex is a hybrid that reflects activation of both the left and right ventricles. While variable and determined by programming, the following features may be seen:

- Lead V1 typically shows a dominant R wave.
  - Comment: This pattern is different from isolated RV pacing that characteristically produces a dominant S wave in lead V1.
- Lead I typically shows a negative deflection.
- Separate left followed by right ventricular stimulus artifacts may be visible.
  - Comment: The right ventricular stimulus artifact is often hidden within the QRS complex.

Pacemaker malfunction, failure to capture either the atrium or ventricle appropriately
- A pacemaker stimulus that fails to capture the appropriate chamber when nonrefractory.

Pacemaker malfunction, failure to sense either atrial or ventricular complexes appropriately
- A pacemaker output that fails to be appropriately inhibited by an intrinsic depolarization in either the atrium or the ventricle.

Pacemaker malfunction, failure to fire appropriately on demand
- A pacemaker stimulus that does not appear when it would normally be expected.

▶ II. AV CONDUCTION ABNORMALITIES

AV block, first-degree
- Sinus rhythm in which every P wave is followed by a QRS complex.
- The PR interval is prolonged >0.2 seconds.

AV block, second-degree, Mobitz type I
- Sinus rhythm with at least two consecutively conducted complexes.
- Intermittent failure of AV conduction when expected.
  - A single P wave is not followed by a QRS complex.
- A nonconducted P wave that ends the sequence is preceded by at least one or more sinus complexes with a prolonged PR interval relative to the first conducted complex.
  - Classic form:
    - Progressive PR prolongation exhibiting the Wenckebach phenomenon.
    - The shortest PR interval is the first in a sequence.
    - The maximal prolongation of the PR intervals occurs between the first and second conducted complexes in a sequence.
    - The incremental change in PR prolongation decreases with each conducted complex. This results in progressively shorter R-R intervals.
    - The R-R interval containing the nonconducted P wave is less than the sum of two P-P intervals.
  - Common form:
    - Variable PR prolongation without a progressive pattern.
    - The shortest PR interval is the first in a sequence.
- Supporting criteria:
  - The conducted QRS complexes are usually narrow.

AV block, second-degree, Mobitz type II
- Sinus rhythm with at least two consecutively conducted complexes.
- Intermittent failure of AV conduction when expected.
  - A single P wave is not followed by a QRS complex.
- The PR interval is constant in the complexes before and after the nonconducted P wave.
- The R-R intervals are constant, with those straddling the nonconducted P wave equal to the sum of two P-P intervals.
- Supporting criteria:
  - The QRS complex is usually wide (≥0.12 seconds).

AV block, second-degree, 2:1
- Sinus rhythm is present.
- Conducted P waves alternate with those that are nonconducted.

AV block, high-grade or advanced second-degree AV block
- Sinus rhythm is present.
- The atrial rate must be greater than the ventricular rate.
- Two or more P waves fail to conduct to the ventricles (the conduction ratio is 3:1 or greater, typically in even numbers).
- Comment: The presence of any conducted complexes indicates the block is high grade rather than complete.

AV block, third-degree or complete
- There is an absence of AV conduction with P waves and QRS complexes completely dissociated.
- The atrial rate must be greater than the ventricular rate.
- Comment:
  - The rhythm may be a supraventricular rhythm other than sinus, such as atrial fibrillation, atrial flutter, or another supraventricular arrhythmia.
  - An escape rhythm may be present, originating either in the AV junction or ventricles.

Ventricular preexcitation (WPW pattern)
- Short PR interval (<0.12 seconds).
- Normal P wave morphology.
- Slurring of the initial QRS complex (delta wave).
- Wide QRS complex (usually >0.12 seconds).
- Secondary ST segment and T wave abnormalities.
- Comment: The size of the delta wave, the degree of PR interval shortening, and the amount of QRS complex prolongation, all depend on the relative amount of myocardium activated by the accessory pathway versus normal conduction.

Enhanced AV conduction (isolated short PR interval)
- Sinus rhythm with a short PR interval of <0.12 seconds.
- Normal P wave morphology.
- Normal QRS complex duration and morphology.

▶ III. MISCELLANEOUS AV RELATIONSHIPS

Concealed conduction
- The phenomenon of partial penetration of atrial, AV junctional, or ventricular impulses into any portion of the specialized conduction system.
- The evidence is not visible on the surface ECG (concealed), but manifests its effect by altering the conduction of a following impulse.
- Most often seen as partial antegrade penetration of the AV junction by a supraventricular impulse or partial retrograde penetration by a ventricular impulse.

Ventriculophasic sinus arrhythmia
- A form of sinus arrhythmia in which the sinus cycles that contain ventricular depolarizations are shorter than those cycles that do not.
- Typically associated with complete heart block.
- May be observed whether the origin of the ventricular complex is from the native myocardium or via an electronic pacemaker.

AV dissociation

- The presence of independent atrial and ventricular rhythms.
- The mechanisms include (alone or in combination):
  - A slowing or default of the sinus impulse with the emergence of a subsidiary pacemaker.
  - Abnormal acceleration of a normally latent pacemaker that usurps control.
  - AV block that prevents transmission of the atrial impulse from reaching the ventricles.

Reciprocal (echo) complex

- A reentry-based complex resulting from a depolarization that originates in one chamber and returns to reactivate the same chamber.

Retrograde atrial activation from a ventricular focus

- A ventricular impulse that conducts retrograde to depolarize the atrium.

Fusion complex

- A complex that represents the combined activation from more than one focus.
- The resulting hybrid complex demonstrates a morphology intermediate between the baseline morphology of the two independent depolarizations.

Ventricular capture complex

- During a period of AV dissociation, a supraventricular impulse that conducts to the ventricles.
- Comment: Usually refers to a sinus impulse that captures the ventricle during a period of ventricular tachycardia.

Interpolation of ventricular premature complexes

- Ventricular premature complexes that are interposed between two sinus complexes.
- The normal sinus rhythm is undisturbed.
- Comment: A prolonged PR interval typically follows the VPC, which is a result of concealed retrograde conduction into the AV junction.

▶ IV. P WAVE ABNORMALITIES

Right atrial abnormality/enlargement

- Increased P wave amplitude >2.5 mm in leads II, III, and aVF.
- Tall initial P wave amplitude >1.5 mm in lead V1.
- Normal P wave duration <0.12 seconds.
- Supporting criteria:
  - P wave axis shifted rightward of +75 degrees.

Left atrial abnormality/enlargement

- Prolonged and notched P wave with duration ≥0.12 seconds in leads I, II, aVF, V5, V6.
- Abnormal P terminal force ≥0.04 mm-sec in lead V1.
- Supporting criteria:
  - P wave axis leftward of +15 degrees.

Bi-atrial abnormality/enlargement

- In lead V1, a tall initial P wave amplitude >1.5 mm and an abnormal P terminal force ≥0.04 mm-sec.
- In the limb leads, a notched and prolonged P wave ≥0.12 seconds with an amplitude >2.5 mm.

Nonspecific atrial abnormality/Intraatrial block

- A wide P wave ≥0.12 seconds without other criteria for atrial abnormalities.

PR segment abnormalities

- PR segment depression below the baseline of ≥0.8 mm.
- PR segment elevation above the baseline of ≥0.5 mm.

▶ V. ABNORMALITIES OF QRS AXIS OR VOLTAGE

Left axis deviation

- A mean frontal plane QRS axis between −30 and −90 degrees.
- Comment: Some electrocardiographers further characterize left axis deviation as either moderate (between −30 and −45 degrees) or marked (between −45 and −90 degrees).

Right axis deviation

- A mean frontal plane QRS axis between +90 degrees and +180 degrees.
- Comment: Some electrocardiographers further characterize right axis deviation as either moderate (between +90 and +120 degrees) or marked (between +120 and +180 degrees).

Extreme axis deviation

- A mean frontal plane axis between −90 degrees and ±180 degrees.
- Comment: This may represent either extreme right or left axis deviation.

Indeterminate axis

- The mean QRS axis is directed out of the frontal plane resulting in equiphasic complexes in multiple leads.

Poor R wave progression

- R waves are present and increase in voltage from leads V1-V3, but the R wave amplitude in V3 is ≤3 mm.
  - Reverse R wave progression is as above, except that R wave voltage decreases from leads V1-V3.
- Comment: Not applicable when there is low voltage in the precordial leads, left bundle branch block and preexcitation (WPW pattern).

Low voltage, limb leads

- The amplitude of the entire QRS complex (R wave + S wave) in each of the limb leads is <5 mm.

Low voltage, precordial leads

- The amplitude of the entire QRS complex (R wave + S wave) in each of the precordial leads is <10 mm.

Electrical alternans

- Beat-to-beat voltage changes in the P wave, QRS complex, and T wave, alone or in combination.

▶ VI. INTRAVENTRICULAR CONDUCTION ABNORMALITIES

Right bundle branch block, complete
- QRS duration ≥0.12 seconds.
- rsr´, rsR´, rSR´, or M-shaped pattern in leads V1 or V2.
- The secondary R´ wave is usually wider and of greater amplitude than the initial r wave.
- Secondary ST segment and T wave abnormalities in the right precordial leads directed opposite to that of the dominant R wave.
- Supporting criteria:
  - Prolonged R peak time (time to the intrinsicoid deflection) >0.05 seconds in lead V1.
  - Broad S waves in leads I, aVL, and V5-V6.

Right bundle branch block, incomplete
- Criteria for right bundle branch block, but with a QRS duration >0.10 and <0.12 seconds.

Left anterior fascicular block
- Left axis deviation between −45 and −90 degrees.
- QRS duration <0.12 seconds.
- A positive terminal deflection in leads aVL and aVR with the peak of the terminal R wave in aVR occurring later than in aVL (reflecting a counterclockwise vector loop).
- No other cause of left axis deviation (eg, left ventricular enlargement, inferior wall MI, congenital heart disease).
- Supporting criteria:
  - qR complex in leads I and aVL.
  - rS complex in leads II, III, aVF, and an S wave in lead III, deeper than lead II.
  - Prolonged R peak time (time to the intrinsicoid deflection) ≥0.045 seconds in lead aVL.

Left posterior fascicular block
- Right axis deviation between +90 and +180 degrees in adults.
- QRS duration <0.12 seconds.
- rS pattern in leads I and aVL.
- qR pattern in leads II, III, and aVF (Q wave width <0.04 seconds).
  - Comment: R wave in lead III usually equals or exceeds the R wave in lead II.
- No other cause of right axis deviation (eg, extensive lateral wall MI, right ventricular enlargement, pulmonary disease).
- Comment: Usually associated with right bundle branch block.

Left bundle branch block, complete
- QRS duration ≥0.12 seconds.
- Broad, notched, or slurred R waves (rR´, RR´) in leads I, aVL, and V5-V6.
- Absent Q waves in leads I, V5-V6 (may be present in lead aVL).
- Secondary ST segment and T wave abnormalities in the left precordial leads directed opposite to that of the dominant R wave (also leads I and aVL).

- Supporting criteria:
  - Prolonged R peak time (time to the intrinsicoid deflection) >0.06 seconds in leads V5-V6.
  - Broad S waves in leads V1-V2 with rS or QS pattern.

Left bundle branch block, incomplete
- Criteria for left bundle branch block, but with a QRS complex duration >0.10 and <0.12 seconds.

Nonspecific intraventricular conduction delay
- The QRS complex duration is prolonged >0.10 seconds, but without diagnostic criteria for either right bundle branch block or left bundle branch block.

Aberrant intraventricular conduction
- A transient intraventricular conduction delay due to partial refractoriness of the conduction system associated with variances in cycle length.
- May accompany any supraventricular complex or rhythm including sinus, AV junctional, supraventricular tachycardia, atrial flutter, and atrial fibrillation.

▶ VII. VENTRICULAR ENLARGEMENT/ HYPERTROPHY

Left ventricular enlargement/hypertrophy
A variety of different criteria exist, each with strengths and weaknesses.

Precordial lead based
- S wave in lead V1 + R wave in lead V5 or V6 is >35 mm (age >40).
- S wave in lead V1 + R wave in lead V5 or V6 is >40 mm (age 31-40).
- S wave in lead V1 + R wave in lead V5 or V6 is >60 mm (age 16-30).

Limb lead based
- R wave in lead I + S wave in lead III is >25 mm.

Combined precordial and limb lead based
- In men, R wave in lead aVL + S wave in lead V3 is >28 mm.
- In women, R wave in lead aVL + S wave in lead V3 is >20 mm.

Scoring system based (4 = "probable" and ≥5 = "definite")
- R wave or S wave in any limb lead ≥20 mm (3 points).
- S wave in lead V1 or V2 ≥30 mm (3 points).
- R wave in lead V5 or V6 ≥30 mm (3 points).
- Left ventricular strain pattern.
  - Without digitalis (3 points).
  - With digitalis (1 point).
- Abnormal P terminal force lead V1 (3 points).
- Left axis deviation ≥−30 degrees (2 points).
- QRS duration ≥0.09 seconds (1 point).
- R wave peak time (time to the intrinsicoid deflection) in lead V5 or V6 ≥0.05 seconds (1 point).

Right ventricular enlargement/hypertrophy

- Right axis deviation (in the absence of other causes).
- R/S ratio in V1 >1.
- R/S ratio in lead V5 or V6 ≤1.
- R wave in lead V1 ≥7 mm.
- qR pattern in lead V1.
- rSR′pattern in lead V1 with R′wave ≥10 mm (normal QRS duration).
- Supporting criteria:
  - ST segment depression and T wave inversion in the right precordial leads.
  - Right atrial abnormality.
  - R wave peak time (time to the intrinsicoid deflection) in lead V1 ≥0.04 seconds.

Combined, right and left ventricular enlargement/hypertrophy

- The criteria for left and right ventricular enlargement/ hypertrophy occur together.

▶ VIII. Q-WAVE MYOCARDIAL INFARCTION

General features

- Acute or recent myocardial infarction (MI) is characterized by diagnostic Q waves (or developing Q waves) in conjunction with ST segment abnormalities of acute myocardial injury. These include horizontal or concave down (coved) ST segment elevation in the affected contiguous leads (ST segment depression in leads V1-V2 for posterior MI).
- Old or of indeterminate age MI is identified when there are diagnostic Q waves without associated ST segment or T wave abnormalities to suggest acute or recent injury. Q (or QS) waves are considered diagnostic when they have a width of ≥0.04 seconds wide with an amplitude ≥1 mm deep. Diagnostic accuracy is increased when the depth of the Q wave exceeds 25% of the corresponding R wave.
- Recent (subacute) MI is characterized by resolving ST segment abnormalities associated with T wave inversion in the affected contiguous leads (upright T wave for posterior infarction).
- Comment: It is often impossible to definitively determine the timing of the infarction without clinical correlation and serial tracings. Multiple patterns exist, including those that do not conform exactly to the following diagnoses.

Anteroseptal

- Leads V1-V3.

Anterior

- Leads V3-V4 ± V2.

Anterolateral

- Leads V4-V6 ± I, aVL.

Extensive Anterior

- Leads V1-V5 ± V6.

Lateral or High Lateral

- Leads I, aVL.

Inferior (diaphragmatic)

- Leads II, III, aVF.

Posterior

- Tall R waves ≥0.04 seconds with R>S waves in leads V1-V2.

Suggestive of ventricular aneurysm

- ST segment elevation in leads containing Q waves that persist for at least 2 weeks after MI.

▶ IX. ST SEGMENT, T WAVE, QT INTERVAL, AND U WAVE ABNORMALITIES

Normal variant, isolated J point elevation (early repolarization pattern)

- Upward displacement of the ST segment at the J junction from 1 to 4 mm above the isoelectric line. The ST segment demonstrates upward concavity and is associated with upright T waves that are tall, broad, and symmetrical in shape.

Isolated J-point depression

- Upsloping ST segment depression at the J junction associated with an otherwise normal QRS complex and T wave.

Normal variant, RsR′ (or rsR′) pattern

- The RsR′ complex is of normal duration.
- The primary R wave in lead V1 is ≤8 mm.
- The secondary R′ wave is <6 mm.
- The R′/S ratio is <1 in any right precordial lead.

Normal variant, persistent juvenile T wave pattern

- Asymmetrical T wave inversion in two or more leads, V1-V3 in an otherwise normal adult ECG. T waves remain upright in leads I, II, V5, and V6.

ST segment or T wave abnormalities suggesting acute or recent myocardial injury

- Horizontal or concave downward (coved) ST segment elevation with or without associated T wave inversion.
  - For posterior wall injury, horizontal ST depression with an upright T wave in leads V1-V2.

ST segment or T wave abnormalities suggesting either reciprocal change or myocardial ischemia in the setting of acute myocardial injury

- Horizontal or downsloping ST segment depression with or without T wave abnormalities in leads opposite to those with ST segment elevation.

ST segment or T wave abnormalities suggesting myocardial ischemia in the absence of acute myocardial injury
- Horizontal or downsloping ST segment depression with or without T wave abnormalities without concomitant ST segment elevation in additional leads.

ST segment or T wave abnormalities secondary to ventricular enlargement/hypertrophy
- Left ventricular enlargement/hypertrophy.
  - ST segment depression and T wave inversion in the left precordial leads where the QRS complex is upright (eg, leads V5, V6).
    - Comment: May also be present in leads I and aVL with a horizontal axis and in leads II, III, and aVF with a vertical axis.
  - Slight ST segment elevation and upright T waves in precordial leads where the QRS complex is negative (eg, leads V1, V2).
- Right ventricular enlargement/hypertrophy.
  - ST segment depression and T wave inversion in leads V1, V2.
    - Comment: May also be present in leads II, III, and aVF.

ST segment or T wave abnormalities secondary to ventricular conduction abnormality.
- Left bundle branch block.
  - ST segment depression and T wave inversion in the left precordial leads where the QRS complex is upright (eg, leads V5, V6).
    - Comment: Also commonly present in leads I and aVL.
- Right bundle branch block.
  - ST segment depression and T wave inversion in the right precordial leads where the QRS complex is upright (eg, leads V1, V2).

ST segment or T wave abnormalities suggesting acute pericarditis
- Diffuse, concave upward ST segment elevation.
- Typically in multiple leads, but most common in leads I, II, and V5-V6.
- Supporting criteria:
  - Reciprocal changes and concomitant T wave inversion are absent, helping to distinguish pericarditis from acute myocardial injury.
  - The T wave remains concordant with the direction of the ST segment in early pericarditis.
  - PR segment depression in leads with ST segment elevation.
  - PR segment elevation may in seen in lead aVR.

Nonspecific ST segment or T wave abnormalities
- Slight ST segment depression or elevation, isolated T wave inversion, or other findings that cannot be determined to be secondary to a specific abnormality.

Post ventricular premature complex T wave abnormality
- An alteration of the baseline T wave morphology of the complex that follows a ventricular premature complex.

Peaked T waves
- The T wave amplitude is >6 mm in the limb leads or >10 mm in any precordial lead.

Prolonged QT interval for heart rate (QTc)
- The normal QT interval varies by heart rate and gender, termed the corrected QT interval (QTc).
- The most common correction method is the Bazett formula, which is the QTc = QT interval (measured in seconds) divided by the square root of the R-R interval (measured in seconds). The formula assumes a stable R-R interval and is most valid between the heart rates of 60 and 100 bpm.
- The normal QTc for men is >390 msec and <450 msec.
- The normal QTc for women is >390 msec and <460 msec.
- Comment: A quick way to evaluate for QT prolongation, valid between a heart rate of 60 to 100, is to assess whether the QT interval is less than half of the R-R interval. A simple method is to count the number of small boxes for each interval and determine whether the number of boxes for the QT interval is less than half those of the R-R interval. A QT interval more than half of the R-R interval is potentially abnormal and a more formal mathematical calculation is warranted.

Prominent U wave
- The maximum U wave amplitude is usually 1.0 mm, rarely reaching 2.0 mm.
- The amplitude of the U wave is proportional to that of the T wave, but should be <25% of the T wave amplitude.

Inverted U wave
- The U wave generally follows the direction of the T wave.
- U wave inversion in leads with a normally upright T wave should be considered abnormal.

▶ X. TECHNICAL PROBLEMS

Technical errors or artifacts are present
- Incorrect electrode placement or lead reversal.
- Artifact due electrical interference.
- Artifact due to tremor.
- Standardization change (specify half or double standardization).

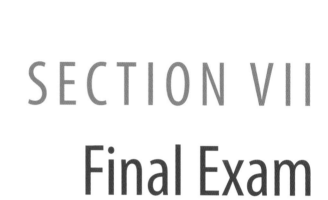

SECTION VII
Final Exam

Final Exam

In this section you will find twenty-five, 12-lead electrocardiograms for you to interpret. The clinical history is presented above each tracing. Apply the method of interpretation you learned in Chapter 24 and the criteria found in Chapter 25. Use the concept of structured reporting to measure, identify, and then synthesize the findings into a comprehensive interpretation. Include all of the items from the list below in your report.

Technical quality:

Rhythm:

Atrial rate:

Ventricular rate:

PR interval:

QRS duration:

QT interval:

Axis:

Abnormalities:

Synthesis:

ECG #1 A 65-year-old man seen for a routine yearly physical.

RHYTHM STRIP: II 25 mm/sec; 1 cm/mV

▶ ECG #1

Interpretation

Technical quality: Satisfactory

Rhythm: Sinus

Atrial rate: 79 bpm

Ventricular rate: 79 bpm

PR interval: 0.14 seconds

QRS duration: 0.08 seconds

QT interval: 0.38 seconds

Axis: −75 degrees

Abnormalities: Axis leftward of −30 degrees. Abnormal P terminal force, lead V1. R wave voltage in leads V1-V3 <3 mm.

Synthesis: Sinus rhythm. Left axis deviation. Left atrial abnormality. Left anterior fascicular block. Poor R wave progression.

Comment: Marked left axis deviation is present indicative of left anterior fascicular block. Poor R wave progression is commonly seen in left anterior fascicular block as the loss of anterior forces in the horizontal plane reduces R wave voltage in leads V1-V3. Left atrial abnormality is present with abnormal P terminal force in lead V1. The notched P waves in leads II, III, and aVF support this diagnosis.

ECG #2 An 80-year-old woman with congestive heart failure.

RHYTHM STRIP: II 25 mm/sec; 1 cm/mV

► **ECG #2**

Interpretation

Technical quality: Satisfactory

Rhythm: Sinus

Atrial rate: 69 bpm

Ventricular rate: 69 bpm

PR interval: 0.20 seconds

QRS duration: 0.16 seconds

QT interval: 0.40 seconds

Axis: −15 degrees

Abnormalities: Prolonged QRS complex duration. Wide, notched QRS complex associated with ST segment depression and T wave inversion in leads I, aVL, V5-V6.

Synthesis: Sinus rhythm. Left bundle branch block with secondary ST segment and T wave abnormalities.

Comment: Left bundle branch block is frequently a marker for significant myocardial disease, left ventricular systolic dysfunction, and congestive heart failure.

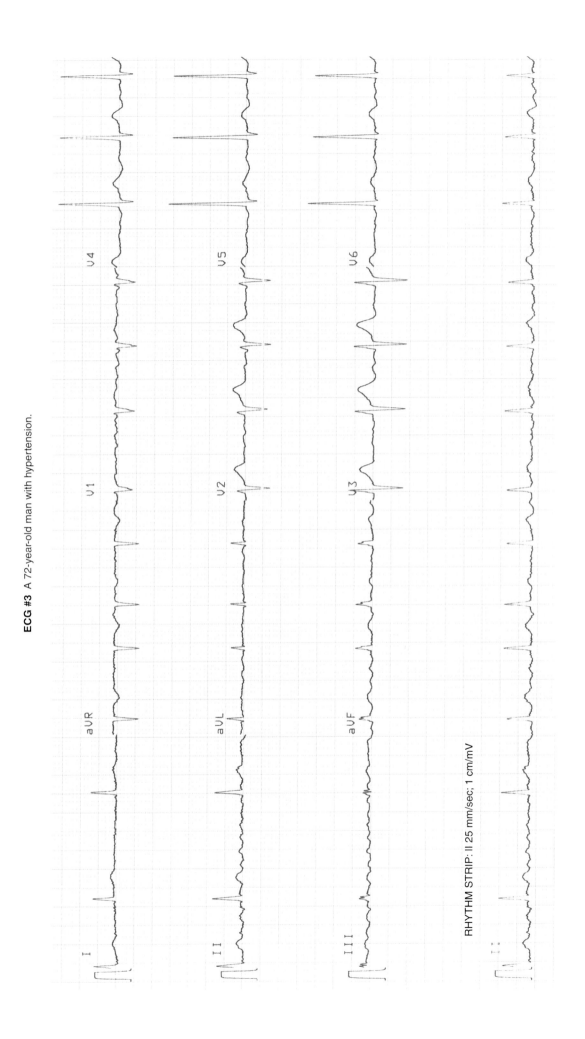

ECG #3 A 72-year-old man with hypertension.

RHYTHM STRIP: II 25 mm/sec; 1 cm/mV

▶ **ECG #3**

Interpretation

Technical quality: Satisfactory

Rhythm: Atrial fibrillation

Atrial rate: N/A

Ventricular rate: 81 bpm (average)

PR interval: N/A

QRS duration: 0.08 seconds

QT interval: 0.36 seconds

Axis: +30 degrees

Abnormalities: P waves replaced by fibrillatory waves.

Synthesis: Atrial fibrillation with a controlled ventricular response. Otherwise normal tracing.

Comment: Atrial fibrillation is the most common sustained arrhythmia. In this patient, the ventricular response was controlled with the use of long-acting diltiazem, a calcium channel blocker that has both antihypertensive and AV-blocking properties.

ECG #4 An 85-year-old man with sepsis.

RHYTHM STRIP: II
25 mm/sec;1 cm/mV

▶ **ECG #4**

Interpretation

Technical quality: Satisfactory

Rhythm: Sinus tachycardia

Atrial rate: 124 bpm

Ventricular rate: 124 bpm

PR interval: 0.14 seconds

QRS duration: 0.08 seconds

QT interval: 0.32 seconds

Axis: –15 degrees

Abnormalities: Heart rate >100 bpm. Q waves in leads II, III, aVF. Slight ST depression in leads I, aVL, V6. Flat T waves in leads I, II, III, aVL, aVF, V5-V6.

Synthesis: Sinus tachycardia. Inferior wall myocardial infarction, old or of indeterminate age. Nonspecific ST segment and T wave abnormalities.

Comment: Sinus tachycardia is commonly present in sepsis, presenting as a physiologic response to fever, dehydration, and hypotension. This patient also had a history of coronary artery disease with evidence of a prior inferior wall MI. The ST segment and T wave findings are nonspecific and should not be reported as suggestive of an acute coronary syndrome.

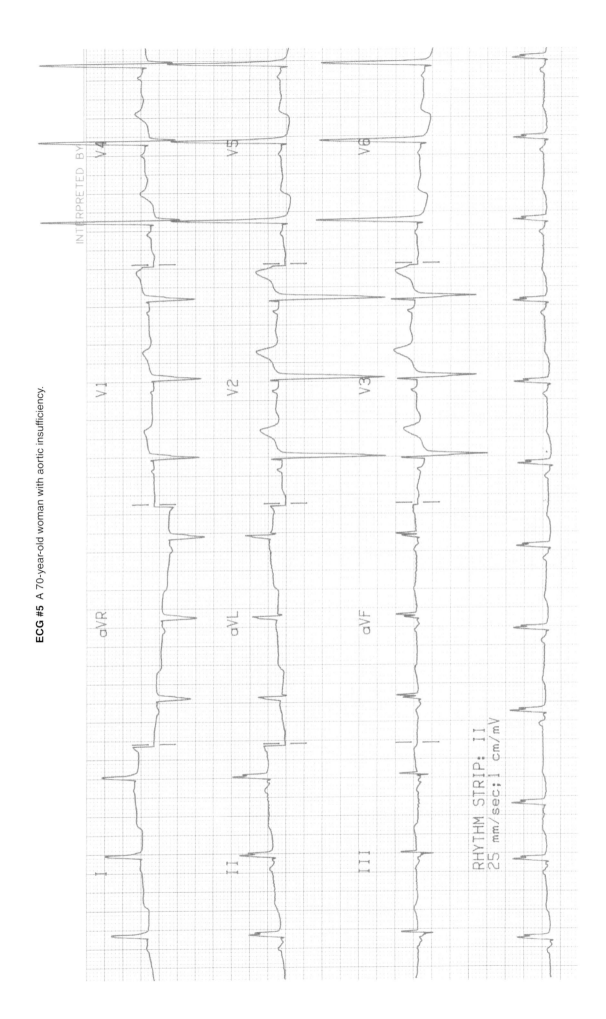

ECG #5 A 70-year-old woman with aortic insufficiency.

I aVR V1 V4

II aVL V2 V5

III aVF V3 V6

RHYTHM STRIP: II
25 mm/sec; 1 cm/mV

▶ ECG #5

Interpretation

Technical quality: Satisfactory

Rhythm: Sinus with occasional atrial premature complex

Atrial rate: 69 bpm

Ventricular rate: 69 bpm

PR interval: 0.16 seconds

QRS duration: 0.08 seconds

QT interval: 0.40 seconds

Axis: +30 degrees

Abnormalities: Narrow premature complex. S wave in lead V1 + R wave in lead V5 >35 mm. ST segment depression in leads I, aVL, V4-V6. Biphasic T waves in leads I, aVL, V5-V6. Low T wave voltage in leads II, aVF.

Synthesis: Sinus rhythm. APC. Left ventricular enlargement/hypertrophy with secondary ST segment and T wave abnormalities. Additional nonspecific T wave abnormalities.

Comment: Severe aortic insufficiency can result in a marked increase in left ventricular mass. Note that the ST segment and T wave abnormalities in the lateral limb and precordial leads are likely repolarization findings secondary to ventricular enlargement. The relatively low T wave voltage in leads II and aVF are best considered nonspecific.

ECG #6 A 60-year-old man with symptoms of palpitation.

RHYTHM STRIP: II 25 mm/sec; 1 cm/mV

I aVR V1 V4

II aVL V2 V5

III aVF V3 V6

II

▶ **ECG #6**

Interpretation

Technical quality: Satisfactory

Rhythm: Sinus with atrial premature complexes

Atrial rate: 95 bpm

Ventricular rate: 95 bpm

PR interval: 0.16 seconds

QRS duration: 0.10 seconds

QT interval: 0.34 seconds

Axis: 0 degrees

Abnormalities: Narrow premature complexes with occasional change in QRS complex morphology.

Synthesis: Sinus rhythm. Frequent atrial premature complexes with occasional aberrant conduction. Otherwise normal tracing.

Comment: Frequent atrial premature complexes are present. Most are conducted normally with the QRS complex unchanged significantly from the baseline. Although not readily evident on the lead II rhythm strip, aberrant conduction of one of the APCs is seen in lead V1. Do not mistake this wide complex as a VPC. On close inspection, evidence of a P wave is present on the downslope of the preceding T wave. Also don't be confused by the fully compensatory pause after the premature complex, which is more common with a VPC. Here, it reflects the fact that the premature atrial depolarization did not reset the sinus node. Note the rsR´ (RBBB-type) morphology of the wide complex that appears after a long-short sequence, a pattern highly suggestive of aberrant conduction. Somewhat surprising is that the next long-short sequence conducts normally. Although not obvious on the surface ECG, one can theorize that there was a slight delay in transmission of this premature impulse through the AV node, allowing recovery of the right bundle branch and explaining the narrow complex.

ECG #7 An 81-year-old man seen in preoperative consultation.

aVR   V1   V4

aVL   V2   V5

aVF   V3   V6

I

II

III

II

40 Hz   25.0 mm/s   10.0 mm/mV   4 by 2.5s + 1 rhythm ld   MAC55 010A   12SL

▲ ECG #7

Interpretation

Technical quality: Satisfactory

Rhythm: Sinus

Atrial rate: 75 bpm

Ventricular rate: 75 bpm

PR interval: 0.18 seconds

QRS duration: 0.14 seconds

QT interval: 0.42 seconds

Axis: +75 degrees

Abnormalities: Wide, notched P wave in lead II and abnormal P terminal force in lead V1. Prolonged QRS complex duration with rSR′ pattern accompanied by ST segment abnormalities and T wave inversion in leads V1 and V2.

Synthesis: Sinus rhythm. Left atrial abnormality. Right bundle branch block with secondary ST segment and T wave abnormalities.

Comment: Note the rSR′ pattern in lead V1 and V2 with ST segment and T wave findings that are diagnostic of right bundle branch block. There is also a broad S wave in leads I, aVL, and V4-V6, which record the electrical findings from a perspective looking away from the right-sided terminal conduction delay.

ECG #8 A 55-year-old man in the emergency department with chest discomfort.

I

aVR

V1

V4

II

aVL

V2

V5

III

aVF

V3

V6

RHYTHM STRIP: II
25 mm/sec;1 cm/mV

▲ ECG #8

Interpretation

Technical quality: Satisfactory

Rhythm: Sinus bradyarrhythmia

Atrial rate: 56 bpm

Ventricular rate: 56 bpm

PR interval: 0.16 seconds

QRS duration: 0.08 seconds

QT interval: 0.40 seconds

Axis: +15 degrees

Abnormalities: Heart rate <60 bpm. Phasic variability of P-P intervals that vary from the shortest to longest cycle by >0.12 seconds. ST segment elevation in leads II, III, aVF, V5-V6. ST segment depression in leads aVL, V1-V3.

Synthesis: Sinus bradyarrhythmia. Inferior wall myocardial infarction with ST segment elevation suggestive of acute myocardial injury. ST segment depression in leads V1-V2 compatible with either acute posterior wall myocardial infarction or reciprocal changes.

Comment: The findings of an acute inferior wall myocardial infarction are obvious on this tracing. There are no standard ECG leads that look directly at the posterior wall, therefore one cannot determine with certainty whether the findings in leads V1-V2 represent concomitant posterior wall MI versus reciprocal inferior wall changes. This patient was taken immediately to the catheterization laboratory and found to have an occlusion of a dominant right coronary artery and underwent intervention. The dramatic results are seen in the next tracing.

ECG #9 A 55-year-old man 2 hours after receiving a right coronary artery stent.

▲ ECG #9

Interpretation

Technical quality: Satisfactory

Rhythm: Sinus bradycardia

Atrial rate: 52 bpm

Ventricular rate: 52 bpm

PR interval: 0.16 seconds

QRS duration: 0.08 seconds

QT interval: 0.42 seconds

Axis: +15 degrees

Abnormalities: Heart rate <60 bpm.

Synthesis: Sinus bradycardia. Otherwise within normal limits. Compared with the prior tracing of [date/time], the previous findings of acute ST elevation inferior wall (and possible posterior wall) myocardial infarction have resolved.

Comment: Here we have a prior tracing for comparison. It's important to mention the new findings, whether favorable as in this case or if progressively abnormal. When reporting a comparison, remember to specify the date and time of the previous tracing.

ECG #10 A 63-year-old man with heart palpitations.

40 Hz   25.0 mm/s   10.0 mm/mV   4 by 2.5s + 1 rhythm ld   MAC55 010A   ⚌₀ 12SL™

▲ **ECG #10**

Interpretation

Technical quality: Satisfactory

Rhythm: Supraventricular tachycardia

Atrial rate: 152 bpm

Ventricular rate: 152 bpm

PR interval: N/A

QRS duration: 0.08 seconds

QT interval: 0.30 seconds

Axis: 0 degrees

Abnormalities: Heart rate >100 bpm. No P waves evident. ST depression in leads V3-V5.

Synthesis: Supraventricular tachycardia. Nonspecific ST segment abnormalities.

Comment: The most likely diagnosis is AV nodal reentrant tachycardia (AVNRT). Note the "pseudo s waves" in leads II, III, and aVF that represent the inverted, retrograde P′ waves that appear just after the QRS complex. This is characteristic of a slow-fast, short RP′ interval AVNRT.

ECG #11 A 44-year-old asymptomatic man.

RHYTHM STRIP: II
25 mm/sec; 1 cm/mV

aVR   V1   V4

aVL   V2   V5

aVF   V3   V6

I

II

III

▲ ECG #11

Interpretation

Technical quality: Satisfactory

Rhythm: Sinus with occasional ventricular premature complex

Atrial rate: 78 bpm

Ventricular rate: 78 bpm

PR interval: 0.10 seconds

QRS duration: 0.12 seconds

QT interval: 0.42 seconds

Axis: +15 degrees

Abnormalities: Short PR interval. Delta wave leading to wide QRS complex with ST segment depression and flat or biphasic T waves, most prominent in leads II, III, aVF, V2-V6. Wide premature complex. Notched P wave in leads II, aVF and abnormal P terminal force in lead V1.

Synthesis: Sinus rhythm with preexcitation (WPW pattern). Occasional ventricular premature complex. Left atrial enlargement.

Comment: At first glance at the precordial leads, the large R wave voltage in lead V5 might lead one to mistakenly consider a diagnosis of left ventricular enlargement/hypertrophy. The tall R waves in leads V2-V3 also appear abnormal. On closer inspection, the short PR interval and delta wave are easily seen in multiple leads, indicating preexcitation. The WPW pattern is one of the great "imitators" of other ECG diagnoses.

ECG #12 A 54-year-old man seen in clinic.

25mm/s   10mm/mV   40Hz

▲ ECG #12

Interpretation

Technical quality: Satisfactory

Rhythm: Sinus with second-degree AV block, Mobitz type I

Atrial rate: 66 bpm

Ventricular rate: 53 (average) bpm

PR interval: Variable

QRS duration: 0.08 seconds

QT interval: 0.44 seconds

Axis: +15 degrees

Abnormalities: Progressive prolongation of the PR interval until failure to conduct.

Synthesis: Sinus rhythm with second-degree AV block, Mobitz type I. Otherwise normal tracing.

Comment: On the rhythm strip, note the "classic" Wenckebach sequence. The PR interval immediately after the pause is the shortest of the sequence, with a subtle, progressive increase in the PR interval and shortening of the R-R interval until a QRS is "dropped." The conduction delay of Mobitz type I, second-degree AV block is typically at the level of the AV node, and is unlikely to progress to higher degrees of block.

ECG #13 A 53-year-old woman with decompensated asthma who is receiving a bronchodilator.

RHYTHM STRIP: II
25 mm/sec; 1 cm/mV

► ECG #13

Interpretation

Technical quality: Satisfactory

Rhythm: Accelerated AV junctional rhythm

Atrial rate: N/A

Ventricular rate: 78 bpm

PR interval: N/A

QRS duration: 0.08 seconds

QT interval: 0.36 seconds

Axis: +45 degrees

Abnormalities: Absent P waves. S wave in lead V1 + R wave in lead V5 >35 mm. ST segment depression leads I, V4-V5. Biphasic T wave lead aVL.

Synthesis: Accelerated AV junctional rhythm. Left ventricular enlargement/hypertrophy with secondary ST segment and T wave abnormalities.

Comment: The natural, intrinsic rate of the AV junction is 40 to 60 bpm. The rate seen here is greater; therefore, it is categorized as an *accelerated* AV junctional rhythm. The hyperautomatic junctional focus has usurped control of the normally dominant sinus depolarization, likely due to bronchodilator therapy.

ECG #14 A 58-year-old man in the coronary care unit with chest discomfort.

I   aVR   V1   V4

II   aVL   V2   V5

III   aVF   V3   V6

RHYTHM STRIP: II
25 mm/sec;1 cm/mV

▲ ECG #14

Interpretation

Technical quality: Satisfactory with some fine baseline artifact

Rhythm: Sinus with occasional ventricular premature complex

Atrial rate: 101 bpm

Ventricular rate: 101 bpm

PR interval: 0.18 seconds

QRS duration: 0.08 seconds

QT interval: 0.30 seconds

Axis: +30 degrees

Abnormalities: HR >100 bpm. Wide premature complex. Marked ST segment depression leads I, II, aVL, aVF, V4-V6. T wave inversion leads I, aVL, V5-V6. Biphasic T wave leads II, V4. ST elevation lead V1 and borderline elevation lead V2. R wave voltage in leads V1-V3 <3 mm.

Synthesis: Sinus tachycardia with occasional VPC. ST segment and T wave abnormalities in inferior and lateral leads suggestive of myocardial ischemia. ST segment abnormalities in leads V1-V2 suggestive of posterior myocardial ischemia, but cannot exclude acute anteroseptal myocardial injury. Poor R wave progression.

Comment: This example demonstrates the typical findings of a non-ST elevation myocardial infarction with ST segment depression and T wave inversion in the inferior and lateral leads. There is slight segment ST elevation in leads V1-V2 that is likely part of the same process and reflects posterior ischemia. The patient was found to have a severe stenosis in a large obtuse marginal branch of the left circumflex coronary artery and received a coronary stent.

ECG #15 A 90-year-old man with a fractured hip seen in preoperative consultation. Medications include digitalis.

428

▶ ECG #15

Interpretation

Technical quality: Satisfactory

Rhythm: Atrial fibrillation with ventricular pacemaker and fusion complexes

Atrial rate: N/A

Ventricular rate: 85 (average) bpm

PR interval: N/A

QRS duration: 0.08 seconds

QT interval: 0.30 seconds

Axis: +15 degrees

Abnormalities: P waves replaced by fibrillatory waves. Slight ST segment depression lead I. Generalized low T wave voltage. T waves biphasic or inverted in leads I, II, aVF, V4-V6 and flat in leads III, aVL, V1-V3. Ventricular pacemaker complexes. Fusion complexes.

Synthesis: Atrial fibrillation with a moderate ventricular response. Nonspecific ST segment and T wave abnormalities. Ventricular pacemaker on demand. Fusion complexes.

Comment: The native rhythm is atrial fibrillation with a ventricular pacemaker firing on demand. The escape rate and pacing rate are both programmed to 70 bpm. On the rhythm strip, the second from the left and the last complex on the right are fusion complexes. The hybrid QRS complex morphology represents simultaneous ventricular activation from both supraventricular conduction and the pacemaker. You can appreciate this even more clearly by comparing the first three complexes recorded in leads aVL and aVF where the second complex represents fusion of the other two morphologies. The nonspecific T waves abnormalities and relatively short QT interval seen in this tracing are likely due to digitalis effect.

ECG #16 A 62-year-old man who presents to the emergency department eight hours after the onset of chest discomfort.

RHYTHM STRIP: II
25 mm/sec; 1 cm/mV

▶ ECG #16

Interpretation

Technical quality: Satisfactory

Rhythm: Sinus

Atrial rate: 70 bpm

Ventricular rate: 70 bpm

PR interval: 0.14 seconds

QRS duration: 0.08 seconds

QT interval: 0.40 seconds

Axis: 0 degrees

Abnormalities: ST segment elevation in leads I, aVL, V1-V6. T wave inversion in leads I, aVL, V2-V4. Flat T waves in leads V5-V6. QS waves in leads V2-V3.

Synthesis: Sinus rhythm. Extensive anterior and lateral wall myocardial infarction with ST segment and T wave abnormalities suggesting acute myocardial injury.

Comment: The tracing shows an acute, extensive anterior and lateral wall MI. ST segment elevation and T wave inversion indicates acute myocardial injury. Unfortunately, the patient's late presentation has allowed for QS waves to develop indicating the likely presence of substantial myocardial necrosis.

ECG #17 A 55-year-old man in the coronary care unit.

I aVR V1 V4

II aVL V2 V5

III aVF V3 V6

RHYTHM STRIP: II
25 mm/sec: 1 cm/mV

▶ ECG #17

Interpretation

Technical quality: Satisfactory

Rhythm: Atrial flutter with 2:1 AV conduction

Atrial rate: 264 bpm

Ventricular rate: 132 bpm

PR interval: N/A

QRS duration: 0.08 seconds

QT interval: 0.32 seconds

Axis: +15 degrees

Abnormalities: P waves replaced by flutter waves.

Synthesis: Atrial flutter with 2:1 AV conduction. Otherwise, within normal limits.

Comment: A heart rate in the range of ~120 to 175 bpm should always raise the suspicion of atrial flutter with 2:1 AV conduction. Note the "sawtooth" baseline in the inferior limb leads that confirms the diagnosis. One of the two flutter waves is typically "buried" within the QRS complex, but is readily identifiable here in leads aVF and V1. Remember that the 2:1 AV conduction represents a normal physiologic property of the AV node and not pathologic heart block.

ECG #18 A 72-year-old woman with chronic kidney disease.

RHYTHM STRIP: II 25 mm/sec; 1 cm/mV

aVR   V1   V4

I

aVL   V2   V5

II

aVF   V3   V6

III

II

▲ ECG #18

Interpretation

Technical quality: Satisfactory

Rhythm: Sinus bradycardia

Atrial rate: 43 bpm

Ventricular rate: 43 bpm

PR interval: 0.18 seconds

QRS duration: 0.10 seconds

QT interval: 0.48 seconds

Axis: 0 degrees

Abnormalities: HR <60 bpm. Generalized, tall, symmetrically shaped T waves.

Synthesis: Sinus bradycardia. T wave abnormalities suggesting hyperkalemia.

Comment: Note the tall, "tent-shaped" T waves throughout the tracing that are typical for hyperkalemia. This patient with chronic kidney disease was home with an infection and missed two sessions of dialysis. She eventually presented with severe sepsis, acidosis, and a potassium level of 7.1 mEq/L. The ECG findings normalized with correction of the metabolic and electrolyte abnormalities. The QT interval is normal when corrected for the slow heart rate.

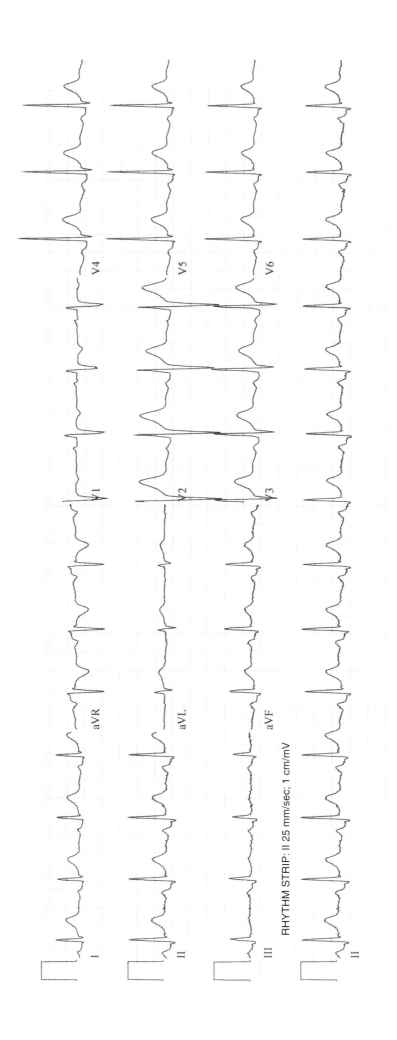

ECG #19 A 33-year-old man with chest discomfort.

RHYTHM STRIP: II 25 mm/sec; 1 cm/mV

I

II

III

aVR

aVL

aVF

V1

V2

V3

V4

V5

V6

II

▲ ECG #19

Interpretation

Technical quality: Satisfactory

Rhythm: Sinus

Atrial rate: 85 bpm

Ventricular rate: 85 bpm

PR interval: 0.16 seconds

QRS duration: 0.08 seconds

QT interval: 0.36 seconds

Axis: +60 degrees

Abnormalities: Concave upward ST segment elevation in leads I, II, III, aVF, V2-V6. PR segment depression in leads I, II, aVF, V2-V6. PR segment elevation lead aVR.

Synthesis: Sinus rhythm. ST segment elevation and PR segment findings suggesting acute pericarditis.

Comment: Note the diffuse, concave upward (smiling) ST segment elevation that is present in virtually every lead. Along with the accompanying PR segment abnormalities, these findings are pathognomonic of acute pericarditis. In contrast, the ST segment abnormalities of an acute MI are typically concave downward (coved) and are present in contiguous leads that face the area of infarction.

ECG #20 A 48-year-old man in the emergency department complaining of lightheadedness.

▲ **ECG #20**

Interpretation

Technical quality: Satisfactory

Rhythm: Wide complex tachycardia consistent with ventricular tachycardia

Atrial rate: N/A

Ventricular rate: 130 bpm

PR interval: N/A

QRS duration: 0.22 seconds

QT interval: N/A

Axis: −150 degrees

Abnormalities: Wide, notched QRS complex associated with ST segment and T wave abnormalities at a heart rate >100 bpm.

Synthesis: Wide complex tachycardia consistent with ventricular tachycardia.

Comment: This rapid, wide complex rhythm "checks all the boxes" for ventricular tachycardia based on multiple criteria. These include (1) northwest axis, (2) dominant R wave in lead aVR, (3) RBBB-type complex with a Rr′ morphology in lead V1, (4) RBBB morphology with QRS duration >0.14 seconds, (5) precordial lead RS duration >100 msec, and (6) initial deflection time in lead II >50 msec. Remember that the clinical status of the patient does not help you differentiate ventricular tachycardia from supraventricular tachycardia with aberrant conduction. In this case, the relatively slow ventricular rate averted hemodynamic collapse.

ECG #21 A 64-year-old man with chronic pulmonary disease.

I aVR V1 V4

II aVL V2 V5

III aVF V3 V6

II

0.32-40 Hz   ZPD   25.0 mm/s   10.0 mm/mV   60Hz   4 by 2.5s + 1 rhythm 1d   MAC55 010Bsp2   12SL™

440

▲ **ECG #21**

Interpretation

Technical quality: Satisfactory

Rhythm: Multifocal atrial tachycardia

Atrial rate: 130 bpm (average)

Ventricular rate: 130 bpm (average)

PR interval: 0.12 seconds

QRS duration: 0.08 seconds

QT interval: 0.32 seconds

Axis: +15 degrees

Abnormalities: Atrial rhythm with ≥3 consecutive P′ waves with different morphologies at a rate >100 bpm. Generalized low T wave voltage limb leads.

Synthesis: Multifocal atrial tachycardia. Nonspecific T wave abnormality.

Comment: Multifocal atrial tachycardia is a hyper-automatic arrhythmia commonly associated with chronic pulmonary disease or acute hypoxia from any etiology. A single dominant atrial pacemaker is absent, with multiple atrial foci producing P′ waves with different morphologies and variable P′R intervals.

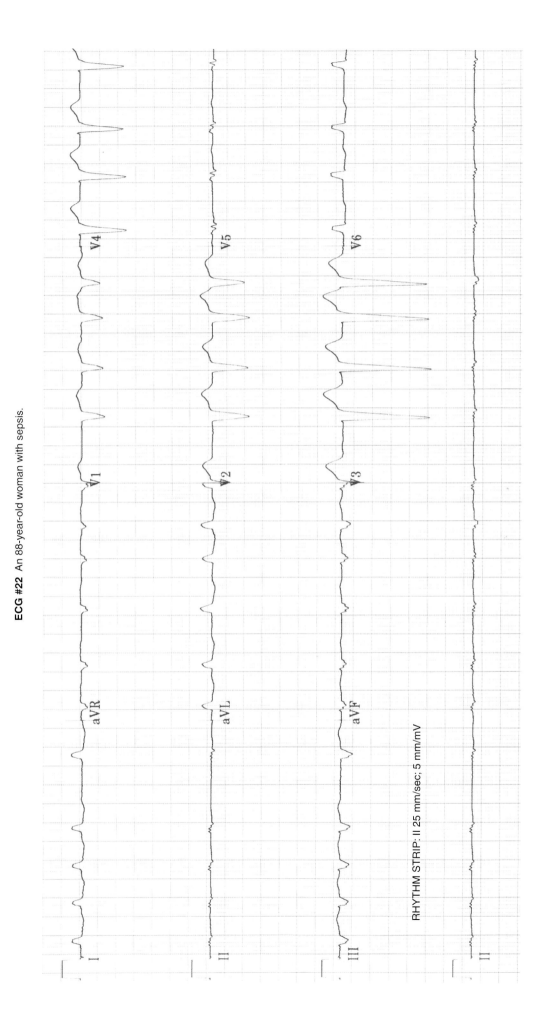

ECG #22 An 88-year-old woman with sepsis.

RHYTHM STRIP: II 25 mm/sec; 5 mm/mV

▲ ECG #22

Interpretation

Technical quality: Tracing recorded at one-half standardization

Rhythm: Atrial fibrillation

Atrial rate: N/A

Ventricular rate: 118 bpm (average)

PR interval: N/A

QRS duration: 0.12 seconds

QT interval: 0.36 seconds

Axis: −30 degrees

Abnormalities: Tracing recorded at one-half standardization. Heart rate >100 bpm. P waves replaced by fibrillatory waves. Prolonged QRS complex duration. Wide, notched QRS in leads I, aVL, V6 associated with ST segment depression and T wave inversion.

Synthesis: Atrial fibrillation with a rapid ventricular response. Left bundle branch block with secondary ST segment and T wave abnormalities. Tracing recorded at one-half standardization.

Comment: If not careful, you might make an erroneous diagnosis of low voltage in the limb leads. You might even mistakenly consider a lead reversal as the complexes in lead II look almost flat line. At normal standardization (10 mm = 1 mV), the amplitude of all the complexes in this tracing would be twice that which is recorded here. Always check the standardization and technical quality of each tracing.

ECG #23 A 50-year-old asymptomatic man who is a marathon runner.

RHYTHM STRIP: II 25 mm/sec; 10 mm/mV

▶ ECG #23

Interpretation

Technical quality: Satisfactory

Rhythm: Sinus bradycardia with sinus pause and junctional escape rhythm

Atrial rate: 55 bpm

Ventricular rate: 55 bpm

PR interval: 0.16 seconds

QRS duration: 0.10 seconds

QT interval: 0.44 seconds

Axis: 0 degrees

Abnormalities: HR <60 bpm. Sinus pause with narrow complex escape rhythm.

Synthesis: Sinus bradycardia with sinus pause and junctional escape rhythm. Otherwise within normal limits.

Comment: Extremely fit individuals have high vagal tone, which is responsible for the slow resting heart rate and periodic sinus pause seen here. A junctional escape rhythm emerges after the pause, as a subsidiary pacemaker in the AV junction responds at a rate of 39 bpm. In the lead II rhythm strip, note the slight negative deflection within the S wave of the junctional complexes, which represents the inverted, retrograde P' wave. After two junctional complexes, the sinus node resumes control.

ECG #24 A 71-year-old man with congestive heart failure.

| I | aVR | V1 | V4 |

| II | aVL | V2 | V5 |

| III | aVF | V3 | V6 |

RHYTHM STRIP: II 25 mm/sec; 10 mm/mV

▶ ECG #24

Interpretation

Technical quality: Satisfactory

Rhythm: Atrial fibrillation with frequent ventricular premature complexes

Atrial rate: N/A

Ventricular rate: 90 (average) bpm

PR interval: N/A

QRS duration: 0.08 seconds

QT interval: 0.38 seconds

Axis: −45 degrees

Abnormalities: P waves replaced by fibrillatory waves. Wide, premature complexes, single and in pairs. Axis leftward of −30 degrees. R waves V1-V3 <3 mm. Generalized low T wave voltage.

Synthesis: Atrial fibrillation with a controlled ventricular response. Frequent VPCs, single and in pairs. Left axis deviation. Left anterior fascicular block. Poor R wave progression.

Comment: The rhythm is atrial fibrillation with frequent VPCs. Long-short sequences are common in atrial fibrillation that may promote aberrant conduction, but the wide complexes in this example are clearly ventricular in origin. On the rhythm strip, note the fixed coupling intervals of the wide complexes. There are also morphologic clues to ventricular ectopy. Look at leads V1 and V2 where the wide complexes have a LBBB-type morphology. The notched and delayed initial downstroke in these complexes all strongly favor ventricular ectopy over aberrancy.

ECG #25 A 53-year-old woman with pulmonary disease.

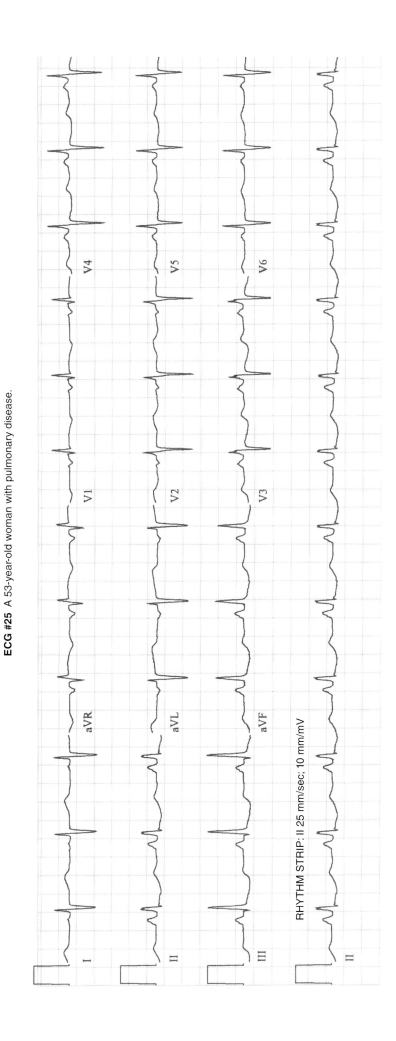

RHYTHM STRIP: II 25 mm/sec; 10 mm/mV

▲ ECG #25

Interpretation

Technical quality: Satisfactory

Rhythm: Sinus

Atrial rate: 73 bpm

Ventricular rate: 73 bpm

PR interval: 0.14 seconds

QRS duration: 0.08 seconds

QT interval: 0.48 seconds

Axis: +120 degrees

Abnormalities: Axis rightward of +90 degrees. P wave voltage >2.5 mm in lead aVF. Abnormal P terminal force, lead V1. qR complex, lead V1. R/S ratio in lead V5 and V6 ≤1. ST depression in leads II, III, aVF, V3-V5. Generalized low T wave voltage. Prolonged QT interval.

Synthesis: Sinus rhythm. Right axis deviation. Probable biatrial abnormality/enlargement. Right ventricular enlargement/hypertrophy. Nonspecific ST segment and T wave abnormalities. Prolonged QT interval.

Comment: The findings in this example are all related to severe pulmonary hypertension and abnormalities of the right heart chambers. Note the right axis deviation, qR complex in lead V1, and deep S wave in lead V6. The patient had marked right ventricular and right atrial dilation by echocardiography. The criteria for both right and left atrial enlargement are borderline, but the diagnoses are worthwhile to report as "probable." The QT interval remains prolonged after correction for the heart rate (QTc = 0.53 seconds).

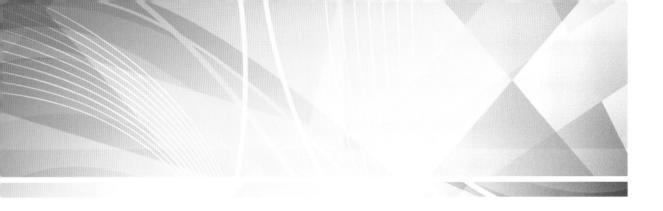

Index

Note: Page numbers followed by *f* indicate figures; those followed by *t* indicate tables.